ANATOMY
PALPATION AND SURFACE MARK...

Acquisitions editor: Heidi Allen
Development editor: Myriam Brearley
Production controller: Chris Jarvis
Desk editor: Jane Campbell
Cover designer: Alan Studholme

ANATOMY
PALPATION AND SURFACE MARKINGS

Third edition

DEREK FIELD Grad Dip Phys, FCSP, Dip TP, SRP
Former Vice Principal, North London School of Physiotherapy, City University, London

OXFORD   AUCKLAND   BOSTON   JOHANNESBURG   MELBOURNE   NEW DELHI

Butterworth Heinemann
Elsevier Science Limited, Robert Stevenson House,
1-3 Baxter's Place, Leith Walk, Edinburgh EH1 3AF
An imprint of Elsevier Science Limited

First published 1994
Second edition 1997
Third edition 2001
Reprinted 2002

British Library Cataloguing in Publication Data
Field, Derek
Anatomy: palpation and surface markings. - 3rd ed.
  1. Physycal diagnosis
  I. Title
  616'.0754

Lybrary of Congress Cataloging in Publication Data
Field, Derek
  Anatomy: palpation and surface markings / Derek Field. 3rd ed.
   p.; cm.
  Includes bibliographical references and index.
  ISBN 0 7506 4618 7
  1. Anatomy, Surgical and topographical.   2. Palpation.   I. Title.
  [DNLM: 1. Palpation – methods.   2. Palpation – methods – Atlases. WB 275 F453a 2001]
  QM531. F53 2001
  611–dc21   2001025848

ISBN 0 7506 4618 7

 your source for books,
journals and multimedia
in the health sciences

www.elsevierhealth.com

Contents

Introduction to Prefaces

It was decided that in this Third Edition of *Anatomy, Palpation and Surface Markings*, it would be of some interest to the student of anatomy to include the preface to the First and Second Editions. This would explain how the book was conceived and some of the reasoning and developments which have taken place in the production of this Third Edition. The basic plan has always been the same; to produce a book which is easy to read with clear photographs and drawings facilitating the accumulation of knowledge of the human body and endeavouring to make the study of anatomy a pleasant and enjoyable assignment.

Preface to the first edition

The aim of this book is to familiarize the student of anatomy with a basic plan of the human body, combining this knowledge with the art of palpation. This is a vital discipline for a true understanding of the relationship of structures with the surface, and provides both students and practitioners with an ability to visualize these structures through the skin.

The book is designed to be an adjunct to the study of anatomy; therefore, only details of bone, joint structure, muscle attachments, nerve origins and distributions which can be palpated or determined from the surface will be included. Nevertheless, the text, with its illustrations on facing pages, where possible, provide the student and practitioner with a source of information which is designed to be clear and easy to understand. It should also stimulate the anatomist to develop the ability to palpate all types of structure below the skin, as well as the quality of movement in joints, and tension and texture in tissues. Finally, with practice, it is hoped that the palpator will develop the ability to identify fine movements, tissue and joint damage and other anomalies which will facilitate patient assessment.

There are five main sections of the book: the upper limb, the lower limb, the head and neck, the thorax and the abdomen. Each is divided into the following subsections: bones, joints, muscles, nerves, arteries and veins. The lymphatic system has been excluded as it is normally impossible to palpate, although the drainage routes can be seen from time to time, particularly when there is an infection in the region drained. The lymph nodes are also difficult to palpate unless they are enlarged as a consequence of pathological reaction.

Wherever possible, the left-hand page of text contains information on palpation, with an outline of the surface markings. The facing page consists of photographs of the region taken from different angles, beside which is a line drawing indicating the underlying structures, together with measurements, where possible, showing the relationship between the structures. Between the photographs and the line drawings is a list of structures of importance, identified by arrows where appropriate.

Much of the information in the following pages has been acquired from the study of the living body, dissections and numerous standard anatomical textbooks. The reader is recommended to refer to as many authors as possible to ensure a broad knowledge and understanding of anatomy.

Preface to the second edition

Due to the popularity and success of the first edition of this book it has been decided to cease reprints and move immediately into the production of a second edition.

The aims and layout of this second edition are very similar to those in the first, with improvements being made to the index and text. Drawings and photographs are, where possible, facing relevant text with the labelling shared between photographs and drawings. Full colour has now been used to give greater clarification to the photographs and in addition the headings of each section have been highlighted. The cover illustration has been altered to portray the palpating hands on the surface of the shoulder.

To improve the accuracy of the identification of structures below the surface and for the benefit of those searching for the structure, small black dots were applied to the surface marking of the structures before the photographs were taken. This, combined with accurate photography, has ensured the portrayal of the exact location of structures not seen below the surface.

These improvements have been incorporated to enhance the clarity and appearance of the book. It is hoped that the reader, whether studying anatomy for medicine, sport or purely for pleasure will derive as much information and interest from this second edition as from the first.

Preface to the third edition

With the continuing popularity and success of the second edition of *Anatomy, Palpation and Surface Markings* there was a great deal of discussion as to whether it was going to be necessary or even helpful to produce a third edition. The second edition has become a 'best seller' in the Butterworth-Heinemann medical books section and appeared to give the reader the information and stimulus that was needed for the application of the art of palpation to the study of living anatomy. The author, however, being presented with the opportunity to develop some of the ideas which had been impossible to use in the first and second editions, due to cost and space, felt that vast improvements could be made.

Much of the text assumed that the student had a basic knowledge of anatomy and that the shape and construction of underlying structures would be known. With the additional space for text it meant that a short description could precede the area to be examined, thus avoiding the necessity of checking in other books. It must be pointed out, however, that only a basic outline of description is given. This extra space for text also allowed the introduction of additional sections on:

Outline descriptions of bones and muscles
Palpation on movement
Functional anatomy
General location and description of organs
Outline of joint structure, etc.

All of these, it is hoped, will increase the quest for further knowledge in the student.

Having the photograph and drawing opposite the relevant text in the first and second editions was a feature which was praised by many readers. It was therefore decided to improve this facility by, where possible, placing the photograph opposite the drawing and labelling them both so that they line up on each page. This allows more labels to be added to the drawings to help with the location of more bony features. It was also felt that being able to locate the labelled point in the text would save time. The relevant word in the text has therefore been highlighted in blue.

The photographs and drawings have been enlarged to improve their clarity and the text has been divided into four separate blocks below, while still maintaining the clear print. The page headers are again highlighted in a blue strip but the sections have been re-ordered to improve their location.

The enlargement of photographs and drawings, the positioning of the text below with highlighted labels, the additional sections and the improved general layout of this third edition should ease the burden of study for the student of anatomy and help to develop an enjoyment in the investigation of anatomical structures which are palpable deep to the skin.

Acknowledgements

I would like to take this opportunity to thank my colleagues, friends and readers from all over the world, who have assisted me in the production of this Third Edition of *Anatomy: Palpation and Surface Markings*.

My thanks go to Anthony B. Ward LBIPP, of Churchill Ward Associates, Long Hanborough, who patiently spent four very full days shooting and perfecting the many colour photographs used in the Third Edition. I would like to thank him for his advice and care and for the hospitality that he and his wife showed us during the photography sessions.

My thanks also go to Tim Brown who gave a great deal of his time and energy holding difficult poses, sometimes hanging from the old oak beams under very exhausting spotlights! I would like to include Sally Ede who posed for most of the face, head and neck shots. Both she and Tim endured the attaching and removal of hundreds of sticky black dots to parts of their anatomy, which never enhance their appearance at any time.

Again, I must express a special thankyou to Caroline Makepeace, Publisher, at Butterworth-Heinemann, who together with her colleagues, made my task more enjoyable by easing my work load wherever possible. Caroline was always on hand to give encouragement and help.

Finally, I would like to express a very special thankyou to Yvonne Ibbott who has spend many hours of organizing schedules and work sessions, reading and editing all sorts of information and research, helping to collate the dots on the photographs with the labels and, most importantly, encouraging me to make this edition better than ever.

Palpation: principles and practice

Palpation: definition, application and practice

DEFINITION

The Shorter Oxford English Dictionary describes the verb to palpate as:

To examine by the sense of touch, to feel, a method of medical examination. Medical examination by feeling.

Here there is an implication that palpation is more than just the use of the hands to feel. *To examine* is defined as an investigation by inspection or manipulation, and even goes as far as to suggest a scrutiny, an investigation or critical inquiry. Further, the word investigate is defined as searching, tracking or tracing out, to examine systematically in detail.

Gould's Medical Dictionary describes the verb to palpate as:

To touch gently. Examination by touch for purposes of diagnosis; application of the hand or fingers ... to detect characteristics and condition of local tissues of the underlying organs or tumors.

If one expands the investigation to include the definition found in this dictionary, there is the additional quality of 'gentleness' and 'for diagnosis'.

Churchill's Medical Dictionary describes palpation as being:

From the Latin *palpare* – to stroke, caress. To explore or examine by touching and probing with the hands and fingers.

This dictionary adds such terms as, to 'stroke' or 'caress' and the 'use of the hands to explore'.

Application

Palpation uses one of the primary senses, that of touch, in order to investigate and provide information or to supplement that already gained by other means, such as sight. It is the earliest system to become functional in the human being and is also thought to be the last of the senses to be lost immediately prior to death. It is used continuously throughout life, but in the conscious human is often, in part, subjugated in favour of other sensory modalities. Only when recognition of change occurs does it return to a conscious level, for example picking up a garment and immediately recognizing, through its texture and 'feel', that it is unfamiliar or being aware of the materials of trousers touching the legs immediately after a long period of wearing shorts.

Palpation appears to be a combination of touch, feel, examination, sensory feedback and interpretation through previous experience. It involves utilizing certain skills in a methodical way to enable specific information to be acquired. It may be used, for example, to acquire everyday information such as the warmth of water. A thermometer could be used to determine the temperature, but direct testing, by using the sensory endings in the skin, is often easier. The response may at first appear to be crude, but in fact provides a range of meaningful descriptions; for example, burning, scorching, boiling, extremely hot, very hot, fairly hot, hot, quite hot, very warm, blood heat, warm, fairly warm, slightly warm, cool, cold, quite cold, very cold, bitterly cold, freezing and icy cold which are all terms used in everyday life to pass on information about temperature. A temperature of 42°C read from a thermometer has little meaning as to whether something is too hot or too cold to touch.

All areas of the skin are normally able to perceive sensations of pain, touch, pressure, heat and cold to a greater or lesser degree. Some areas are more sensitive to stimuli than others. For example, in the lumbar region, two points can only be perceived separately if they are more than approximately 70 mm apart. However, the tips of the fingers can distinguish two separate points even when they are as close as 1–2 mm. This is referred to as the 'Two Point Discrimination Test' (Guyton, 1991; Sunderland, 1978). This means that only fairly large objects can be recognized using the lumbar area, but fine point discrimination can be achieved using the fingertips.

The ability to read Braille, for example, depends on this sensitivity. With sufficient practice, sighted as well as visually impaired individuals can read Braille with their fingers. The quality of touch and discrimination developed can be of great benefit to the practitioner who wishes to 'read' information lying deep to the skin. The controlled use of pressure and movement, coupled with feedback and experience, unlocks a vast quantity of information unavailable to the eye.

The art of palpation is one which is not fully appreciated until it is needed, perhaps to compensate for the loss of another sense, e.g. sight or hearing, which may be completely lost or impaired. To extend the practice of palpation to its full potential involves a two-way passage of information, often creating physical or sometimes psychological reactions. These reactions may take the form of pleasure or pain, relaxation or tension and even love or hate. For example, gently squeezing the hand may imply love, whereas gripping the hand could imply anger. The young seem to have a desire to have manual contact with others close to them. Their psychological and physical development appears to depend to some extent, on this contact. Ashley Montague (1978), in his book 'Touching', summarizes the observations of many researchers to conclude that:

Cutaneous stimulation in the various forms in which the newborn and young receive it is of prime importance for their healthy physical and behavioural development... It appears probable that for human beings, tactile stimulation is of fundamental significance for develop- ment of healthy, emotional and affectional relationships.

He quotes examples of cases that were studied by another researcher, Lorna Marshall, who spent much time between 1950 and 1961 living among the Bushmen of the Kalahari Desert in Botswana, South West Africa, where the development of the new born, infant, adolescent and adult appeared to be influenced by the way the child was handled in early life. He also refers to accounts by Margaret Mead, who compares the Arapesh and Mundugumor societies in New Guinea, as they were in the 1930s. In the former the child was in contact with its mother for most of the day. The adults of the tribe were kind, happy peace-loving people. In the second tribe the child had little human contact, being kept in a rough plaited basket which was usually suspended from the mother's forehead. The adults of this tribe, at this time, grew to be unattractive, aggressive and cannibalistic.

In some nationalities and cultures in adulthood there is a tendency to avoid this type of contact which has been so important in their development. Montague draws certain obvious conclusions: 'There exists not only cultural and national differences in tactile behaviour but also class differences.' He cites the English upper class as a good example of non-tactile social behaviour in comparison to other nationalities, for example, the French and Italians who are far more open with their greetings and make more contact with one another.

In the latter end of the 20th century, manual contact with others appears to have changed. It has now become much more acceptable for male and female to express their love, admiration and appreciation by physical contact with each other. Male and female will readily embrace each other, hold hands or even kiss in public. Sportsmen and sportswomen will readily throw their arms around one another or even kiss each other on the cheek after a winning achievement.

Women often embrace each other in victory or defeat. This has, fairly recently, been adopted by male sportsmen who will willingly embrace each other on achieving victory. Watch any football match when a goal is scored. Several players may wrap their arms around the scorer so enthusiastically that they may fall to the ground in a heap. During the 2000 Olympic Games in Sydney, Australia, how pleasing it was to see both successful and unsuccessful competitors embracing one another and how satisfying it is to know that this warmth crosses many of the traditional barriers of creed, class and ethnic backgrounds.

Practice

The improvement or perfection of an art is achieved by its continual practice and use. The study and practice of manual contact techniques over a long period of time provides the practitioner with an additional skill for receiving information concerning that particular patient. Many years of experience of palpating in a careful and controlled manner will allow the moving, stretching and compression of tissues to be applied with precise control. Thus the therapist will be able to receive information from the patient, allowing him or her to adjust their technique accordingly. Fine palpable changes in tension, temperature, dampness, movement and swelling, for example, will be observed, noted and acted upon. Grieve (1986) states:

> Of the entire objective examination of the vertebral column, the palpation examination of accessible tissues is probably the most informative and therefore the most valuable.

The person being palpated is fully aware of the skill and ability of the palpator. During an initial examination both the palpator and the person being palpated progress through a learning process in which each is assessing the other by the giving and receiving of information. Little information can be gained if one of the participants is reluctant to communicate.

The learning process takes time, and often a true picture of the problem does not appear until much later. This is partly due to a mutual relaxation of tension in both parties, but mainly to the beginning of the two-way passage of information between them, each benefiting from the knowledge being gained. This skill is therefore not just a crude touching or contact; it is an investigative examination providing information to both participants. In the author's experience, palpation is only 10% gift–the other 90% is practice.

Sighted Braille transcribers have been known to master the Braille system and codes in only 3 weeks. This is, of course, totally dedicating themselves to the task. On the other hand, using the fingertips, it is estimated that it would take a regular user, on average, around $1^{1}/_{2}$–2 years to reach a speed suitable for serious study. This is not due to lack of knowledge of the system, but because the palpation and recognition of the signs using this sense of touch need time and practice to develop. As in all skills, the speed and quality of reading depends on the amount of use. The ability to palpate with any finger or fingers can be developed, the use of the index finger being the most popular. In rare instances, people who have been unable to use their fingers have developed the same ability to read Braille in their toes or even their lips! This means that regardless of the method by which this is achieved, the ability to palpate can, given the time and desire, be improved. With enough practice, the ability to increase the information being received by the fingers and hands can be maximized.

EFFECTS OF PALPATION ON THE PATIENT

Many patients are still reluctant to consult a professional concerning personal problems, particularly those associated with their own body. Both parties may put up barriers, but both must contribute towards breaking these down if closer co-operation is to be achieved.

The patient normally presents with a combination of questions, problems and information, having no particular order of priority except perhaps the overriding presence of pain. Much of this information may be quite irrelevant, but it is a vital part of the investigation and must be thoroughly evaluated before it can be discarded.

The investigator must be sympathetically receptive to all forms of information, trying to analyse the facts and producing a full assessment of the situation. Sometimes a set plan will be used to facilitate the compilation of the facts into some sort of order. This will help lead the investigator to a conclusion or diagnosis. Care must be taken, however, that this set plan does not interfere with the information given by the patient and contaminate the final picture.

The initial investigation must be handled with great care and sensitivity, as it may influence both parties in the examination which is to follow. The physical examination needs the same degree of tact and diplomacy, employing care, precision and gentleness. Physical or verbal clumsiness at this stage could lead to a complete block and reluctance to co-operate on the part of the patient. Palpation begins at the first contact with the patient and information concerning further examinations must be acquired efficiently. The author has found that most patients expect to be examined and would feel poorly treated if palpation was omitted. Some indication of the patient's reaction to contact should be gained immediately, and the act of shaking hands or helping the patient from or to a chair can provide the investigator with a great deal of information concerning the need for assistance or the reluctance to accept help. Of course, this contact with the patient is only one of the many examinations and assessment techniques being performed at the time. Observation, hearing and even the sense of smell also provide useful sources of information concerning the patient.

During the period of questioning it is beneficial to make careful contact with the area of pain, which encourages both parties to focus attention as to the reason for the consultation. Movements should be tested with great care, palpating and observing continuously, monitoring any reluctance to move, tension, muscle spasm, joint anomalies and pain. Inadvertently causing the patient acute pain is one of the easiest ways of losing his or her confidence, with vital information also being lost.

The patient will gradually gain confidence. Much of the fear of meeting will have passed at the first contact. By the time movement is examined, there should already be some feeling of trust, and if the handling was careful but firm, a great deal of tension may be reduced. A feeling of co-operation and confidence overcomes that initial reluctance to the seeking of medical advice.

Palpation continues throughout the examination and subsequent treatment. If it is carried out with care and feeling, it provides information concerning the physical problems of the patient and may also 'unlock' psychological problems, which until this relationship was established were either purposely hidden or not recognized as having any relevance to the physical aspect. Many practitioners will have experience of patients who will allow a minor physical problem to be the reason to contact a therapist, and then during the examination or treatment will refer to their underlying problem. All practitioners must be aware of this possibility and should note any odd comments that may creep into the conversation. Physical contact with the patient appears to be the link necessary for this process, but the ability to recognize the sign is dependent on the skill, training and sensitivity of the observer.

The patient must have confidence in the palpator, which should promote the offering of information either verbally or non-verbally. Additional information concerning the patient's condition should be continuously received during treatment. Even the simplest of treatments should promote the feeling of care, confidence and understanding. The patient will often contribute as much to the treatment as he or she receives, provided that encouragement is given and information is genuinely being sought.

TECHNIQUES OF PALPATION

It is not enough merely to place the hands on the patient's body and hope to receive the information required. Positive steps must be taken to search for the data. Palpation is a seeking of information (see page 2) and must be approached in a rational and planned manner. Very little can be gained by contacting a surface with the hands and remaining stationary. Movement of the hands is required so that structures can pass under the fingers in a controlled manner in order to determine and take note of changes in surface, pressure and temperature, for example. The speed of movement can be adjusted so that the maximum information is read. If the fingers are run over Braille script too quickly, dots can be felt but no information is read, while at the correct speed for that individual the mass of dots become an intelligible text.

Sometimes the palpation needs to be deep and slow, at other times light and quick. For example, palpation of the transverse processes of the lumbar region or the hook of the hamate needs careful application of deep pressure, combined with slow movement and sensitivity to the reactions of the patient. Palpation of the spines of the thoracic vertebrae, particularly when counting down, is much easier if the fingertips are gently moved up and down three or four centimetres at a time, marking each spine with the finger of the other hand and holding it until the position of the next spine is confirmed. This type of palpation works in a similar fashion to a scanner using a beam to build up a clearer picture. The technique can be used for obtaining a clearer picture of the rib cage, particularly from the posterior aspect.

Using one or even two complete palms and fingers gives more information regarding movement below the surface and about the reaction of the patient to contact. The application of just the fingertips, for example, would be used for palpating a pulse. Generally, if the objects below the surface are stationary, the hands will have to be used in a controlled movement, whereas if the objects are mobile, the hands should remain stationary. The finer the movement below the surface, the more delicate must be the palpation – this is clearly shown in searching for a faint pulse.

If joints are being manipulated to examine quality of movement, and to assess limiting factors, the hands should be moved as little as possible so as to avoid any feedback from the palpator's own tissues obscuring information from the patient's tissues. In fact, with this type of palpation a minimum of all other movements, with the exception of the joint being examined, is required. This involves adopting a stance which will avoid movement of the feet, applying a hold which will allow the full range of movement without change, and reducing all skin sliding by firm contact. Finally, the palpator must be absolutely sure that the patient's position is stable and that the movement being tested is localized to the joint being examined and is in the plane around the axis required. It is not uncommon, when testing the movements of the upper or lower limb, for a 'clicking' or crepitus to occur and neither the patient nor examiner are able to locate its source. Conversely, if the examiner's thumb nails touch when pressure is being applied to the posterior aspect of the lateral mass of the atlas (C1), the patient may, erroneously, report a grinding sound located in the atlanto-occipital joint.

When examining the end-range of a joint, all variations must be known in advance so that movement, normal and accessory, is tested correctly, noting the range available and the limiting factors. This is a highly skilled form of palpation, needing a great deal of practice on normal joints in order to perfect the technique, considerable experience with abnormal joints to be able to recognize the variations, and an expert knowledge of the various conditions to assess how much or how little testing should be done. It is not suggested that this form of palpation should be done only by an expert; on the contrary, it should be practised at the earliest opportunity and based on palpation of normal anatomy. Gradually, if care is taken and limits set, considerable skill can be gained.

Unfortunately, many palpators either feel little and try to compensate by observation, or feel enthusiastically but do not interpret what they feel. Some may also feel what they believe they are meant to feel. It is easy to be persuaded by an eager patient, by prior knowledge or by a more experienced observer that one can feel changes that are not really there. Honesty is essential: remember Hans Andersen's story of the Emperor's new clothes!

IMPROVING THE ART OF PALPATION

As with the example of the Braille reader, improvement in palpation techniques can only be achieved with practice. The desire to learn is of the utmost importance. This is dependent upon the need to know what lies beneath the surface and the desire to find some means of offering help. How often is it said by a practitioner, 'If only I could see what is happening inside'? Because of this need, the development of all skills which may help to fulfil this desire must be developed, including the sensitivity of the hands.

The involvement of the hands in all forms of observation, often enhanced by reducing the input of other senses and increasing the use of touch, can be improved by closing the eyes and using the hands to recognize different textures, weights, surfaces, liquids, coins, etc. The palpator must endeavour to gain as much information as possible. Different objects can be placed in a bag and recognized only by the hands. As the skill improves, the objects can be chosen so that they are less distinctive and smaller. All of the objects should be handled sensitively, recognizing any blemishes or distinctive features. Progression would be made so that the same objects can be palpated and recognized through the material of the bag, beginning with a plastic bag and gradually changing to a thicker material, thereby increasing the difficulty of palpation. Practice should be applied continuously in everyday life, and as often as possible, always noting the technique which is most useful for each object. Make a habit of checking the change you have in your pocket or purse before removing the correct amount for a purchase. The recognition of coins is fairly easy and one should be confident enough to pay out the correct change without looking at the coins. Take care – this could prove to be an expensive way to learn the art of palpation if enough practice is not allowed! Also, try each day to select the clothes you wish to wear by touch rather than sight. Keep in mind that a person without sight will have to utilize these skills every day.

The development of the sense of touch needs to be nurtured. Each contact with another object should be treated as if one has no sight or hearing, and as much information as possible must be gained. Those who have the privilege of handling patients professionally possess a constant source of practice in their study of structure and function, and examination of the normal and abnormal. They are even more fortunate if they also use massage, movement, mobilizations and manipulations. Those who have formally studied and practised the art of massage are indeed already well versed in the knowledge, skills and abilities, and education necessary, and must do all in their power to restore their talent to its full capacity in the interpretation of what they feel.

The continuation and enhancement of the formal study of anatomy is essential, as there is little gained if the expert palpator is unaware of what is to be palpated.

CARE OF THE HANDS

In all skills where the hands are used to achieve precise movements with fine tactile sensitivity, positive steps must be taken to maintain their mobility, sensitivity and dexterity.

Cleanliness is essential and contributes enormously to the sense of touch. Traces of grease, cream, dirt, dust, etc., will place another interventional layer between the sensory receptor organs and nerve endings and the object or subject to be palpated. Most Braille readers will try to keep their hands clean while reading Braille and tend to avoid eating anything sticky to prevent their fingers losing sensitivity. A routine of washing the hands in gentle soap, drying them thoroughly and avoiding any additional cream unless absolutely necessary, should be practised. A good hand cream can be used at night to maintain the smooth, soft condition of the skin, but the hands must be thoroughly washed before any palpation is attempted. In addition, the nails should be clean and short, cutting down the risks of

injury or infection, and allowing them to be used as tools. The quality of the palpation depends, to a great extent, on the texture and suppleness of the hands. They should look and feel good, promoting the patient's confidence in the palpator. Poorly maintained hands which are dirty, stiff and covered with hard skin will only promote a reluctance to be touched and act as a barrier to the passage of information from the body of the patient to the receptors of the palpator.

The joints of the hands must all be maintained in a supple condition with the musculature firm and strong. Regular exercises should be practised, maintaining mobility and increasing strength. Contact with all abrasive surfaces and detergents should be avoided and gloves must be worn at all times when manual work is performed, particularly during activities such as gardening, car mechanics or building. Many liquids, certain soaps and detergents remove the natural greases from the skin and these therefore should be avoided. Any activity which will lead to the production of blisters or hard skin, such as rowing, climbing ropes, gripping handles, etc., should also be avoided and, most importantly, great care must be taken in using sharp instruments or engaging in any activity which will cause trauma and infection of the skin. Any of these circumstances may reduce the ability to perform high-quality palpation.

PALPATION OF DIFFERENT TISSUES

Normal palpation by the lay person, and even by many professionals, is sometimes crude and of little value. It may denote the difference between bone, muscle or tendons, etc., but often does little more. The skilled student will be able to distinguish different parts of bones, differing shapes and texture of muscle, their connections to tendons, and be able to trace them to their attachments. Such students will also be able to count vertebrae, palpate lumbar transverse processes and other deep bony structures, locate certain ligaments, palpate elusive pulses and determine abnormalities, such as different types of swelling, misalignment and rupture. The highly skilled palpator must go far beyond this concept of palpation and must complete the picture that is hidden within the body. Bony landmarks should be studied, linking them together and obtaining a clear mental image of the skeletal layout. This should include angles of ribs, transverse processes and spines of all vertebrae including their differing features; for example, the bifid spinous processes in the cervical region, in contrast to the pointed spines in the thoracic and the rectangular-shaped spines of T12 and in the lumbar region.

Alignment of one bone to another is more easily examined in the upper and lower limbs, but much more difficult in the vertebral column. Defects in the contour of a bone can be located and possible avulsions recognized.

Variations in muscle texture should be recognizable and note taken of differences occurring in normal muscle, enabling the examiner to recognize any abnormal variations. Some muscles, such as gluteus maximus and the middle fibres of deltoid, have a coarse structure due to the type of muscle fibres involved, whereas muscles such as the oblique abdominals and quadratus lumborum have a smoother texture. Fibrous tissue between the muscle fibres may give a stringy feel, while local areas of spasm are hard but regular in shape. The former tend to remain in the same position irrespective of what is done to them; the latter will often disappear on applying either heat or massage. Often both types can be found in the rhomboid muscles between the scapula and spinous processes of the vertebral column.

Careful palpation will reveal where each muscle joins its tendon, and where and how the tendon is attached. Palpation can also determine how tightly the muscle is bound down by fascia and whether the tendon is maintained in its position by a retinaculum. The extent of retinacula can be examined and a study made of those structures which pass under or over them.

Swellings in muscle are often caused by bruising (haematoma) and bleeding between the muscle fibres. These are normally contained within a localized area and become hard and painful, often warm to the touch and possibly producing redness over the area. There is nearly always a history of trauma to the region. However, care should be taken when palpating any area of swelling as it could be caused by other more serious conditions. It is important to be aware of local changes in temperature, whether higher or lower than expected. Note must be taken of the structures lying below and a knowledge of reasons for such variations may contribute to the diagnosis and treatment of the condition.

When palpating joints, other considerations must be taken into account. The precise location of the joint line is essential, being based on the accurate identification of bony landmarks and measurements, taking into account the general size and shape of other bones and the posture at the time. A detailed knowledge of the structure and extent of the adjacent joint surfaces, as well as where ligaments may hide the joint space, is imperative. The presentation of tissue-filled joint spaces under differing circumstances, for example whether fluid is contained within the joint capsule or within a bursa, together with a detailed knowledge of the surrounding tendons, is also necessary when examining joints.

Examination of how the bones of a joint move on each other, the range and smoothness of movement, whether the axis varies according to its position and how movement is limited are all noteworthy features. Using great care and skill, movement of joints can be examined indirectly through the bones of either side of that joint. The feeling of smooth movement or grinding of joint surfaces felt through the bones on either side and the restriction felt at the end of a joint range, 'end feel', can give the palpator additional information about the condition of the joint. Sometimes, the joint comes to a sudden halt caused by bony contact, but normally joints have a certain amount of springiness as ligaments and muscles become taut.

Most joints possess additional movements, which are of small range and not under voluntary control, which are essential for the efficient functioning of the joint. These are known as accessory movements. A simple example of this type of movement would be found in the axle of a bicycle wheel. On each side the axle is surrounded by a ring of ball-bearings maintained in position by a cone which screws on to the axle. When the cones are loose they allow the wheel to be moved slightly from side to side, but when tight there is no side-to-side or accessory movement. When there is side-to-side movement, the wheel is free to turn, but as the cones are tightened, the ball-bearings become 'close packed' and more difficult to turn, finally locking the wheel. The side-to-side (or accessory) movement is thus essential for the free turning of the wheel, since its elimination results in no movement.

Accessory movements are most demonstrable in human joints within a certain range of the joint movement; that is, when the ligaments allow joint surfaces to be parted or when the surfaces are not congruent. This is termed the 'loose packed' position. When the ligaments of a joint become taut and its surfaces are congruent, there is no further movement, either normal or accessory. The joint is now said to be in a position termed 'close packed' (Williams *et al.*, 1995). If the accessory movements of a joint are lost, then the joint becomes extremely difficult to move, similar to the cones of the wheel being tightened. If, however, accessory movement is restored, as in loosening the cones in the bicycle wheel, see above, then normal movement is also restored. The restoration of accessory movements is an important aim underlying the use of mobilization and manipulation techniques to restore movement in joints. With care and expertise, using a combination of accessory and *normal* movements, joint function can be assessed and the treatment varied accordingly. The use of 'quadrant' techniques (combined movements at the end of range) is a good example of this testing. For further study and information on the application of these types of examination and techniques, see Grieve (1986) and Maitland (1991).

Swelling around a joint deforms its shape and contour according to the amount of swelling involved. The bony features can usually be identified between the areas of swelling. In some instances the swelling is so profuse that it is difficult to find bony landmarks, whereas in others the amount of fluid is so small that precise techniques have to be employed to palpate the swelling which is interfering with normal joint function. Most joint swelling is contained within the capsule, causing a build-up of pressure with increasing pain. The swelling may have to be removed surgically, although this usually is deferred until absolutely necessary because of the risk of infection into the joint. Blood can also escape into a joint space (haemarthrosis), resulting in a similar appearance, but this is usually accompanied by some discoloration and an increased local temperature. Any swelling can lead to severe damage to the mechanics of the joint, which may vary according to the type of fluid involved.

Careful palpation of the swelling can produce more information than at first thought. It may appear soft and movable with the application of pressure – this often gives a fluid feel as it passes from one part of the joint cavity to another. Alternatively it may appear thick and pliable, but difficult to move unless sustained pressure is applied. Swelling may appear to be a solid mass, pitting under pressure from the fingers but taking a considerable time before signs of movement are evident.

SUMMARY

Palpation is a detailed examination using the hands which allows the palpator to elicit information about structures beneath the skin and fascia. It is, in the author's view, very much under-used and undervalued, mainly because of lack of practice and understanding. In addition, it is time-consuming, requiring a conscious effort and a keen interest and inquisitive nature. Its techniques can be practised and developed as long as the desire and patience to succeed are present; however, expertise takes time to acquire.

Palpation is more than just a desire to 'see' through the skin and understand the anatomy; it can be developed in such a way that information can be given to the patient through the hands. It is not hard to understand how the expert can use palpation and touch for persuasion, caring and the unlocking of hidden emotions, even going as far as using touch as therapy in itself, and the 'laying on of hands' to give confirmation to religious beliefs and spiritualism.

Palpation must be learned, practised and developed before it can be applied. The study of anatomy and the added information gained by the correct use of the hands are excellent ways of learning the art of palpation. Anatomy will become clearer and more understandable as the hands become more sensitive to what lies below the skin, leading to an enhancement of knowledge and improvement in assessment – an asset in therapeutic application.

Finally, and perhaps most importantly, the skilled palpator should be aware of the patient's reaction to movement. By observing the patient's face, listening to the patient's comments and being sensitive to all reactions in muscle and joint movement, a total picture of the patient's condition becomes available. With care and sensitivity, a great deal of information can readily be obtained.

The following pages contain a detailed study of the surface markings of many of the body's structures, including a guide to the palpation of certain structures. A quest for knowledge can be used to develop your skill in palpation. Eventually, you will know that what you feel exists and what exists is important.

2

The upper limb

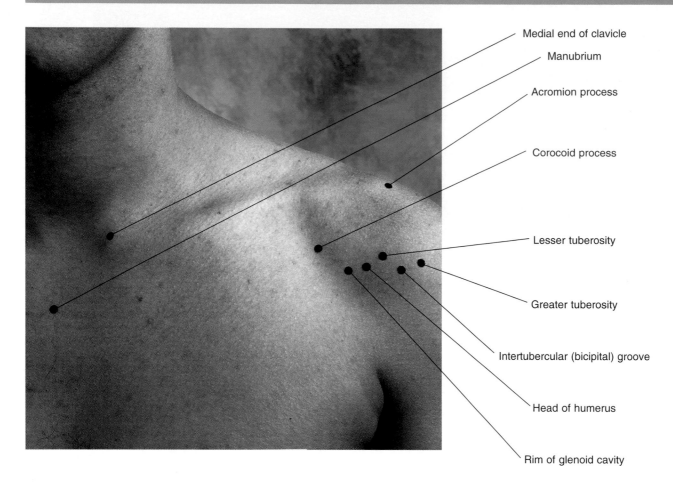

- Medial end of clavicle
- Manubrium
- Acromion process
- Corocoid process
- Lesser tuberosity
- Greater tuberosity
- Intertubercular (bicipital) groove
- Head of humerus
- Rim of glenoid cavity

Fig. 2.1 (a)
The left shoulder (anterior view)

BONES

The pectoral region

The bones in this region are the clavicle and scapula, forming the pectoral girdle, with the upper end of the humerus situated vertically under its lateral margin. The clavicle is situated on the upper part of the anterolateral aspect, and the scapula on the upper part of the posterolateral aspect of the chest wall. The humerus is the upper bone of the arm articulating with the glenoid [*glene* (Gk) = a socket] cavity of the scapula at the shoulder (glenohumeral) joint.

The clavicle [Fig. 2.1]

The clavicle [*clavis* (L) or *kleis* (Gk) = key; also, *clavis* (L) was an S-shaped bar for striking a gong) is about 10 cm long and situated between the manubrium sterni medially and the acromion process of the scapula laterally (Fig. 2.1). It is a long bone and has a shallow S-shape when viewed from above. It ossifies in membrane, which means that its articular surfaces are covered with fibrocartilage and it has no medullary cavity.

Palpation

At the lower boundary of the front of the neck, locate the sternal (jugular) notch centrally. This is formed by the superior border of the manubrium sterni inferiorly, and the medial end of each clavicle on either side. Articular cartilage together with an interarticular disc and interclavicular ligament are interposed between the medial ends of the clavicles and the skin.

Moving laterally, the medial third of the bone is convex forward with a superior and anterior surface, both of which are easily palpable despite giving attachment to the sternocleidomastoid superiorly and pectoralis major anteriorly. Below, the anterior end of the first rib is palpable, particularly where it articulates with the lateral border of the manubrium sterni. Further laterally, the middle third of the clavicle begins to curve backwards, being a little more rounded in cross-section. Posterior to the superior surface a depression, the supraclavicular fossa, can be palpated containing the cord-like structures of the trunks of the brachial plexus running downwards and laterally towards the upper limb. If deep, but careful, pressure is applied in this notch in an inferomedial direction, the upper surface

Acromion process
Lateral end of clavicle
Superior angle of scapula
Greater tuberosity
Head of humerus
Corocoid process
Lesser tuberosity
Medial end of clavicle
Sternal notch
First rib
Anterior surface of scapula
Rim of glenoid cavity
Manubrium
Intertubercular sulcus (bicipital groove)
Second rib
Third rib

CLAVICLE
HUMERUS
SCAPULA

Fig. 2.1 (b)
Bones of the left shoulder (anterior
view)

of the first rib, over which the trunks of the brachial plexus pass, can be recognized. The lateral third of the clavicle becomes flattened from above down and its sharper anterior border is concave forward. Its subcutaneous superior surface can readily be palpated through the skin, becoming thicker at the **lateral end** toward the acromioclavicular joint. Below the anterior border is a depression, the infraclavicular fossa, situated between deltoid laterally and pectoralis major inferomedially. Here the tip of the **coracoid** [*korax* (Gk) = a crow and *oeides* (Gk) = shape] process can readily be palpated lying approximately 3 cm below the junction of the middle and lateral thirds of the anterior border and just medial to the anterior fibres of the deltoid. Both anterior and posterior borders of the clavicle give attachment to muscles, deltoid anteriorly and trapezius posteriorly. The lateral end of the clavicle can be identified by a small tubercle on its superior surface which lies just medial to the acromioclavicular joint (see joints of upper limb).

The upper end of the humerus

This comprises the head, the greater tuberosity and the lesser tuberosity. The head is slightly more than half a sphere, smooth and being directed medially, slightly backwards and upwards. The greater tuberosity lies laterally and the lesser tuberosity projects forwards with the intertubercular groove running vertically between the two tuberosities.

Moving lateral to the coracoid process, a slightly pointed projection, the **lesser tuberosity of the humerus** [*humerus* (L) = the shoulder] can be palpated. This forms the medial border of the **intertubercular groove**, through which passes the tendon of the long head of biceps. The groove can easily be palpated at this point as it runs vertically downwards (Fig. 2.1). Lateral to the tendon of biceps, the anterior surface of the **greater tuberosity** may be difficult to palpate as it is covered by the deltoid muscle. However, with your fingers on the anterior aspect, bring the thumb in just below and lateral to the angle of the acromion, and the greater tuberosity can be grasped between the thumb and fingers between the separate fibres of deltoid. The greater tuberosity accounts, in part, for the rounded bulge of the shoulder region.

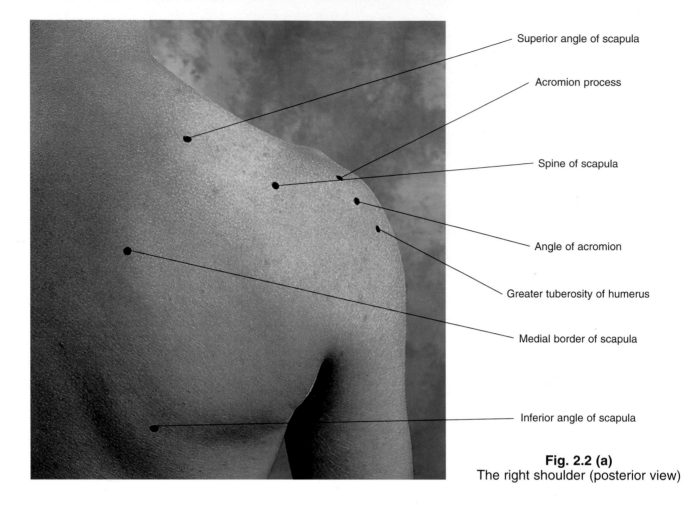

Superior angle of scapula

Acromion process

Spine of scapula

Angle of acromion

Greater tuberosity of humerus

Medial border of scapula

Inferior angle of scapula

Fig. 2.2 (a)
The right shoulder (posterior view)

The scapula [Fig. 2.2]

The scapula [*scapulae* (L) = shoulder blades], (Fig. 2.2) is a flat triangular bone situated on the postero-lateral aspect of the upper chest wall. It has three angles, three borders and costal and dorsal surfaces, the latter being marked by a ledge-shaped spine running almost horizontally.

The spine is wider laterally where it joins the acromion process, but narrows as it passes medially. Its upper and lower borders diverge as it meets the medial border forming a small smooth triangular area. Above the spine there is a deep hollow called the supraspinous fossa and below a larger but shallower depression called the infraspinous fossa.

The lateral angle is expanded and forms the glenoid cavity for articulation with the head of the humerus at the shoulder joint. It also has a sharp bony projection passing forward just below the lateral end of the clavicle called the coracoid process, which is roughened for the attachment of muscle.

Palpation

The whole length of the spine can be palpated between the acromion process laterally and the medial border of the scapula medially. Its upper and lower lips can be recognized easily, even though they give attachment to the trapezius and deltoid muscles, respectively. The posterior surface is clearly palpable and visible, being narrow medially but gradually broadening as it passes laterally to become the superior surface of the acromion. At this point it is covered by a bursa (the supra-acromial bursa), enabling the skin to move easily over this bone. The bone then appears to form a large quadrilateral surface, which is directed upwards and slightly backwards having a posterior, lateral and short anterior border. On its medial side can be palpated the lateral end of the clavicle and the small gap produced by the acromioclavicular joint. The smooth triangular area at the medial end of the spine is also covered by a bursa and can be palpated through the tendinous lower fibres of the trapezius.

The medial border of the scapula is approximately 5 cm lateral to the spines of the second to eighth thoracic vertebrae. Its full length can only be palpated with difficulty, except in lean subjects, as it gives attachment to levator scapulae above and rhomboid major and minor below, as well as being mostly cov-

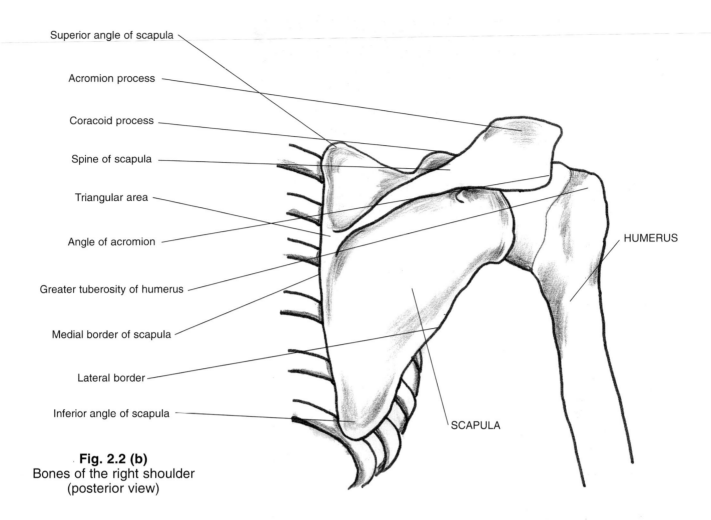

Superior angle of scapula

Acromion process

Coracoid process

Spine of scapula

Triangular area

Angle of acromion

Greater tuberosity of humerus

Medial border of scapula

Lateral border

Inferior angle of scapula

HUMERUS

SCAPULA

Fig. 2.2 (b)
Bones of the right shoulder
(posterior view)

ered by the trapezius muscle. The superior angle is buried in muscle and is tender on deep palpation, but the inferior angle can be identified lying on the posterolateral parts of the seventh and eighth ribs. When the upper limb is raised above the head, the inferior angle can be seen and felt moving laterally around the chest wall as far as the mid-axillary line. The lateral border is very difficult to palpate as it is embedded in thick muscle (teres major and minor). It is by far the thickest of the borders and acts as a lever for its strong muscles to pull it laterally in rotation of the scapula.

Anteriorly, in the infraclavicular fossa, 3 cm below the junction of the lateral and middle thirds of the clavicle, the coracoid process can be palpated despite it giving attachment to three muscles, the short head of the biceps, coracobrachialis and pectoralis minor. Just lateral to the coracoid process running downwards and laterally for approximately 3 cm, the concave anterior rim of the glenoid cavity can be palpated with the head of the humerus lying on its lateral side.

Palpation on movement

Once the boundaries of the scapula have been recognized by palpation, it is important to be able to follow its movements around the chest wall during activities of the shoulder girdle and upper limb.

Place your right hand on the point of the model's right shoulder and place your left hand on the inferior angle and the lower part of the medial border. Get the model to pull the shoulder girdles forward as in hunching the shoulders (protrusion). The scapula is observed moving forwards around the chest wall but staying in its vertical position. Now get the model to brace back the shoulder girdles. The scapula is observed moving backwards and again not changing its vertical position.

Keeping your hands in the same positions, ask the model now to raise (elevation) and lower the shoulder girdles as in shrugging. The scapula will be observed rising and lowering (depression), but still holding its vertical position.

Now ask the model to raise the right arm above the head. When the upper limb reaches 20 degrees the scapula will be observed rotating around an axis just below the spine nearer to its medial end. The superior angle will rise moving medially and the inferior angle will be observed moving laterally and slightly upwards around the chest wall (lateral rotation). In fact, the inferior angle will reach as far as the mid-axillary line on full elevation of the humerus.

When the arm is lowered the scapula will be seen to return to its original position (medial rotation). If, however, the arm is taken behind the chest, medial rotation continues and the inferior angle will come close to the spines of the vertebrae.

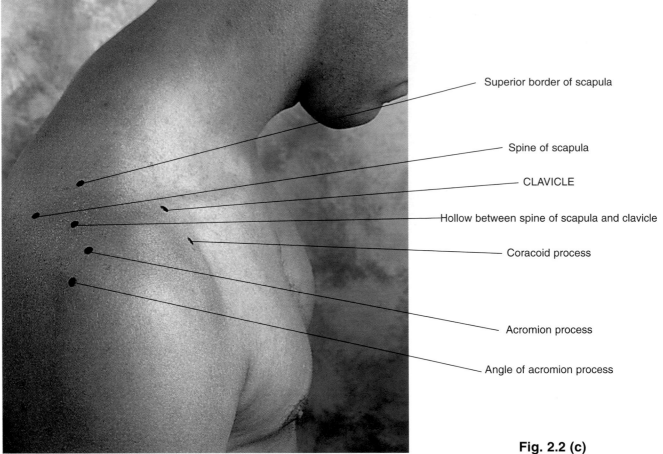

— Superior border of scapula

— Spine of scapula

— CLAVICLE

—Hollow between spine of scapula and clavicle

— Coracoid process

— Acromion process

— Angle of acromion process

Fig. 2.2 (c)
The right shoulder (upper lateral view)

Anatomy

Viewed from above and slightly laterally with the upper limb in about 45 degrees of abduction, the shoulder girdle forms a 'V' shape with the **clavicle** being the anterior and the **spine of the scapula** the posterior stem. They form an angle with each other of approximately 70 degrees and are joined at the acromioclavicular joint. The greater tuberosity of the humerus is now tucked underneath the arch of the **acromion**. Below the junction of the middle with the lateral third of the clavicle lies the **coracoid process** and below the lateral third of the clavicle lies the head of the humerus. The acromion appears quadrilateral from above and continues medially and backwards as the spine of the scapula. The **upper third of the scapula** lies above and anterior to the spine with the superior angle being most medial and the **superior border** passing laterally, presenting the **suprascapular notch** and continuing to the **base of the coracoid process**.

The anterior border of the lateral third of the clavicle continues laterally with the short anterior border of the acromion process, which is again continuous with the lateral border and its posterior border. This continues as the inferior border of the spine.

The posterior border of the lateral third of the clavicle is in the same line as the superior border of the spine of the scapula but acutely angled.

Palpation

Run your fingers from the anterior border of the clavicle across the acromioclavicular joint where the anterior border of the acromion process of the scapula continues in line for approximately 1.5 cm. It then passes backwards as the lateral border of the acromion [*akros* (Gk) = summit and *omos* = shoulders] for a further 5 cm before turning medially (**acromial angle**) to become the inferior lip of the spine of the scapula, all of which is palpable and gives attachment to the deltoid muscle.

Palpation on movement

Place the fingers and thumb of your right hand on the medial end and the fingers and thumb of the left hand on the lateral end of the right clavicle.

As the model draws the shoulder girdle forward (protraction), the lateral end will move forward accompanying the sliding of the scapula around the chest wall. The medial end, however, will be felt gliding backwards in the clavicular notch of the sternum. The axis around which this occurs is approximately 3 cm from its medial end, where the costoclavicular ligament attaches to the under surface of the clavicle. If the shoulder is now drawn backwards (retraction), the lateral end of the clavicle will move backwards, but the medial end will move forwards and become proud of the sternum.

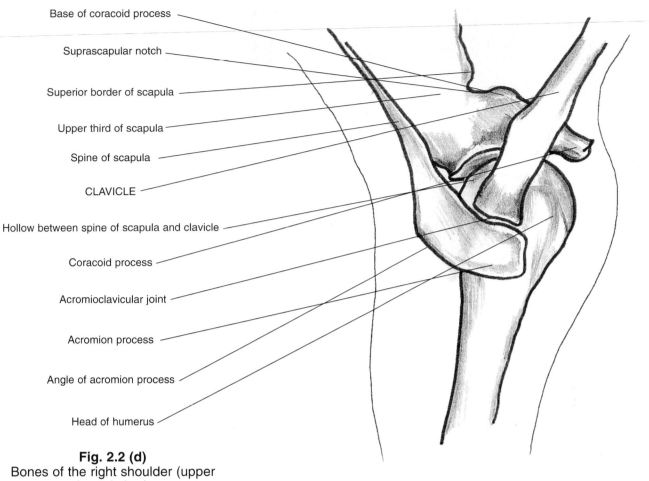

Base of coracoid process

Suprascapular notch

Superior border of scapula

Upper third of scapula

Spine of scapula

CLAVICLE

Hollow between spine of scapula and clavicle

Coracoid process

Acromioclavicular joint

Acromion process

Angle of acromion process

Head of humerus

Fig. 2.2 (d)
Bones of the right shoulder (upper
lateral view)

If the model now raises the shoulder girdle (elevation), the lateral end will rise and the medial end will move down, rolling into the clavicular notch of the sternum using the same fulcrum as above. When the shoulder girdle is lowered the lateral end will drop, and the medial end will rise to its original position or even protrude upwards if the girdle is further depressed.

If the arm is now raised above the head the clavicle will first of all move as in elevation but will, in the final stage, rotate as a whole with the anterior surface moving upwards. This movement accompanies lateral rotation of the scapula. Lowering the arm will return the shoulder girdle to its original position.

Movements of the clavicle, scapula and humerus and the joints between them are highly complex and should be studied in *Anatomy and Human Movement* (Palastanga *et al.*, 1998).

Functional anatomy

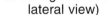

The clavicle acts as a rigid lever bracing the shoulder girdle backwards, allowing the upper limb to move freely away from the chest wall. With the powerful upper fibres of the trapezius muscle raising or supporting its lateral end and the adjoining acromion process, it helps to transmit weight from the upper limb to the vertebral column via the manubrium sterni and the upper ribs. The clavicle moves around an axis close to its medial end at the attachment of the costoclavicular ligament and is tightly bound to the coracoid laterally by the coracoclavicular ligament. Fractures of the bone may occur due to a fall on the shoulder, as in horse riding, motorcycling and rugby. Normally the fracture will take place where the medial two-thirds joins the lateral third, medial to the coracoclavicular ligament. The shoulder girdle may protrude forwards and a large hard swelling can be palpated and seen at the site of the fracture. Complications can occur from fractures of this bone if it is more central and the sharp bone ends are forced backwards, thus damaging the brachial plexus and/or the subclavian artery. Provided there are no serious complications the fracture will unite readily in approximately six weeks, although movements of the upper limb and shoulder girdle can begin in two weeks or when the sharp pain has subsided.

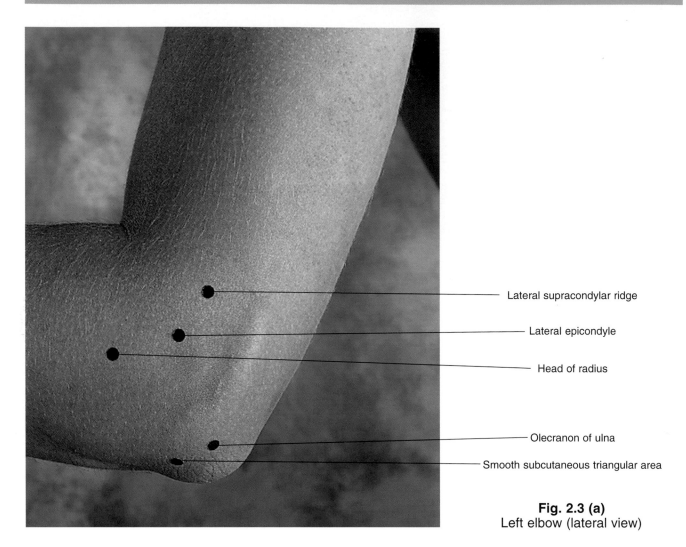

Lateral supracondylar ridge

Lateral epicondyle

Head of radius

Olecranon of ulna

Smooth subcutaneous triangular area

Fig. 2.3 (a)
Left elbow (lateral view)

The elbow region [Fig. 2.3]

This region is made up of the lower end of the humerus, and the upper ends of the radius and ulna.

The lower end of the humerus is composed of a medial and lateral condyle, having two articular surfaces, the trochlea and the capitulum respectively. Above these surfaces anteriorly are two fossae, the coronoid medially and radial laterally. Posteriorly there is a larger depression called the olecranon fossa. On the lateral side of the lateral condyle is a prominence called the lateral epicondyle, which lies at the lower end of the lateral supracondylar ridge.

The upper end of the radius is composed of a head, button-shaped and articular on its upper surface and on the medial third of its rim, a neck, which is cylindrical, joining the head to the upper end of the shaft, and a large tuberosity (bicipital tuberosity), which projects from its medial side at the base of the neck and is roughened on its posterior aspect for the attachment of the tendon of the biceps brachii.

Palpation

Just below the lower attachment of deltoid, halfway down the lateral side of the arm, the humerus can be palpated. It is crossed laterally by the radial nerve running downwards and forwards. Trauma in this area can cause pain, tingling and, sometimes, numbness of the posterolateral aspect of the hand. Inferiorly, the bone can be palpated as a sharp border, the lateral supracondylar ridge, terminating at the large lateral epicondyle. The posterior surface of this epicondyle is subcutaneous and with the elbow flexed can be traced medially across the back of the humerus to the commencement of the olecranon [*olekranon* (Gk) = the point of the elbow] fossa. With the elbow extended, the lateral side of the button-shaped head of the radius [*radius* (L) = spoke of a wheel] can be felt immediately below the epicondyle. The narrow groove running horizontally between the two is the radiohumeral part of the elbow joint. Palpate around the lateral half of the radial head, posteriorly as far as the posterior aspect of the superior radioulnar joint. Just below the head, laterally, the narrowed neck can be identified, being hidden by muscles anteriorly and posteriorly.

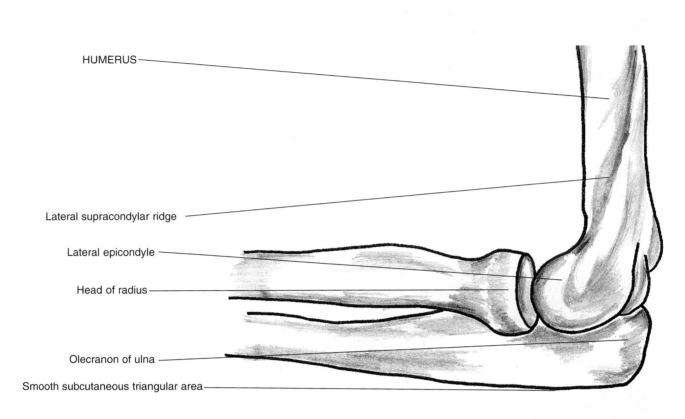

HUMERUS

Lateral supracondylar ridge

Lateral epicondyle

Head of radius

Olecranon of ulna

Smooth subcutaneous triangular area

Fig. 2.3 (b)
Bones of the left elbow (lateral view)

The large bony formation of the olecranon (Fig. 2.3a,b) can be palpated, particularly when the elbow is flexed. Its superior surface is more difficult to feel as it is covered by the tendon of triceps, as it inserts into its posterior aspect. With your fingers now placed on the posterior triangular surface of the olecranon, the skin and superficial fascia can easily be moved owing to the presence of the subcutaneous olecranon bursa. If pressure is applied for some time to this area, as in leaning on the elbows, the bursa can become inflamed and swollen (bursitis). The narrow triangular surface has its apex downwards and is continuous with the posterior border of the ulna, which is subcutaneous as far as its head. The medial and lateral surfaces of the olecranon can readily be palpated; however, lower down they become covered by muscle.

The olecranon is much more difficult to palpate when the elbow is extended, as it moves into the olecranon fossa of the posterior surface of the distal end of the humerus.

Palpation on movement

With the right elbow flexed to 90 degrees, place the fingers of your left hand on the superior surface of the olecranon, which will be at the back of the elbow. Now, with your right hand place the fingers on the medial epicondyle and the thumb on the lateral epicondyle of the humerus. When the model extends the elbow you will observe that the olecranon will virtually disappear into the olecranon fossa on the posterior aspect of the humerus.

With the right elbow again in flexion, find the lateral epicondyle of the humerus. At its lower end there is a small space and then the outer edge of the disc-like head of the radius. If the model now pronates and supinates the forearm you will feel the head of the radius rotating below your fingers.

Finally, stand in front of the fully flexed elbow. Take the arm in your left hand and the forearm in your right. If the model now extends the elbow joint you will observe that the forearm, which was slightly medial to the line of the humerus, now moves more to the lateral side forming an angle with the upper part of the arm. This is termed 'the carrying angle'.

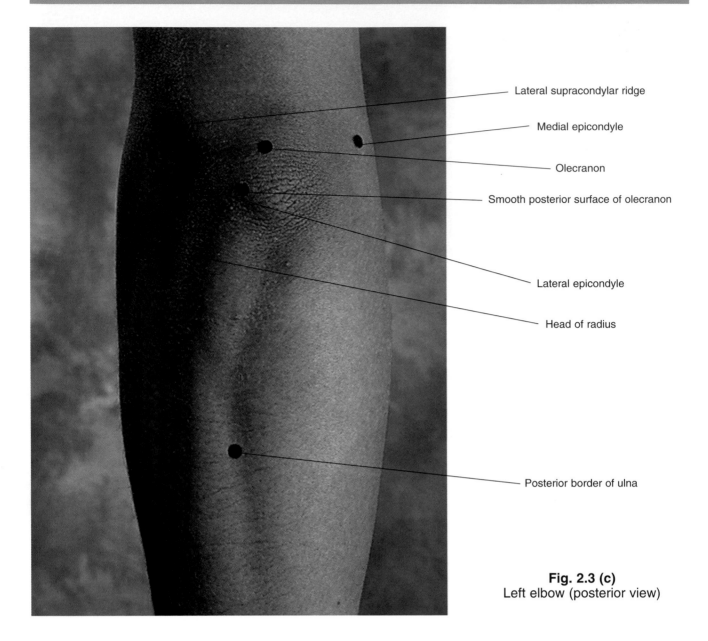

— Lateral supracondylar ridge

— Medial epicondyle

— Olecranon

— Smooth posterior surface of olecranon

— Lateral epicondyle

— Head of radius

— Posterior border of ulna

Fig. 2.3 (c)
Left elbow (posterior view)

Bones

On the medial surface of the medial condyle of the humerus there is a large projection called the **medial epicondyle**, being slightly hollowed posteriorly. Above this is the **medial supracondylar ridge** which passes up to the medial side of the shaft.

The pulley-shaped trochlea is articular and covers the anterior, inferior and posterior aspect of the bone. Its medial flange is lower than the lateral and accounts for the angle at the elbow joint.

The upper end of the ulna, lying below the trochlea of the humerus, is composed mainly of a hook-shaped process called the **olecranon** and a shelf-like process projecting forwards from the upper end of the shaft called the coronoid process. The two form a socket shape facing forwards and called the trochlear notch. This articulates with the trochlea of the humerus in the elbow joint.

Palpation

On the medial side of the elbow, the sharp medial supracondylar ridge can be palpated and traced upwards for approximately the lower quarter of the humerus. At its lower end a large, bony prominence can be palpated 2 cm above the elbow joint and approximately 1 cm below the level of the lateral epicondyle. This is the medial epicondyle behind which there is a deep groove for the ulnar nerve. Palpation of this area may be quite tender and could cause tingling or even numbness on the medial side of the hand due to pressure on the ulnar nerve. This is often referred to as the 'funny bone', owing to the strange sensation when it is compressed.

With the elbow fully flexed, it is just possible to feel the depression of the olecranon fossa through the tendon of the triceps. From the posterior, locate the medial and lateral epicondyles. At a point midway between the two, press your thumb onto the back of the triceps tendon – it will sink slightly into the olecranon fossa. Just below your thumb you will palpate the bony olecranon.

Medial supracondylar ridge

Lateral supracondylar ridge

Medial epicondyle

Olecranon

Smooth posterior surface of olecranon

Lateral epicondyle

Head of radius

Posterior border of ulna

Fig. 2.3 (d)
Bones of the left elbow (posterior
view)

With the right elbow fully extended and the forearm fully supinated, examine the anterior of this region. Place the flat surface of your right hand 2.5 cm below and 2.5 cm lateral to the medial epicondyle. You will feel a hard bony projection deep to the mass of flexor muscles. This is the coronoid [*corone* (Gk) = crown; also the name given to the pointed front of a ship or plough] process. The contrast can be observed by placing your left thumb in a similar position laterally.

Functional anatomy

The title 'carrying angle' at the elbow joint must have been given when the carrying of pails of water was common. In fact most objects carried in the hand with the elbow extended are normally accompanied by the forearm being held in the mid prone position. This eliminates the angle at the elbow. You

will also observe that when the elbow is fully flexed the hand does not oppose the shoulder joint but locates itself to mid clavicle position.

If the shoulder is now flexed you will observe that the hand is taken first to the chin and then to the mouth, thus facilitating feeding. Keeping the arm in this position, if the forearm is now fully pronated and the fingers extended, the hand now becomes a protection to the face.

Injuries and degeneration of the elbow and superior radioulnar joint often lead to loss of flexion or extension or both. This results in serious dysfunction of the upper limb, with its ability to shorten and position the hand impeded. In one elbow this is perhaps acceptable, but if this dysfunction is present in both elbow complexes it may be devastating to a person's quality of life. Not only is dressing and eating affected, but the use of the hands when visiting the toilet may be impossible

Terminal phalanx of middle finger

Middle phalanx of index finger

Proximal phalanx of index finger

Head of metacarpal bone of index finger

Metacarpal of index finger

Hook of hamate

Tubercle of scaphoid

Pisiform

Head of ulna

Fig. 2.4 (a)
Right hand (anterior view)

The wrist and hand

The lower ends of the radius and ulna form a shallow mortice into which three of the four bones of the proximal row of carpals – scaphoid, lunate and triquetral – fit. The fourth bone in the proximal row, the pisiform, lies anterior to the triquetral. Distally, the proximal row of carpal bones forms another concavity for the reception of the second row of carpal bones – the trapezium, trapezoid, capitate [*capitate* (L) = head-shaped] and hamate. The capitate is the largest of the four and fits snugly into the deepest part of the concavity, being in contact with all the carpal bones except the pisiform, triquetral and trapezium (Fig. 2.4b).

The metacarpals are miniature long bones lying distal to the carpals: that for the thumb articulating with the trapezium; the second mainly articulating with the trapezoid; that for the middle finger mainly articulating with the capitate; and the fourth and fifth articulating with the hamate.

Each metacarpal head articulates with a proximal phalanx.

Each finger has a middle and a distal phalanx, the thumb just a distal phalanx.

Anterior, medial and lateral aspects

Palpation

The bones of the wrist and hand are more difficult to locate on the anterior surface as they tend to be hidden by the muscles which arise and insert in the hand.

Return to the wrist joint and locate the head of the ulna on its medial side (Fig. 2.4). Immediately distal to this, the medial and posterior surfaces of the triquetral [*triquetrus* (L) = having three corners] can be palpated with the pea-shaped pisiform [*pisum* (L) = a pea] lying on its anterior surface, being easily recognizable owing to its prominence, and by the attachment of the tendon of flexor carpi ulnaris to its proximal side.

Deep pressure applied with the tip of the thumb 1 cm distal and slightly lateral to the pisiform reveals a small but distinct bony prominence. This is the hook of the hamate [*hamatus* (L) = hooked]. If the thumb is moved from side to side, two small nerves, the superficial terminal branches of the ulnar nerve, can be compressed against this prominence.

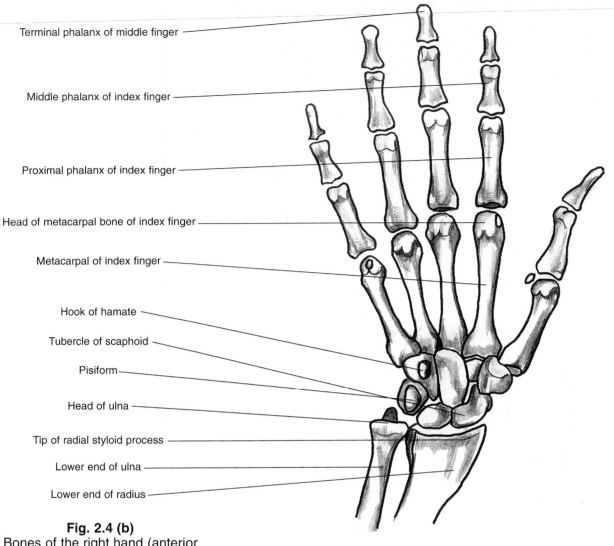

Terminal phalanx of middle finger

Middle phalanx of index finger

Proximal phalanx of index finger

Head of metacarpal bone of index finger

Metacarpal of index finger

Hook of hamate

Tubercle of scaphoid

Pisiform

Head of ulna

Tip of radial styloid process

Lower end of ulna

Lower end of radius

Fig. 2.4 (b)
Bones of the right hand (anterior
view)

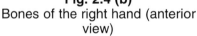

On the lateral side of the wrist, locate the **tip of the radial styloid process**. It lies within a space termed the 'anatomical snuff box'. The styloid process can be traced upwards for a short distance, its anterior border continuing as the sharp anterior border of the shaft. Just medial to this crest lies the radial artery. Distal to the styloid process are the lateral surface of the scaphoid [*skaphe* (Gk) = a skiff], the trapezium [*trapezion* (Gk) = an irregular four-sided figure] and the base of the first metacarpal, marked by a small tubercle. Its shaft leads distally to its head. The base, shaft and the head of the proximal phalanx are clearly palpable, as also are the base and shaft as far as the nail of the distal phalanx [*phalanx* (Gk) = a band of soldiers]. You should note that the posterior surface of the bones of the thumb face laterally due to the thumb lying at right angles to the palm. Medially, the anterior surfaces are difficult to determine due to the presence of muscle and tendon.

The **tubercle of the scaphoid** can be found at the proximal end of the thenar eminence, on the front of the carpal region, 1 cm medial to the tip of the radial styloid process. It is often quite difficult to palpate, although this is made easier if the wrist is extended. The vertical ridge of the trapezium is just palpable with deep pressure 1 cm distal to the scaphoid tubercle. This can often be a painful area for deep palpation, which is best done sparingly. The tubercle is prominent enough to be damaged by falls on the outstretched hand and a fracture may cause pain and dysfunction of the hand for many months due to its poor blood supply leading to a long healing time (see next page).

The anterior surfaces of the remaining carpal, metacarpal and phalangeal bones are difficult to palpate as they lie deep to the muscle and fascia. Only if the fingers are fully extended can the anterior surfaces of the heads of the metacarpals be felt in line with each finger, 2 cm proximal to the web between the fingers. The heads of each phalanx are also palpable in full or hyperextension, being just proximal to the creases of the interphalangeal joints. They normally present a small tubercle on either side, palpable if the lateral sides of the head are gripped between finger and thumb.

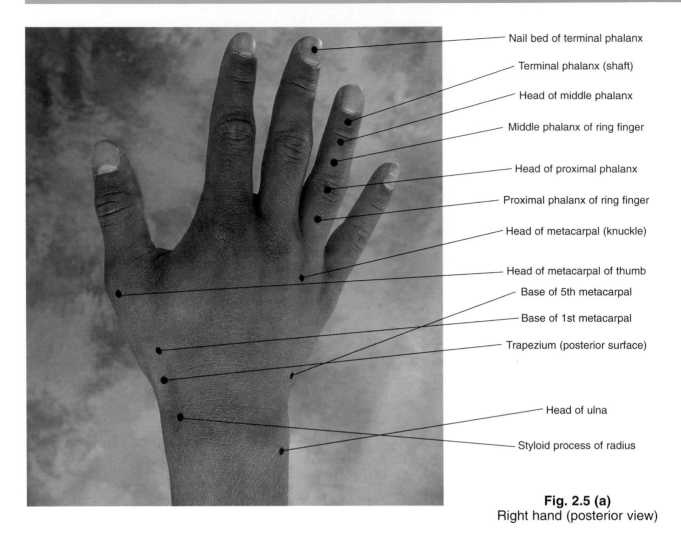

Nail bed of terminal phalanx

Terminal phalanx (shaft)

Head of middle phalanx

Middle phalanx of ring finger

Head of proximal phalanx

Proximal phalanx of ring finger

Head of metacarpal (knuckle)

Head of metacarpal of thumb

Base of 5th metacarpal

Base of 1st metacarpal

Trapezium (posterior surface)

Head of ulna

Styloid process of radius

Fig. 2.5 (a)
Right hand (posterior view)

Posterior aspect [Fig. 2.5]

Palpation

Place your finger on the button-shaped head of the ulna, clearly palpable posteromedially, but hidden by the tendon of flexor carpi ulnaris anteriorly. On its posteromedial aspect, a small projection, the ulnar styloid process, can be palpated, although it is partially hidden by the tendon of the extensor carpi ulnaris. If the wrist is radially deviated, the head of the ulna and its styloid process become much easier to identify.

On the lateral side of the wrist, the radial styloid process can be identified, having tendons running in front and behind. If traced upwards, the lower half of the lateral side of the radius can be palpated before being covered by the bulk of the brachioradialis muscle. This region may be quite tender to palpate as it is often crossed by the superficial terminal branch(es) of the radial nerve.

On the posterior aspect of the distal end of the radius, just above the level of the styloid process, the dorsal tubercle of the radius can be palpated, with the tendon of the extensor pollicis longus grooving its medial side and using it as a pulley. Below the level of the dorsal tubercle and the head of the ulna is a hollow, limited 2 cm below by the bases of the metacarpal bones. With the subject's wrist flexed,

the posterior surfaces of the scaphoid, lunate [luna (L) = the moon] and triquetral can be identified in a line distal to the tips of the radial and ulnar styloid processes. Just beyond these the trapezoid, at the base of the second metacarpal, the capitate, at the base of the third, and the hamate, at the base of the fourth and fifth metacarpals, can all be identified if the bones are gripped between the fingers posteriorly, and the thumb anteriorly. The lower limit of this area is marked by the bases of the metacarpal bones with their shafts running distally to end in rounded heads, all of which are easily palpable. The base, shaft and head of each phalanx are again readily palpable posteriorly, particularly when the subject's fingers are flexed. Anteriorly, they are hidden by tendons and the pulp of the fingers.

Palpation on movement

With the wrist in extension, locate the tubercle of the scaphoid and the pisiform bone. As the wrist is taken into flexion they appear to move backwards and become indistinct. Keeping the wrist in flexion, the posterior aspect of the carpal bones can be palpated just below the ulna and radius. If the wrist

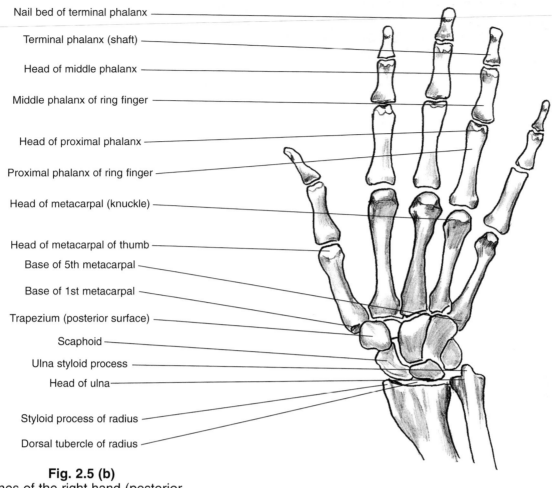

Nail bed of terminal phalanx

Terminal phalanx (shaft)

Head of middle phalanx

Middle phalanx of ring finger

Head of proximal phalanx

Proximal phalanx of ring finger

Head of metacarpal (knuckle)

Head of metacarpal of thumb

Base of 5th metacarpal

Base of 1st metacarpal

Trapezium (posterior surface)

Scaphoid

Ulna styloid process

Head of ulna

Styloid process of radius

Dorsal tubercle of radius

Fig. 2.5 (b)
Bones of the right hand (posterior
view)

is taken back into extension, they appear to move forwards and become indistinct.

With the model's index finger in extension, grip the base of the proximal phalanx with your thumb anteriorly and the fingers posteriorly. When the model now flexes the finger you will note that the phalanx moves round to the front of the head of the metacarpal leaving the head prominent (the knuckle). This is common to all the fingers, but more obvious in the index finger. Apply the same procedure to the base of the proximal phalanx of the thumb and you will note that only half the movement is available and the head of the metacarpal is only partially exposed.

If the same procedure is carried out on the interphalangeal joints, the head of the most proximal of the two bones becomes palpable as a small 'knuckle' shape.

Functional anatomy

Fractures of the carpal bones are rare except in the case of the scaphoid, which is sometimes damaged by a fall on the outstretched hand. Palpation of the area will normally identify swelling and a rise in temperature around the area, but may elicit acute pain. It is more common in young adults and may need 2–3 months in plaster before healing occurs. As the blood supply to the tubercle of the scaphoid passes through its neck, if the fracture occurs at this point there may be delayed or even non union and a prolonged period in plaster or even an operation may have to be performed. (See orthopaedic literature for further information.)

Fractures of the metacarpal bones is fairly common at all ages and is often due again to a fall on the outstretched hand or a longitudinal force along the metacarpal, as in punching. Displacements are easily palpable combined with the swelling and increase in temperature. Only if there is displacement is there a need for intervention.

Injuries to the phalanges are usually due to direct violence such as trapping the fingers in a door. Displacement is easily palpable, along with the swelling, increase in temperature and acute pain. Alignment must be restored and minimal splinting should be used, perhaps just to the adjoining finger.

All splinting of the hand should be kept to a minimum due to the serious complication of stiffness.

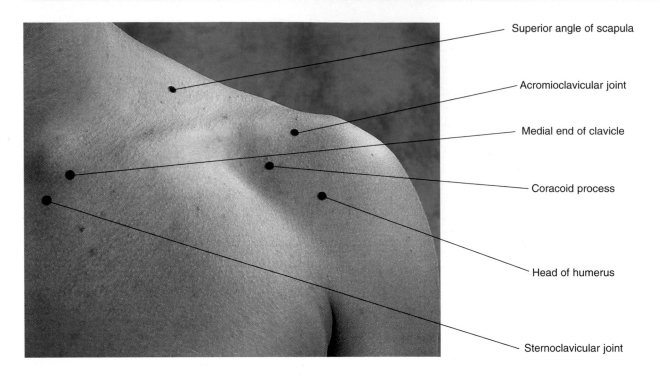

Superior angle of scapula

Acromioclavicular joint

Medial end of clavicle

Coracoid process

Head of humerus

Sternoclavicular joint

Fig. 2.6 (a)
The shoulder region (anterior view)

JOINTS

Joints of the pectoral girdle

The sternoclavicular joint [Fig. 2.6]

At its medial end the clavicle articulates with the clavicular notch of the manubrium. The joint is synovial, being surrounded by a capsule lined with synovial membrane, except where it is attached to the edges of a fibrous disc which divides the joint space into two separate cavities. It is a modified saddle (sellar) joint and its capsule is supported by ligaments, the intercostal above and medially, the costoclavicular laterally below the clavicle and the anterior and posterior across the front and back of the joint. It is subcutaneous, allowing easy palpation of the joint line and a reasonable examination of joint movement.

Surface marking

The sternoclavicular joint can be palpated at the upper lateral corner of the manubrium sterni, as a curved line concave laterally. It is approximately 1 cm in length, extending over the lower half of the medial surface of the clavicle, passing inferolaterally for approximately 0.5 cm.

Palpation

Run your fingers down the front of the neck until you reach the sternal notch. Below you will feel the manubrium sterni and laterally the medial end of the clavicle with the sternoclavicular joint between the two.

Immediately lateral to the joint, between the clavicle and the first rib, is the costoclavicular ligament. This is not palpable, but acts as the fulcrum for movements of the clavicle at the joint. Thus when the lateral end of the clavicle is drawn backwards (retraction), the medial end can be observed gliding forward, projecting anterior to the plane of the

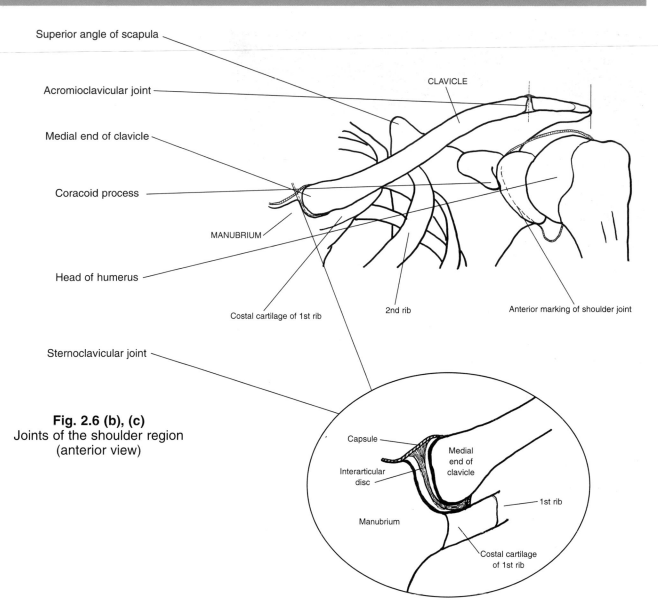

Fig. 2.6 (b), (c)
Joints of the shoulder region
(anterior view)

manubrium. Similarly, when the lateral end of the clavicle is brought forwards (protraction), the medial end can be palpated moving backwards behind the plane of the manubrium. If the pectoral girdle is raised (elevation), the medial end of the clavicle glides downwards on the clavicular notch of the manubrium until it is level with the superior border of the manubrium. If the pectoral girdle is pulled downwards (depression), the medial end of the clavicle rises on the clavicular notch. All these movements can be observed occurring around the attachment of the costoclavicular ligament.

When the upper limb is raised above the head, the scapula laterally rotates against the chest wall, and the lateral end of the clavicle is elevated until, during the final few degrees of movement, it is accompanied by a backward rotation of the whole clavicle so that the anterior surface faces more superiorly. This rotation is due to the tension developed in the coracoclavicular ligament.

Accessory movements

Gliding of the medial end of the clavicle either forwards, backwards, upwards or downwards, or rotating its articular surfaces upwards, are all normal movements. Pressure applied to the medial end of the clavicle will produce little movement, as the stress is taken by the costoclavicular ligament which usually remains taut and reasonably inflexible. If, however, similar pressures are applied to the medial end of the clavicle, with the pectoral girdle in an appropriate position to aid the movement, then additional movement can be achieved. For example, if the pectoral girdle is protruded, pressure applied anteroposteriorly will augment the movement of the medial end of the clavicle. Pressure to raise the anterior surface of the medial end of the clavicle, as in the final stages of elevation, is best applied when the upper limb is as near to full elevation as possible.

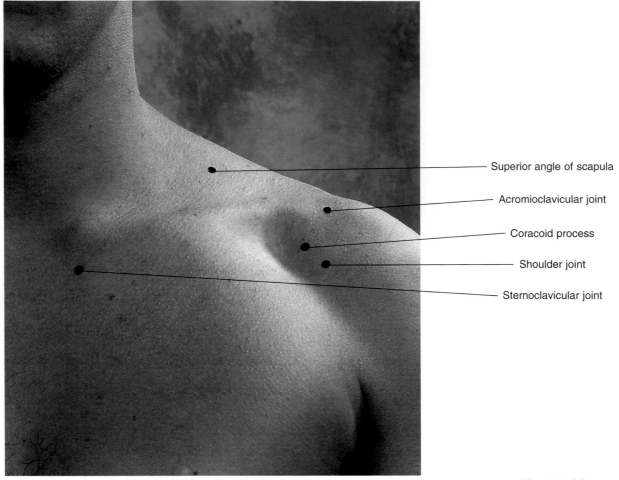

Superior angle of scapula

Acromioclavicular joint

Coracoid process

Shoulder joint

Sternoclavicular joint

Fig. 2.7 (a)
The acromioclavicular joint
(anterior view)

The acromioclavicular joint [Fig. 2.7]

The acromioclavicular joint is immediately lateral to the anterior concavity at the lateral one-third of the clavicle, approximately 1.5 cm medial to the lateral border of the acromion process. It can be marked from above by drawing a line in an antero-posterior direction just lateral to a small tubercle on the upper surface of the lateral end of the clavicle. It is a plane synovial joint lying in a paramedian plane of the body. It is surrounded by a joint capsule supported above by the superior acromioclavicular ligament. It does rely for its stability, however, on the costoclavicular and the coracoclavicular ligaments which act as accessory ligaments to this joint. The two oval facets, one on the lateral end of the clavicle and the other on the medial aspect of the acromion process, are not congruent and rely on a small disc or part of a disc which fills the upper part of the joint space.

Palpation

Stand facing the model's left shoulder. Run your right hand up over the beautiful shape of the deltoid muscle on the lateral aspect of the shoulder. At the top you will feel the lateral border of the acromion process marked posteriorly by its angle. Now trace along the anterior border of the acromion for 1.5 cm and you will feel a small indentation where the clavicle joins the acromion. A very faint groove passes posteriorly to another small indentation on the posterior surface. The joint is quite difficult to palpate unless movement is occurring. Slight twisting or gapping of the acromion against the clavicle can be identified with movements of the pectoral girdle, but even then only with careful palpation. On full elevation of the pectoral girdle the acromion process rotates backwards against the lateral end of the clavicle until the final few degrees of elevation when the clavicle also rotates backwards, producing an upward movement of the anterior surface of the

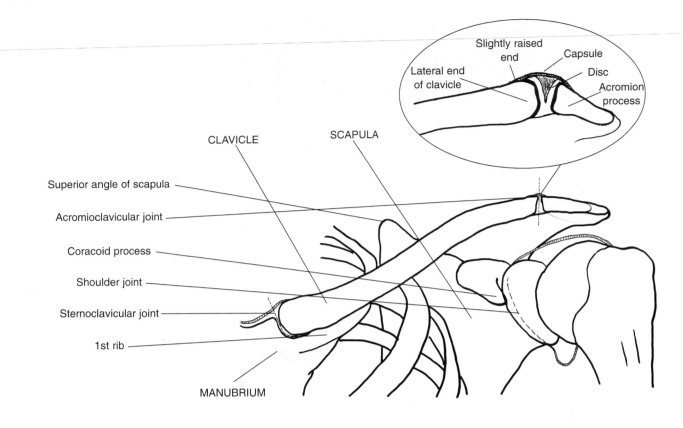

Fig. 2.7 (b), (c)
The acromioclavicular joint
(anterior view)

clavicle in its entire length. This is partly due to the tension of the coronoid part of the coracoclavicular ligament pulling down the posterior aspect of the clavicle, and partly due to the costoclavicular ligament at the medial end of the clavicle attaching to its posterior aspect. This movement is also facilitated by the thickness of the disc in the sternoclavicular joint allowing a longitudinal rotation to occur.

The superior surface of the acromioclavicular joint is usually quite tender on palpation, due to pressure on the superior acromioclavicular ligament. This tenderness is increased after prolonged activity involving the pectoral girdle or after carrying heavy loads on the shoulder.

Accessory movements

This joint is capable of slight gliding movements, these being forwards, backwards, upwards and

downwards. It is also able to rotate, with one surface pivoting on the other, as well as allowing a certain amount of gapping anteriorly and posteriorly. All these movements are normal but, as with the sternoclavicular joint, the end-range can be increased by addition of pressure in the appropriate direction. These again are best performed at the end of normal range, so that, for example, an increase in posterior gliding of the acromion is best achieved with the pectoral girdle retracted. Movement can be achieved by applying pressure, with the thumbs, either to the lateral end of the clavicle or the anterior aspect of the acromion. The former appears to be easier to apply.

Although the acromioclavicular and sternoclavicular joints may appear to be insignificant, stiffness of either will reduce the range of movement of the pectoral girdle, resulting in serious functional loss in the range of movement of the upper limb, and may be misdiagnosed as shoulder joint stiffness.

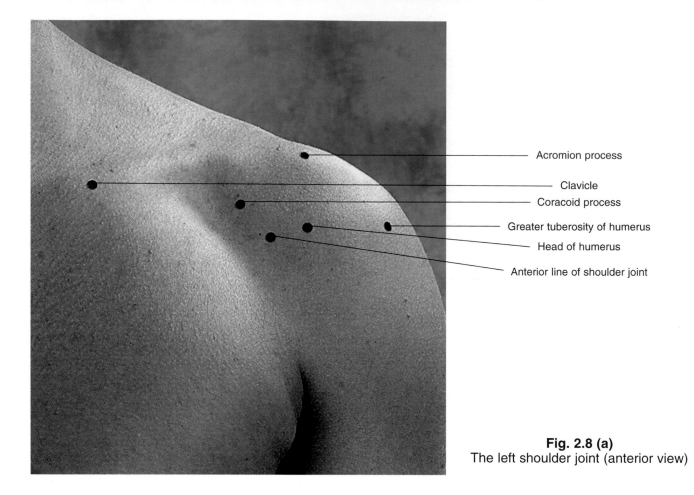

Acromion process

Clavicle

Coracoid process

Greater tuberosity of humerus

Head of humerus

Anterior line of shoulder joint

Fig. 2.8 (a)
The left shoulder joint (anterior view)

The shoulder joint [Fig. 2.8]

This is a synovial joint of the ball-and-socket type. The head of the humerus is slightly less than half a sphere, but is more ovoid in shape. The glenoid cavity is shallow and is estimated to have only one-third the articular surface of the head of the humerus. Both surfaces are covered with articular cartilage. The joint is capable of a large range of movements which are essential for full functional activity of the upper limb. The apparent range of the joint is further increased by the movements of the shoulder (pectoral) girdle, allowing the glenoid cavity to be directed more upwards than laterally.

The joint is surrounded by a loose capsule which is lined by synovial membrane and is supported by ligaments, in front by the glenohumeral, above and posteriorly by the coracohumeral and across the bicipital groove by the transverse ligament. Around the outer rim of the glenoid cavity of the scapula, deep to the joint capsule, is attached a fibrous ring, which is triangular in cross-section and named the glenoidal labrum.

Surface marking

The anterior joint line is a shallow curve concave laterally; its upper boundary is just lateral to and above the coracoid process passing downwards and slightly laterally for approximately 2–3 cm. The head of the humerus can also be identified lying lateral to the joint line.

Palpation

The joint is deep, being surrounded by strong, thick muscles, and is therefore not easy to palpate. Its anterior aspect is the nearest to the surface, and with careful palpation the head of the humerus and the anterior rim of the glenoid fossa can be identified. The rounded anterior part of the head can be palpated with comparative ease; traced upwards it is masked by the anterior part of the acromion, while below it becomes lost in the axilla. Laterally it is bounded by the lesser tubercle, projecting forwards, which forms the medial lip of the bicipital (inter-

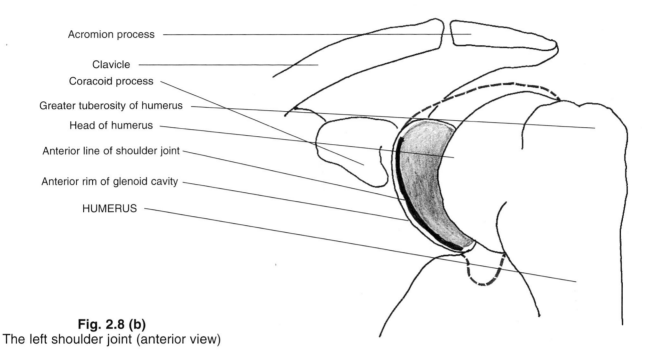

Acromion process

Clavicle

Coracoid process

Greater tuberosity of humerus

Head of humerus

Anterior line of shoulder joint

Anterior rim of glenoid cavity

HUMERUS

Fig. 2.8 (b)
The left shoulder joint (anterior view)

tubercular) groove. The long head of the biceps brachii can be palpated running up the groove and on to the anterolateral aspect of the humeral head.

When the upper limb is laterally rotated, more of the head becomes palpable: on medial rotation it can be felt sliding backwards against the glenoid fossa, eventually disappearing. The lesser tubercle can also be palpated, moving laterally and medially with the movement of rotation of the humerus.

On abduction of the arm, the anterior part of the humeral head can be felt gliding downwards, with the reverse happening when the arm is returned to the side. Palpation of the head in this case, however, is made more difficult by the contraction of the ante-

rior fibres of the deltoid which pass across the anterior aspect of the joint.

Posteriorly (see Fig. 2.8e,f), the shoulder joint is estimated to be at the same level and in the same sagittal plane as it is anteriorly, being just below the spine of the scapula 2–3 cm medial to the angle of the acromion. Laterally (see Fig 2.8c,d), the centre of the joint is approximately 2 cm below the anterior half of the lateral border of the acromion.

Although the lateral border, angle and posterior border are easily palpable and useful for calculating the position of the shoulder joint from the back, the joint itself is set so deeply in muscle that it is impossible to recognise in normal subjects.

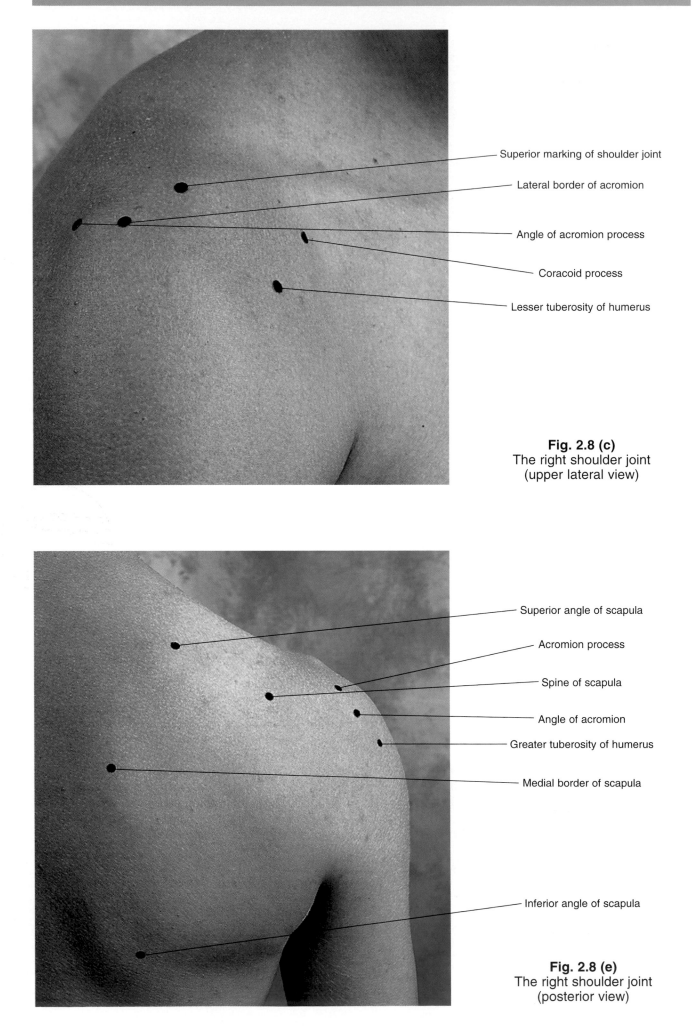

Superior marking of shoulder joint

Lateral border of acromion

Angle of acromion process

Coracoid process

Lesser tuberosity of humerus

Fig. 2.8 (c)
The right shoulder joint
(upper lateral view)

Superior angle of scapula

Acromion process

Spine of scapula

Angle of acromion

Greater tuberosity of humerus

Medial border of scapula

Inferior angle of scapula

Fig. 2.8 (e)
The right shoulder joint
(posterior view)

Spine of scapula

CLAVICLE

Superior marking of shoulder joint

Lateral border of acromion

Angle of acromion process

Coracoid process

Lesser tuberosity of humerus

HUMERUS

Fig. 2.8 (d)
The right shoulder joint
(upper lateral view)

← 2 cm →

Superior angle of scapula

Acromion process

Spine of scapula

Angle of acromion

Greater tuberosity of humerus

Medial border of scapula

Posterior rim of glenoid cavity

Shoulder joint

Head of humerus

SCAPULA

Inferior angle of scapula

HUMERUS

Fig. 2.8 (f)
The right shoulder joint
(posterior view)

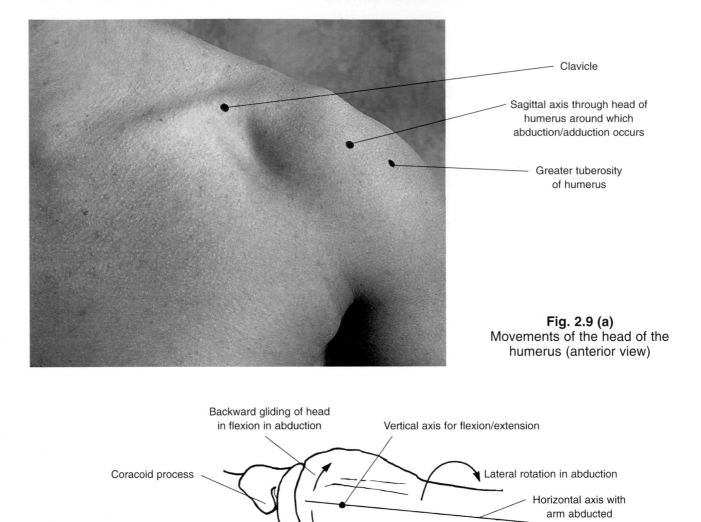

Fig. 2.9 (a)
Movements of the head of the
humerus (anterior view)

Fig. 2.9 (c)
Left humerus in 90° abduction
(superior view)

Movements of the head of the humerus

As the axis of movement of the shoulder joint is through the centre of the head of the humerus (Palastanga *et al.*, 1998), movements of the distal end of the humerus produce an opposite gliding of the head against the glenoid fossa. Thus, abduction causes a downward gliding and an upward rolling of the head of the humerus on the glenoid cavity around a sagittal axis (Fig. 2.9b). Flexion and extension (Fig. 2.9d), however, produce rotation or spin of the head around a frontal axis within the glenoid fossa, similar to that produced by rotating the limb in abduction (Fig. 2.9c). Rotation, with the arm by the side, however, produces a gliding forwards and rolling backwards of the head on lateral rotation and a gliding backwards and rolling forwards on medial rotation around a vertical axis. The combination of rolling in one direction and gliding in the other maintains the position of the centre of axis of the head (Fig. 2.9e). With the subject performing one movement at a time and with your fingers placed over the head of the humerus, these movements can be observed. It becomes even clearer if the palpation is performed with one hand and the humerus is carefully taken through the movement passively.

The shoulder joint has a loose joint capsule and relatively weak associated ligaments, relying to a large extent on muscular activity, especially in the 'rotator cuff' muscles (supraspinatus, infraspinatus, teres minor and subscapularis), for joint stability. It has an extensive range of movement together with a complementary range of accessory movements.

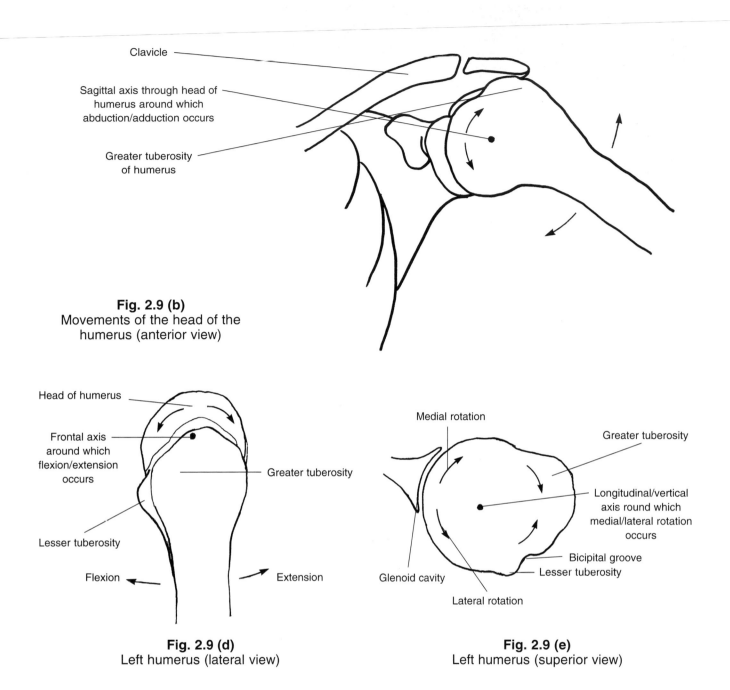

Fig. 2.9 (b)
Movements of the head of the
humerus (anterior view)

Fig. 2.9 (d)
Left humerus (lateral view)

Fig. 2.9 (e)
Left humerus (superior view)

Accessory movements

If the accessory movements are reduced, or lost, normal movement becomes reduced or occasionally eliminated.

The head of the humerus can be drawn laterally away from the glenoid fossa for approximately 1–2 cm, but only when the muscles are completely relaxed (distraction). This is usually possible when the humerus is between 0° and 90° of abduction. To palpate the gapping which occurs, it is best to ask the subject to lie either supine or on his or her side with a colleague actually performing the distraction. Place your fingers on the anterior aspect of the joint where the head and anterior rim of the glenoid fossa can be palpated (see page 30).

Other accessory movements at the joint are: a gliding of the head of the humerus either downwards or upwards by pulling down or pushing up on the arm; and a gliding of the head either forwards or backwards on the glenoid fossa by direct pressure on the upper end of the humerus. Again, it is better to ask a colleague to move the head of the humerus, in the way described above, while you gently palpate using several fingers on the area at the front of the joint where the head and glenoid fossa can be palpated.

HUMERUS

Longitudinal axis of humerus

Medial epicondyle

Coronoid process

Lateral epicondyle

Line of elbow joint

Head of radius

Carrying angle { 10°–15° in men
20°–25° in women

Longitudinal axis of forearm bones

RADIUS

ULNA

2 cm

1 cm

Fig. 2.10 (a), (b)
The right elbow joint (anterior view)

The elbow joint [Fig 2.10]

The elbow joint is basically a hinge joint between the **humerus** above and the **ulna** and **radius** below. The articular surfaces are, medially, the trochlea above and the trochlear notch of the ulna below, and laterally the capitulum above and the upper surface of the **head of radius** below.

The articular surfaces of the trochlea, capitulum, trochlear notch and the head of the radius are all covered with articular cartilage. The joint is surrounded by an extensive capsule which extends up onto the front and back of the humerus above the radial, coronoid and olecranon fossae. It is supported on either side by two strong ligaments. The ulna collateral, triangular, joining the medial epicondyle to the medial side of the olecranon and coronoid processes, and the lateral, again triangular, joining the lateral epicondyle to the annular ligament surrounding the head of the radius. The capsule is lined with synovial membrane.

Surface marking

The joint line is drawn from a point 2 cm below the tip of the **medial epicondyle** to a point 1 cm below the tip of the lateral epicondyle of the humerus (Fig. 2.10a,b). The line passes downwards and medially due to the medial margin of the trochlea projecting down further than the lateral. When viewed from the front, this produces an angle at the elbow where the long axis of the ulna deviates laterally from that of the humerus by approximately 10–15° in men and 20–25° in women (Palastanga *et al.*, 1998). The angle at the elbow is only apparent on full extension and supination of the forearm and is commonly termed the '**carrying angle**' (Fig. 2.10b).

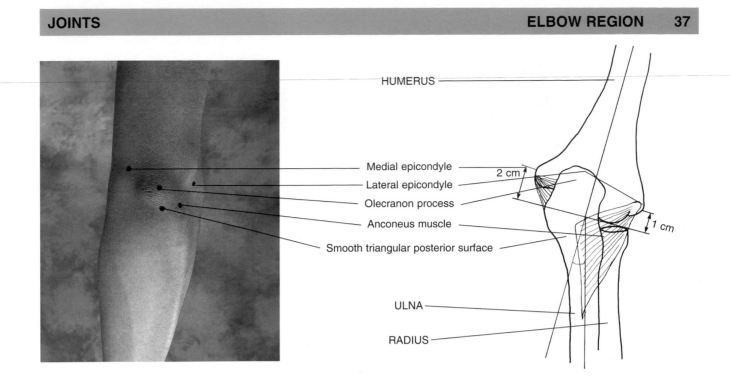

HUMERUS

Medial epicondyle
Lateral epicondyle
Olecranon process
Anconeus muscle
Smooth triangular posterior surface

2 cm

1 cm

ULNA

RADIUS

Fig. 2.10 (c), (d)
The right elbow joint (posterior view)

Palpation

The joint is easily identified on the lateral side
between the lateral epicondyle of the humerus and
the lateral side of the head of the radius (see page
18). However, moving anteriorly the joint line is difficult to follow as it disappears under the superficial
extensor muscles which arise from the lateral epicondyle. Posteriorly, it can be traced as far as the
radial notch of the ulna at the posterior aspect of the
superior radioulnar joint (Fig. 2.10d).

Anteriorly, the elbow joint is not palpable as it lies
deep to muscles: the extensor muscles laterally and
the strong flexor muscles anteromedially, with
brachialis and biceps between. Posteriorly, however,
with the elbow flexed to 90°, the anterior edge of the
olecranon can be palpated and can be traced down
either side until hidden by anconeus laterally and
by the medial collateral ligament medially (Fig.
2.10d).

Accessory movements

With the elbow flexed approximately 15°, the ulna
and radius can be rocked from side to side. This is
achieved by stabilizing the arm just above the
medial and lateral supracondylar ridges with one
hand and applying a side-to-side force just above
the wrist. The correct angle is critical for the movement to take place and varies from individual to
individual.

The elbow can also be distracted, provided that
the muscles are relaxed, by applying a force in the
direction of the long axis of the humerus on a flexed
elbow. This may need considerable force and is best
achieved with the subject lying supine or on their
side.

With the elbow at a right angle and the upper arm
stabilized, the forearm can be moved very slightly in
its long axis, producing a gapping at the anterior
and posterior aspect of the joint. These techniques
are best studied from the mobilization and manipulation literature.

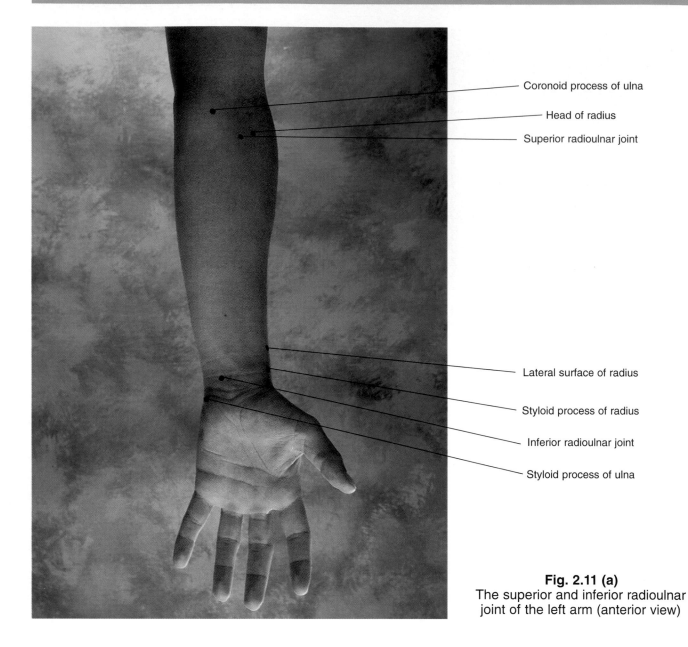

Coronoid process of ulna

Head of radius

Superior radioulnar joint

Lateral surface of radius

Styloid process of radius

Inferior radioulnar joint

Styloid process of ulna

Fig. 2.11 (a)
The superior and inferior radioulnar
joint of the left arm (anterior view)

The radioulnar union

The movements of pronation and supination occur between the radius and ulna. They involve a type of rotation movement at the superior and inferior radioulnar joint and a twisting movement between the shafts of both bones. This latter region is often referred to as the radioulnar union, as the two bones are held together by the interosseous membrane.

The superior radioulnar joint

The superior radioulnar joint is a synovial pivot joint between the medial one-fifth of the head of the radius and the radial notch on the lateral side of the coronoid process of the ulna.

Both surfaces are covered with hyaline cartilage and are reciprocally curved. The head is surrounded by the annular ligament, which is attached in front and behind the radial notch of the ulna and forms the other four-fifths of the ring and is lined with fibrocartilage. The annular ligament is supported from above by the capsule and the triangular radio-

collateral ligament of the elbow joint and from below by the quadrate ligament attaching it to the ulna. The joint is further stabilized by the interosseous membrane which binds the radius and ulna together.

Synovial membrane lines the inner surface of the annular ligament in a double fold attaching to the edges of the articular facets of ulna and radius and emerges just below the annular ligament as a loose fold. It is continuous with that of the elbow joint, although functionally it is a completely separate joint.

Surface marking

The surface marking for the joint anteriorly and posteriorly is a vertical line, 1 cm long, drawn downwards from the line of the elbow joint (see page 36), 2 cm medial to the lateral edge of the head of the radius (Fig. 2.11).

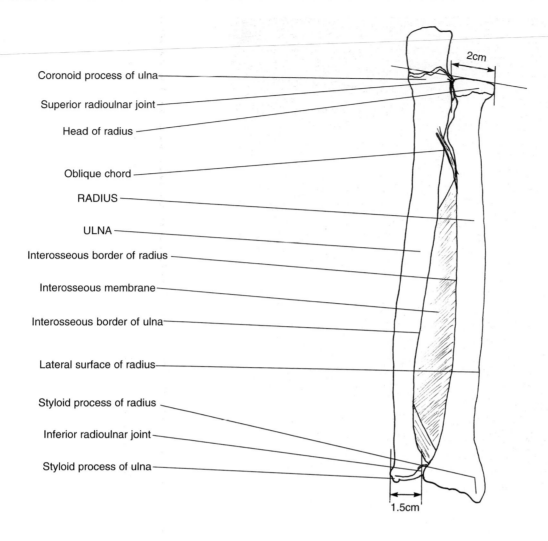

Coronoid process of ulna
Superior radioulnar joint
Head of radius
Oblique chord
RADIUS
ULNA
Interosseous border of radius
Interosseous membrane
Interosseous border of ulna
Lateral surface of radius
Styloid process of radius
Inferior radioulnar joint
Styloid process of ulna

2cm

1.5cm

Fig. 2.11 (b)
The superior and inferior radioulnar
joint of the left arm (anterior view)

Palpation

Locate the head of the radius just below the
lateral epicondyle of the humerus. Trace backwards
around the radial head until the movement is arrest-
ed by contact with the lateral side of the ulna. The
joint space is usually hidden by the anconeus
muscle. Anteriorly, the surface marking is covered
by muscle and is not palpable.

When the forearm is pronated and supinated, the
head of the radius can be felt rotating under the
fingers.

Accessory movements

If the head of the radius is firmly gripped between
the fingers and thumb of one hand and the upper
end of the ulna is stabilized by the other, slight backwards and forwards gliding of the head can be produced.

Traction on the lower part of the radius can produce a slight gliding up and down of the head of the
radius against the radial notch of the ulna. Note that
if too much traction is applied to the radius in
younger children, as in lifting the child by the forearm, the head of the radius may dislocate out of the
annular ring causing much pain and discomfort.

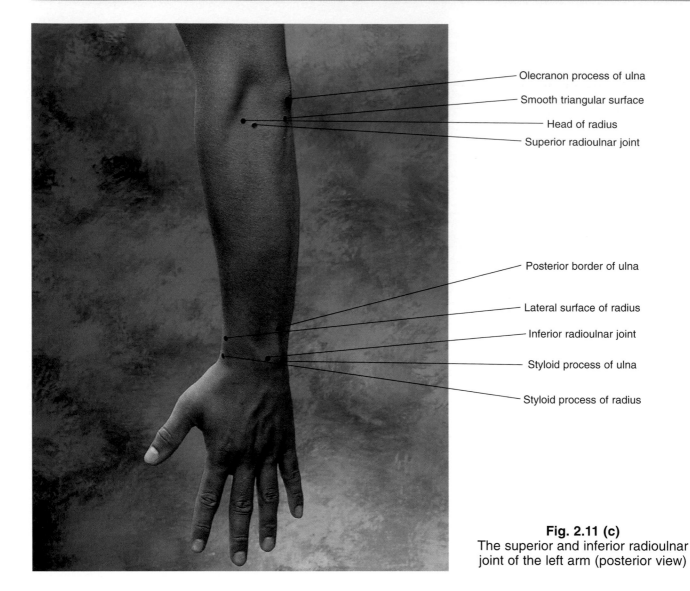

Olecranon process of ulna

Smooth triangular surface

Head of radius

Superior radioulnar joint

Posterior border of ulna

Lateral surface of radius

Inferior radioulnar joint

Styloid process of ulna

Styloid process of radius

Fig. 2.11 (c)
The superior and inferior radioulnar
joint of the left arm (posterior view)

The inferior radioulnar joint

This joint is also a synovial pivot joint, being between the ulnar notch on the medial side of the distal end of the radius and the lateral rim of the head of the ulna. Both surfaces are covered with articular cartilage and the joint is surrounded by a capsule which is thicker front and back. A triangular interarticular disc is situated between the lower end of the ulna and the carpus, which attaches medially to the base of the styloid process of the ulna and laterally to the medial edge of the inferior surface of the radius. At this joint, the radius moves around the head of the ulna in conjunction with the rotation of the head of the radius against the ulna at the superior radioulnar joint.

The mid radioulnar union

The radius and the ulna are joined together for most of their length by the interosseous membrane, which attaches to the interosseous borders of both bones, except for a small space at the upper part. This thin collagenous sheet, broader at its middle, is made up of fibres which pass downwards and

medially from the radius to the ulna. Its fibres help to bind the two bones together whilst allowing movement between them. It gives support to the superior and inferior radioulnar joints and, owing to the direction of its fibres, transmits weight from the radius to the ulna. If you examine both the radius and the ulna you will note that the lower end of the radius is large and takes any force transmitted from the carpus, whereas its head is relatively small and obviously transmits very little, if any, force to the capitulum. The ulna, on the other hand, has a very small head at its lower end, which takes very little force from the carpus, whereas its upper end is large and obviously transmits most of the force through to the trochlea of the humerus.

There is an oblique cord running downwards and laterally which attaches the tubercles at the upper part of the ulna with the radius just below its tuberosity. It is distinct from the interosseous membrane.

The interosseous membrane and oblique cord cannot be palpated.

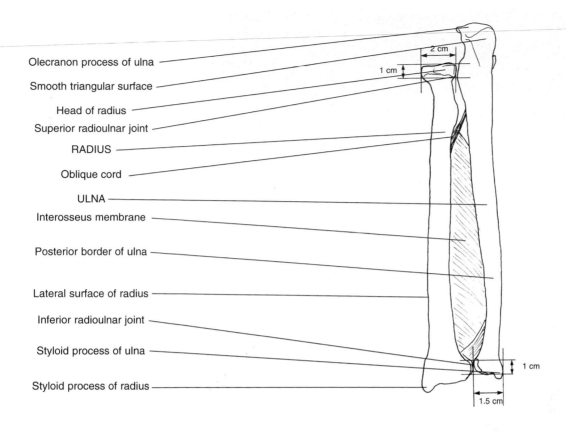

Olecranon process of ulna

Smooth triangular surface

Head of radius

Superior radioulnar joint

RADIUS

Oblique cord

ULNA

Interosseus membrane

Posterior border of ulna

Lateral surface of radius

Inferior radioulnar joint

Styloid process of ulna

Styloid process of radius

2 cm

1 cm

1 cm

1.5 cm

Fig. 2.11 (d)
The superior and inferior radioulnar
joint of the left arm (posterior view)

Surface markings

The joint line is 1.5 cm lateral to the medial rim of the head of the ulna running 1 cm upwards from the line of the wrist joint (Figs 2.11 and 2.12).

Palpation

The joint can more easily be palpated posteriorly, where there is a vertical depression for 1 cm immediately above the line of the wrist joint 1.5 cm lateral to the ulnar styloid process (Fig. 2.11). The tendon of extensor digiti minimi crosses the posterior aspect of the joint and if the little finger is extended it can be identified. Anteriorly the joint is much more difficult to palpate, as the fingers must be slipped under the thick tendon of flexor carpi ulnaris from the medial side.

On pronation and supination the radius can be felt moving around the lateral side of the head of the ulna, which itself in turn moves slightly laterally on pronation and medially on supination.

Accessory movements

If the head of the ulna is gripped firmly between fingers and thumb of one hand and the lower end of the radius is stabilized by the other hand, slight forwards and backwards gliding of the ulnar head can be achieved.

In pronation of the forearm the radius rotates around the head of the ulna. At the same time the lower end of the ulna moves slightly laterally. In supination the reverse occurs. These movements can be observed by holding the forearm in a loose hand, with the elbow flexed, and allowing the model to pronate and supinate. Loss of this movement will limit the range. With the forearm in full pronation, lateral movement can be achieved by applying pressure to the anteromedial aspect of the head of the ulna with the thumbs. With the forearm fully supinated, medial movement of the head of the ulna can be achieved by applying pressure with the thumbs to the posterolateral side of the head of the ulna. Both these manoeuvres achieve slight movement of the head of the ulna.

Pisiform

Tubercle of scaphoid

Wrist joint

Inferior radioulnar joint

Fig. 2.12 (a)
The right wrist joint (radiocarpal
joint) (anterior view)

The wrist (radiocarpal) joint [Fig. 2.12]

The wrist joint is formed by the inferior surface of
the lower end of the radius and an interarticular disc
superiorly, and the proximal surfaces of the
scaphoid, lunate and triquetral inferiorly, which
together with the ulnar and radius styloid processes
form a synovial ellipsoid joint. All joint surfaces are
covered with articular cartilage and the joint is surrounded by a capsule, lined with synovial membrane, and supported by the palmar and dorsal
radiocarpal, ulnocarpal, radial and ulnar collateral
ligaments. The interarticular disc lies between the
inferior surface of the head of the ulna and the triquetral bone.

Surface marking

The surface marking of the wrist joint is a line drawn
between the tips of the two styloid processes, being
slightly concave distally, with the line becoming
increasingly curved as it approaches the styloid
processes (Fig. 2.12).

Palpation

The joint is covered both anteriorly and posteriorly
by tendons running from the forearm into the hand.
There are, however, areas, mainly on the medial
side, where the joint space of the wrist can be palpated.

Locate the ulnar styloid process on the posteromedial side of the wrist and trace along both the
medial and posterior edges of the head of the ulna.
The gap just distal, which is clearly observable
medially, contains the interarticular disc, the inferior
surface of which takes part in the wrist joint articulation.

On the lateral side of the wrist, the joint
line can clearly be palpated just proximal to the
radial styloid process posteriorly and, with a little
more difficulty, anteriorly. If the fingers are pressed
between the extensor tendons, the joint line can be
traced just distal to the dorsal tubercle across the
back of the wrist as far as the head of the ulna. The

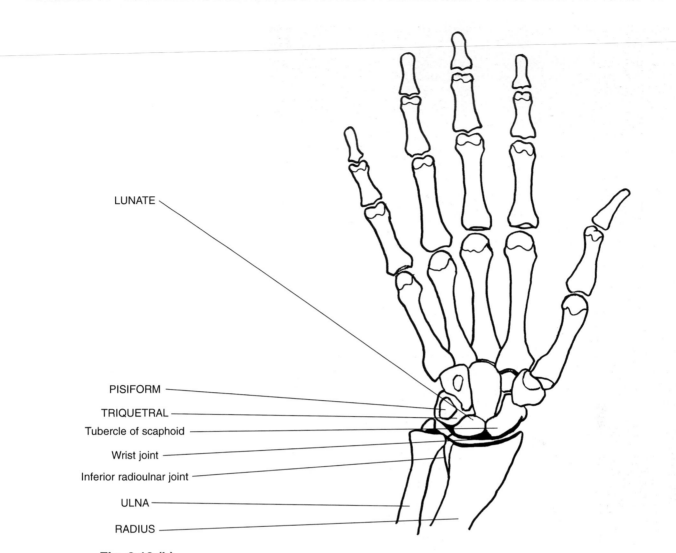

LUNATE

PISIFORM

TRIQUETRAL

Tubercle of scaphoid

Wrist joint

Inferior radioulnar joint

ULNA

RADIUS

Fig. 2.12 (b)
The right wrist joint (radiocarpal
joint) (anterior view)

joint line cannot be palpated anteriorly; however, its line can be drawn horizontally just proximal to the tubercle of the scaphoid. A crease across the anterior of the wrist between the flattened lower end of the forearm and the elevations of the thenar and hypothenar eminences marks the anterior line of the joint. This crease is made more obvious by slight flexion of the wrist.

Accessory movements

With the subject's forearm pronated, grip the dorsum of the lower end of the radius and ulna with one hand and the carpal bones with the other, so that the radial sides of your index fingers and thumbs are nearly touching. The carpus can now be moved forwards and backwards, from side to side and even rotated slightly. Take care not to bend the wrist, but to glide one surface on the other in a transverse plane. It will be difficult to prevent some movement occurring between the bones of the midcarpal joint. As in nearly all joints, distraction is also possible at the wrist. Adopting the same hold as above, draw the two hands apart, taking care to grip the bones tightly, not allowing too much slide of the skin and fascia. Accessory movement at the wrist, if performed correctly, is quite dramatic, producing considerable movement in unusual directions. It must be remembered, however, that some of this occurs at the intercarpal and carpometacarpal joints. It is possible, with practice, to move the bones of the carpus individually on each other or on the lower end of the radius and disc. This is achieved by gripping one bone between finger and thumb of one hand, while stabilizing its neighbour as above, or with the finger and thumb of the other hand.

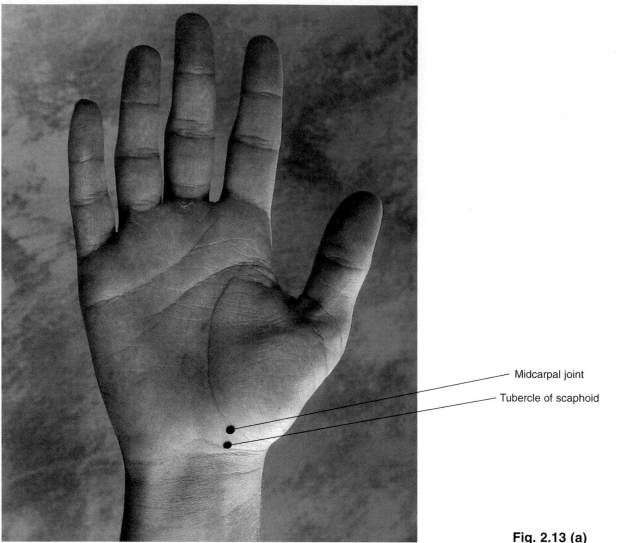

Fig. 2.13 (a)
The intercarpal and midcarpal joints
(anterior view)

The hand

The intercarpal joints [Fig. 2.13]

These are all synovial, plane joints with their surfaces covered with articular cartilage and their capsules lined with synovial membrane. With the
exception of the pisotriquetral joint, the capsule is
supported by the palmar and dorsal ligaments, and
radial and ulnar collateral carpal ligaments. There
are also some interosseous ligaments between the
proximal ends of the proximal row and distal ends
of the distal row of carpal bones.

The pisotriquetral joint is also a synovial plane
joint, but it has a distinct capsule which is supported by the tendon of flexor carpi ulnaris proximally and pisohamate and pisometacarpal ligaments distally.

With the exception of the joint between the
pisiform and triquetral, the joints between the carpal
bones are very difficult to palpate with any degree of
accuracy. The posterior aspects of the carpal bones
can be identified either by relating their position to
the metacarpals or by noting any particular features
(see page 24). Each carpal bone can be gripped

between finger and thumb and moved against the
adjacent bone, but the joint line remains elusive to
the touch.

The pisotriquetral joint. The joint between the
pisiform and the triquetral is easier to identify
medially. The joint line can be palpated by running
the fingers dorsally for 1 cm from the anterior point
of the pisiform on its medial side. Slight movement
of the pisiform will emphasize the joint line.

The midcarpal joint. The joint between the
two rows of carpal bones is known as the
midcarpal joint. It permits gliding forwards, backwards and from side to side, augmenting the movements of flexion, extension, abduction and adduction at the wrist joint. It can be marked by a line
drawn across the carpus just below the tips of the
radial and ulna styloid processes concave downwards, slightly more concave than that of the wrist
joint.

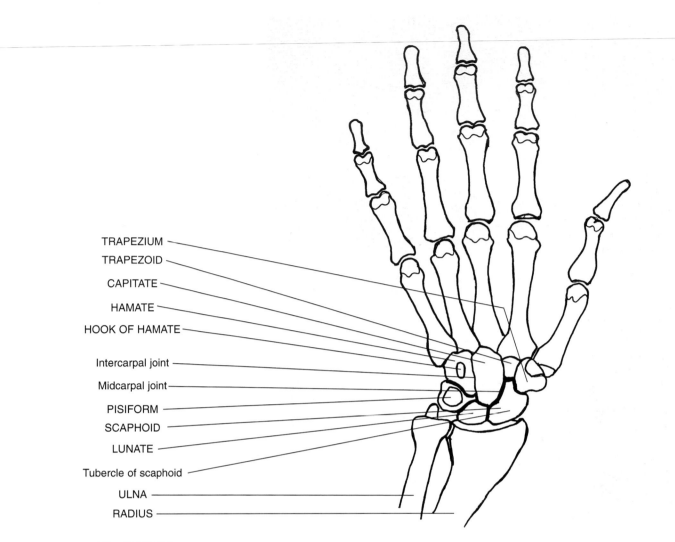

TRAPEZIUM
TRAPEZOID
CAPITATE
HAMATE
HOOK OF HAMATE
Intercarpal joint
Midcarpal joint
PISIFORM
SCAPHOID
LUNATE
Tubercle of scaphoid
ULNA
RADIUS

Fig. 2.13 (b)
The intercarpal and midcarpal joints
(anterior view)

Accessory movements

With the wrist slightly flexed, ulnar deviated, and the flexor carpi ulnaris relaxed, the pisiform can easily be moved from side to side with respect to the triquetral. If the capitate, situated at the base of the third metacarpal, is stabilized, by gripping it between the index finger anteriorly and thumb posteriorly, the surrounding carpal bones can be made to glide anteriorly and posteriorly using a similar grip with the other hand on each bone in turn. The trapezium is clearly palpable at the lateral side of the distal row. Using the same hold as above and stabilizing the rest of the carpus, it can also be moved anteriorly and posteriorly. A good knowledge of the carpal bones is essential, and should be combined with practice of this type of movement. It

is advisable to consult the literature on mobilization and manipulations for therapeutic techniques.

Passive movement can be produced between the two rows of carpal bones (the midcarpal joint) by applying a similar hold to that described for producing accessory movements of the wrist joint, but in this case one hand stabilizes the proximal row while the other moves the distal row. The index finger and thumb of the stabilizing hand should grip the proximal row of carpal bones just distal to the radial and ulnar styloid processes. During the anterior, posterior, lateral and medial gliding, however, it is impossible to prevent some movement occurring in the neighbouring joints.

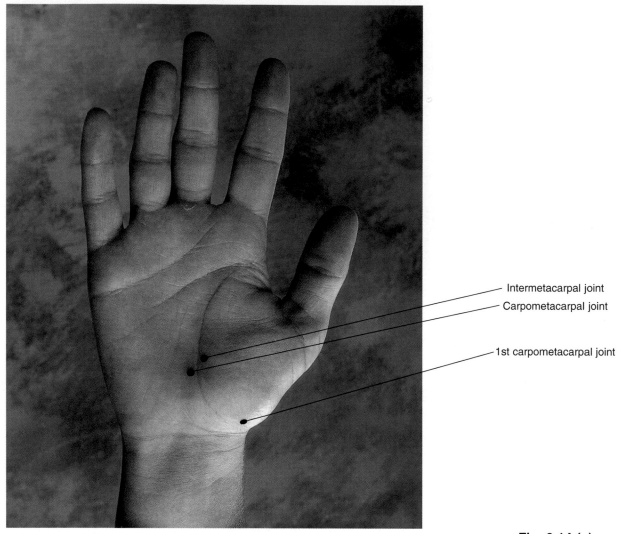

Intermetacarpal joint

Carpometacarpal joint

1st carpometacarpal joint

Fig. 2.14 (a)
Carpometacarpal and intermetacarpal joints (anterior view)

The carpometacarpal joints [Fig. 2.14]

The first metacarpal articulates with the trapezium
by means of a synovial saddle (sellar) joint and is
separate from the remaining carpometacarpal joints
It is surrounded by a capsule which is lined with
synovial membrane and supported by the radial
carpometacarpal, anterior and posterior oblique ligaments. The second articulates mainly with the
trapezoid, having small facets on either side for the
trapezium laterally and the capitate medially. The
third metacarpal articulates only with the capitate,
while the fourth and fifth articulate with the
hamate. Except for that of the thumb, they are all
plane synovial joints having a capsule lined with
synovial membrane and supported by palmar and
dorsal ligaments. As stated previously (see p. 44)
between the distal ends of the hamate, capitate
and trapezoid there is normally an interosseous
ligament.

Palpation

These joints are only palpable from the posterior
aspect. Trace proximally along the back of the first
metacarpal to its enlarged base, beyond which is a
depression. There, the joint line can be palpated
either side of the tendon of extensor pollicis longus.

Dorsally, just proximal to the bases of the second,
third, fourth and fifth metacarpals, 2 cm distal to the
line of the wrist joint, is a line of depressions
between the extensor tendons. These represent the
surface marking of the common carpometacarpal
joint.

On flexion, extension, abduction and adduction of
the thumb, the base of the first metacarpal can be
seen and felt moving on the trapezium. There is
little movement at the common carpometacarpal
joint, except a slight gliding of the surfaces against
each other accompanying movements of the hand.

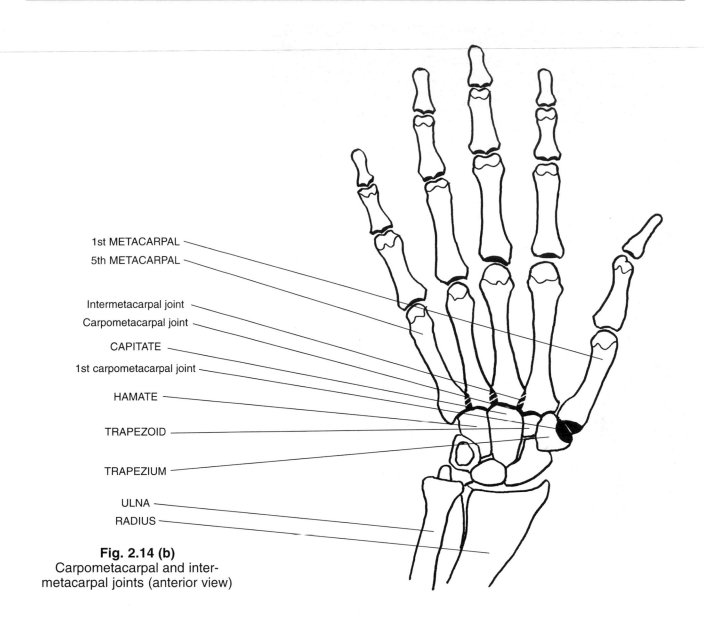

1st METACARPAL

5th METACARPAL

Intermetacarpal joint

Carpometacarpal joint

CAPITATE

1st carpometacarpal joint

HAMATE

TRAPEZOID

TRAPEZIUM

ULNA

RADIUS

Fig. 2.14 (b)
Carpometacarpal and intermetacarpal joints (anterior view)

Accessory movements

With the finger and thumb of one hand stabilizing the trapezium and the other hand gripping the first metacarpal, anterior, posterior, medial and lateral gliding of the metacarpal base against the trapezium can be produced, as can a limited amount of rotation (i.e. rotation of the metacarpal about its long axis). Slight distraction of the joint is possible. If the remaining carpus is stabilized with one hand, and each metacarpal is gripped in turn between fingers and thumb of the other, each metacarpal base can be moved forwards and backwards slightly.

The intermetacarpal joints [Fig. 2.14]

Between the bases of the second to fifth metacarpals are small plane synovial joints surrounded by a capsule lined with synovial membrane and supported by palmar, dorsal and interosseous ligaments. These allow them to be moved individually, giving the hand more mobility and thus more dexterity.

Palpation

On the posterior aspect of the hand, trace proximally up the spaces between the second and third, third and fourth, and fourth and fifth, metacarpal bones until you feel the two bones touching. The joint line can be palpated running vertically for approximately 1 cm from the line of the carpometacarpal joint (see above).

Accessory movements

It is extremely difficult to move the base of one metacarpal against another, except when they are used as levers. With the subject's forearm pronated, grip one metacarpal head between the index finger and thumb of one hand and its neighbour similarly in the other, and move them up and down against each other. There may be up to a centimetre of movement at the level of the heads, with a much smaller twisting movement of one base against its neighbour.

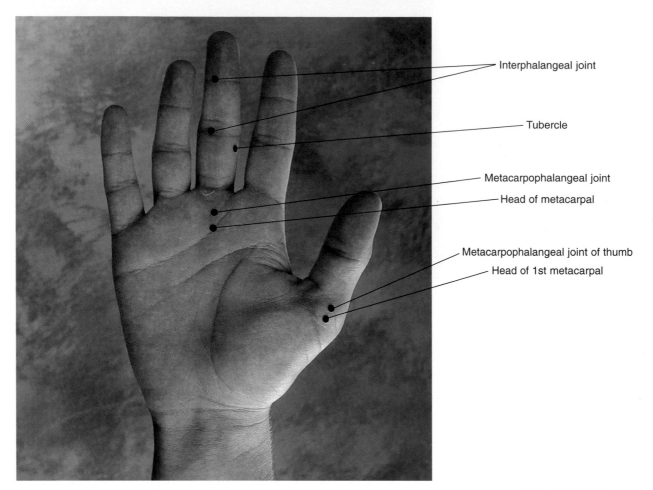

Interphalangeal joint

Tubercle

Metacarpophalangeal joint

Head of metacarpal

Metacarpophalangeal joint of thumb

Head of 1st metacarpal

Fig. 2.15 (a)
The metacarpophalangeal joints and interphalangeal joints of the right hand (anterior view)

The metacarpophalangeal joints

Metacarpophalangeal joints are synovial ellipsoid joints between the head of each metacarpal and the proximal end of each associated proximal phalanx. Each joint is surrounded by a fibrous capsule enclosing the head of the metacarpal and the proximal surface of the phalanx.

The capsule is lined with synovial membrane and is supported by strong, cord-like collateral ligaments and a dense palmar ligament. The posterior of the joint is protected by the dorsal expansion of the extensor digitorum longus tendon. The palmar ligaments of the 2nd to 5th metacarpophalangeal joints are linked by the deep transverse metacarpal ligament. It is worth noting (a) that flexion of the metacarpophalangeal joint of the thumb is only 45°, whereas that of the fingers is 90°, and (b) that this movement occurs at right angles to that in the other metacarpal joints taking the thumb across the palm.

Palpation

The metacarpophalangeal joints of each finger can be palpated just distal to the head of the metacarpal. With the finger flexed to 90°, the joint line appears to be beyond the knuckles, on the anterior surface of the head of the metacarpal (Fig. 2.15). It is easily palpable dorsally on either side of the extensor digitorum longus tendons.

The metacarpophalangeal joint of the thumb is clearly palpable posteriorly, just beyond the metacarpal head.

Accessory movements

With the metacarpal stabilized by one hand and the digit gripped by the other, the base of the proximal phalanx can be moved forwards, backwards and from side to side. The digit can also be rotated about its long axis, producing spin between the two surfaces and distracted sufficiently to produce the 'pop' which some children enjoy doing as a party trick. This is not normally possible at the metacarpophalangeal joint of the thumb.

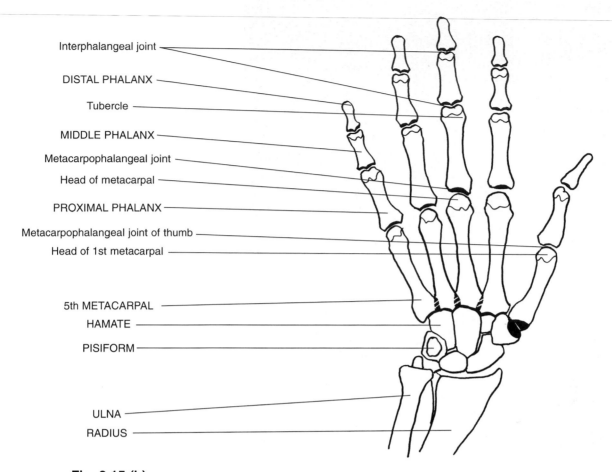

Interphalangeal joint

DISTAL PHALANX

Tubercle

MIDDLE PHALANX

Metacarpophalangeal joint

Head of metacarpal

PROXIMAL PHALANX

Metacarpophalangeal joint of thumb

Head of 1st metacarpal

5th METACARPAL

HAMATE

PISIFORM

ULNA

RADIUS

Fig. 2.15 (b)
The metacarpophalangeal joints and
interphalangeal joints of the right
hand (anterior view)

The interphalangeal joints

Each finger has two interphalangeal joints, whereas the thumb has only one. They are synovial hinge
joints between the head of the more proximal
phalanx and the base of the more distal phalanx
These joints are surrounded by a capsule which is
lined with synovial membrane and supported by
collateral and palmar ligaments.

Palpation

The joints are easier to palpate posteriorly. With the
joint flexed to 90°, trace distally down the back of
each phalanx. Just beyond the slightly expanded
head, the joint line can be palpated, covered centrally by the expansion of extensor digitorum (dorsal
digital expansion).

Accessory movements

With the subject's forearm and hand pronated and
the joint flexed to approximately 30°, stabilize the
more proximal phalanx with one hand and grip the
more distal phalanx between fingers and thumb of
the other. The base of the more distal phalanx can
now be rocked from side to side, often giving rise to
a 'cracking' sound. It is also possible to produce a
slight forwards and backwards gliding of the base
on the head, not easy to palpate, but useful in mobilizing stiff finger joints. Finally, all the interphalangeal joints can be distracted, but owing to their
tight collateral ligaments the space gained between
the articular surfaces is only a fraction of that gained
at the metacarpophalangeal joints.

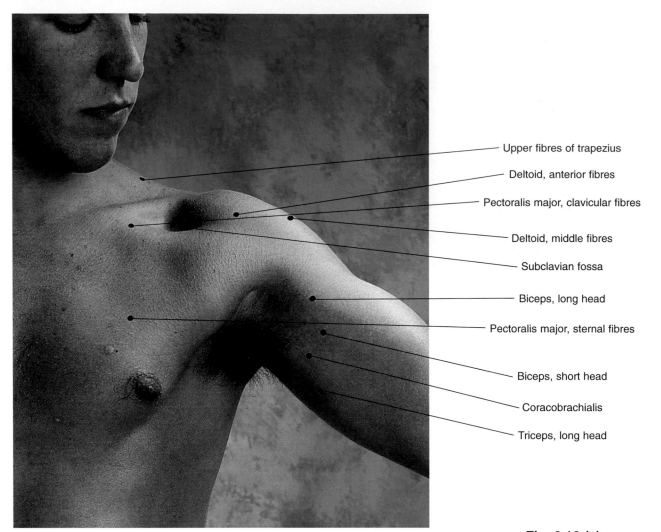

Upper fibres of trapezius

Deltoid, anterior fibres

Pectoralis major, clavicular fibres

Deltoid, middle fibres

Subclavian fossa

Biceps, long head

Pectoralis major, sternal fibres

Biceps, short head

Coracobrachialis

Triceps, long head

Fig. 2.16 (a)
Muscles on the anterior of the left
chest, shoulder and arm

MUSCLES

The muscles that move the arm

Deltoid [Figs 2.16 and 2.17]

The deltoid is a triangular or delta-shaped muscle situated on the lateral aspect of the shoulder joint. It is made up of anterior, middle and posterior sections. These fibres arise above from the lateral end of the anterior border of the clavicle, anterior, lateral and posterior borders of the acromion process, and the lower lip of the spine of the scapula, respectively. They all unite below to attach to the deltoid tubercle on the lateral side of the humerus.

Below the pectoral girdle, the anterior fibres of the deltoid can be seen some 3 cm below the lateral lip of the acromion, level with the greater tuberosity of the humerus. This delta-shaped muscle also covers the anterior and posterior aspects of the shoulder joint and feels thick and well developed. If the upper limb is abducted, its anterior and posterior fibres can be identified as triangular sections with fascial septa separating them from the central fibres.

Palpation

The anterior and posterior fibres feel smooth and strap-like, whereas the middle fibres feel coarse with stringy fibrous bands running vertically. This is due to this middle section of the deltoid being composed of multipennate muscle fibres, which pass obliquely from one vertical tendinous intersection to another. These coarse strips of muscle pass vertically from the lateral border of the acromion downwards to the final common tendon of all three sections halfway down the lateral aspect of the humerus. If the shoulder is flexed or medially rotated, the anterior fibres stand clear and can be traced from clavicle above to humerus below. If the shoulder is extended or laterally rotated, the posterior fibres stand clear and can be traced from the lower lip of the spine of the scapula above to the humerus below.

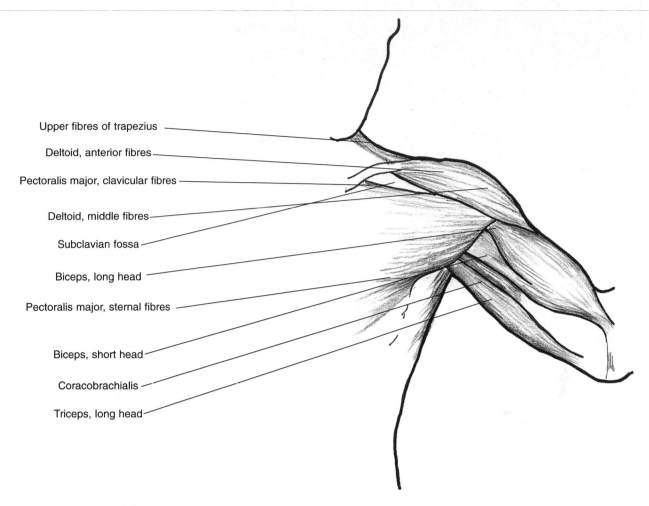

Fig. 2.16 (b)
Muscles on the anterior of the left
chest, shoulder and arm

Labels (top to bottom):
Upper fibres of trapezius
Deltoid, anterior fibres
Pectoralis major, clavicular fibres
Deltoid, middle fibres
Subclavian fossa
Biceps, long head
Pectoralis major, sternal fibres
Biceps, short head
Coracobrachialis
Triceps, long head

Pectoralis major [Fig. 2.16]

Pectoralis major is a thick, strong, triangular muscle, which covers the upper anterior chest wall. It
has its tendinous apex laterally. It comprises two
functionally distinct groups of fibres: clavicular and
sternal. The clavicular section attaches medially to
the anterior surface of the medial half of the clavicle.
The sternal fibres have an extensive attachment
medially to the manubrium, body of the sternum,
anterior surfaces of the upper six costal cartilages
and ribs and the upper part of the aponeurosis of the
external oblique muscle. Laterally, the muscle forms
a broad tendon which attaches to the lateral lip of
the bicipital groove. The lower border of the muscle
appears thickened. This is due to its lower fibres
being folded up behind its upper fibres and forming
a bilaminal tendon at its insertion.

Palpation

If this muscle is traced laterally it passes across, and
forms the anterior wall of the axilla. When the arm
is flexed, its clavicular fibres can be palpated as a
thick muscular column passing from the medial end
of the clavicle to the humerus. If the arm is now
extended, from a flexed position against resistance,
the sternal fibres can be palpated from the lower ribs
and sternum to the same insertion. In women, much
of the muscular section is covered by the breast but
contraction of the muscle is evident to see or palpate. In men, the whole of the muscle is clearly palpable and becomes hard and tense on adduction
and medial rotation of the arm. Laterally a groove
can be palpated between its upper border and the
lower border of the deltoid.

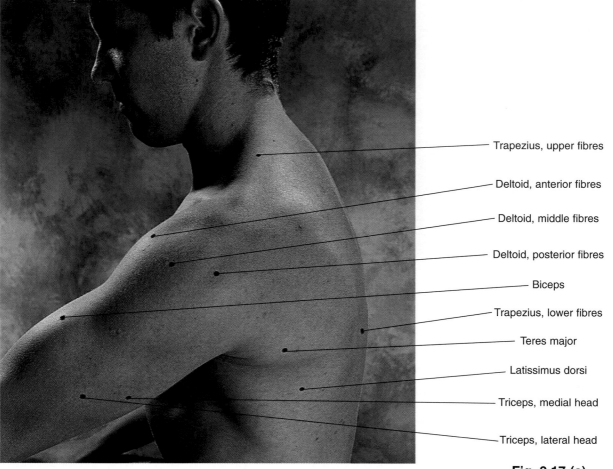

Trapezius, upper fibres

Deltoid, anterior fibres

Deltoid, middle fibres

Deltoid, posterior fibres

Biceps

Trapezius, lower fibres

Teres major

Latissimus dorsi

Triceps, medial head

Triceps, lateral head

Fig. 2.17 (a)
Muscles that move the arm and
forearm (lateral view of left arm)

Biceps brachii [Figs 2.16–2.18]

Biceps brachii is fusiform in shape, situated on the anterior aspect of the upper arm. Its upper end attaches by two heads, as its name implies, one from the supraglenoid tubercle, the other from the tip of the coracoid process of the scapula. Below, it attaches by a strong tendon to the posterior aspect of the radial tubercle on the upper medial aspect of the radius and by an expansion from its medial aspect which blends with the fascia on the medial side of the forearm.

The fusiform shape of biceps brachii can be seen and palpated covering the front of the arm. It can be traced upwards, running deep to pectoralis major and splitting into two parts, both palpable: the long head passing as a tendon in the intertubercular groove, and the short head passing medially to the coracoid process. The tendon of the long head of biceps can be traced up the bicipital groove to pass over the head of the humerus to the supraglenoid tubercle. Below, the muscle forms a well-defined tendon which passes through the cubital fossa giving off an expansion (the bicipital aponeurosis) which blends with the fascia on the medial side of the forearm, reaching as far as the posterior border of the ulna, forming a sickle-shaped edge. On supination of the flexed forearm against resistance, the shape and tendons of biceps become more clearly defined and the aponeurosis can be palpated spreading medially from the tendon. In a well-developed model, the tips of the fingers can be slipped under the posterior border of the bicipital aponeurosis approximately 2 cm anteroinferior to the medial epicondyle (Fig. 2.18).

Brachialis

Brachialis is a thick, triangular muscle situated deep to the lower part of the biceps. It attaches above to the lower half of the anterolateral and anteromedial surfaces of the humerus, crosses the front of the elbow joint and attaches below to the anterior surface of the coronoid process of the ulna.

Palpation

Being deeply situated this muscle is difficult to palpate; however, contraction and relaxation of brachialis, during flexion and extension of the elbow, can be felt on deep palpation either side of the biceps tendon as the subject gently flexes and extends the elbow joint.

Fig. 2.17 (b)
Muscles that move the arm and
forearm (lateral view of left arm)

Trapezius, upper fibres

Deltoid, anterior fibres

Deltoid, middle fibres

Deltoid, posterior fibres

Biceps

Teres major

Latissimus dorsi
Trapezius, lower fibres
Triceps, medial head

Triceps, lateral head

Triceps [Figs. 2.16a,b 2.17a,b]

On the posterior aspect of the arm, the thick muscular mass of the triceps is situated. As its name implies, it arises from three heads: (1) the long head, which is tendinous and passes upwards, below the shoulder joint to attach to the infraglenoid tubercle of the scapula; (2) the lateral head, which attaches to the upper lateral part of the posterior surface of the humerus above and lateral to the radial groove; and (3) the medial head, which attaches to the lower medial part of the posterior surface of the humerus below and medial to the radial groove. All three attach to the posterior part of the superior surface of the olecranon via the triceps tendon.

Palpation

Medially, the long head can be traced upwards as a tendon on the medial aspect of the arm passing up, under the posterior fibres of deltoid, infraspinatus, teres major and minor to lie in front of the posterior wall of the axilla. The medial and lateral heads form a much more fleshy mass down the posterior aspect of the whole of the arm. Just above the elbow joint, the three heads form a strong, thick tendon which attaches to the upper surface of the olecranon process. The muscle and its tendon are more easily palpated if the elbow is slightly flexed and then extended against resistance. The lateral and medial heads can readily be identified, with the former being slightly higher and lateral, while the latter is lower and more medial (Fig. 2.17).

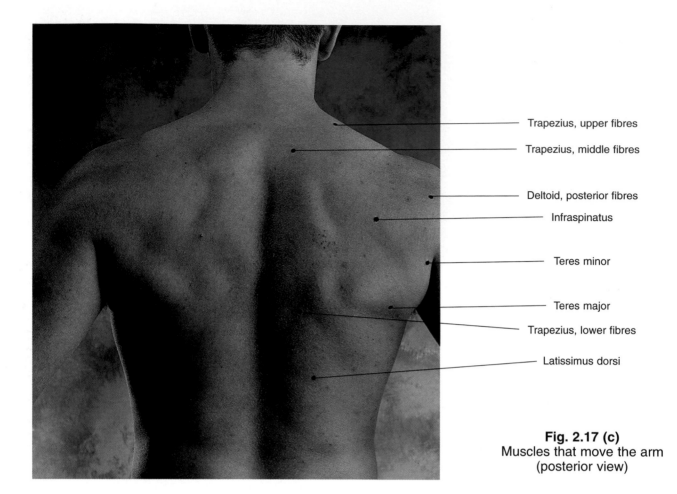

Trapezius, upper fibres

Trapezius, middle fibres

Deltoid, posterior fibres

Infraspinatus

Teres minor

Teres major

Trapezius, lower fibres

Latissimus dorsi

Fig. 2.17 (c)
Muscles that move the arm
(posterior view)

Latissimus dorsi [Fig. 2.17a,b,c and d]

The latissimus dorsi is a large triangular muscle situated on the lower, posterior part of the trunk but passes upwards and laterally to attach to the upper part of the upper limb.

This muscle has an extensive origin from the lower part of the thoracolumbar fascia, the spines of the lower six thoracic, all the lumbar and sacral vertebrae, from the supraspinous and interspinous ligaments which lie between the thoracic and lumbar vertebrae and from the outer lip of the posterior sixth of the crest of the ilium. As it passes upwards it also attaches to the lower three ribs and the posterior aspect of the inferior angle of the scapula.

It attaches above by a flattened tendon, which twists under the axilla and attaches to the floor of the intertubercular groove which lies on the anterior surface of the humerus.

Palpation

The tendon of the latissimus dorsi can be palpated as it passes under teres major, forming the posterior wall of the axilla. If extension and medial rotation of the arm is resisted, the tendon can be traced along the medial side of the humerus towards its insertion into the floor of the intertubercular groove of the humerus. The muscle fibres can also be palpated in the upper lumbar area, particularly if the subject is pulling down on a beam above his/her head (beam heaves) or is asked to cough.

Trapezius, upper fibres

Trapezius, middle fibres

Deltoid, posterior fibres

Infraspinatus

Teres minor

Teres major

Trapezius, lower fibres

Latissimus dorsi

Fig. 2.17 (d)
Muscles that move the arm
(posterior view)

Coracobrachialis [Fig. 2.16a and b]

This is a long thin fusiform muscle situated on the upper medial area of the arm. It attaches above to the tip of the coracoid process by a tendon common to it and the biceps brachii. Below it attaches by a short tendon to a point halfway down the medial side of the humerus.

Palpation

During adduction of the upper limb, the belly of coracobrachialis (see Fig. 2.16a,b) can be palpated high up on the medial side of the arm, passing upwards and forwards towards the coracoid process. If the subject places the hand on the hip and adducts the arm with some force, the tendon can be traced to the posterior aspect of the short head of the biceps and can be identified blending with this tendon. Care must be taken when palpating this area as it contains numerous branches of the brachial plexus and major blood vessels to and from the upper limb.

The posterior aspect of the scapula [Fig. 2.17c and d]

Above the spine of the scapula, the muscle belly of supraspinatus can be palpated, particularly if the upper limb begins to abduct from the side.

Below the spine, the belly of infraspinatus can be palpated passing upwards and laterally to the humerus. This contracts during lateral rotation of the humerus.

The large bulk of muscle covering the lateral border of the scapula is made up of the fibres of teres major and minor and the upper part of latissimus dorsi. These all come into action in adduction of the humerus, the teres minor taking part in lateral rotation of the humerus whilst the teres major and latissimus dorsi take part in medial rotation.

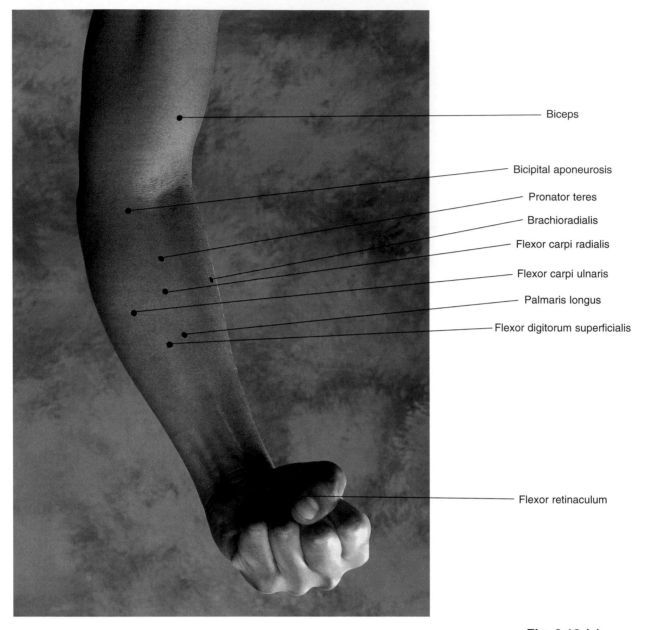

Biceps

Bicipital aponeurosis

Pronator teres

Brachioradialis

Flexor carpi radialis

Flexor carpi ulnaris

Palmaris longus

Flexor digitorum superficialis

Flexor retinaculum

Fig. 2.18 (a)
The right forearm (anterior view)

The anterior aspect of the forearm and wrist

Because of their close proximity, individual identification of the muscles of the forearm is difficult. The point of greatest clarity is where their tendons cross the wrist joint; consequently most muscles will be identified at this point and then traced proximally and distally.

Generally the forearm is greater in circumference in its upper half than in its lower half owing to the presence of the muscle bellies, whereas lower down the muscles give way to tendons (Fig. 2.18).

Brachioradialis is situated most laterally and gives shape to the upper part of the forearm. It appears strap-like and thicker near the elbow, narrowing to a broad tendon towards the lateral surface of the radius. If the elbow is flexed in the mid-prone position against resistance, the muscle

stands clear, showing that its origin attaches to the proximal part of the lateral supracondylar ridge of the humerus (Fig. 2.18).

On the anterior aspect of the wrist, approximately 1 cm medial to the styloid process of the radius, the tendon of flexor carpi radialis can be palpated. Distally, it passes in front of the scaphoid, being lost in the groove on the front of the trapezium. The tendon can, however, be traced halfway up the front of the forearm, becoming muscular in the upper part which attaches to the medial epicondyle of the humerus (Fig. 2.18).

If the wrist is slightly flexed and the base of the thumb and little finger are drawn together, a slim tendon (palmaris longus) can be seen and palpated (if present) medial to the tendon of flexor

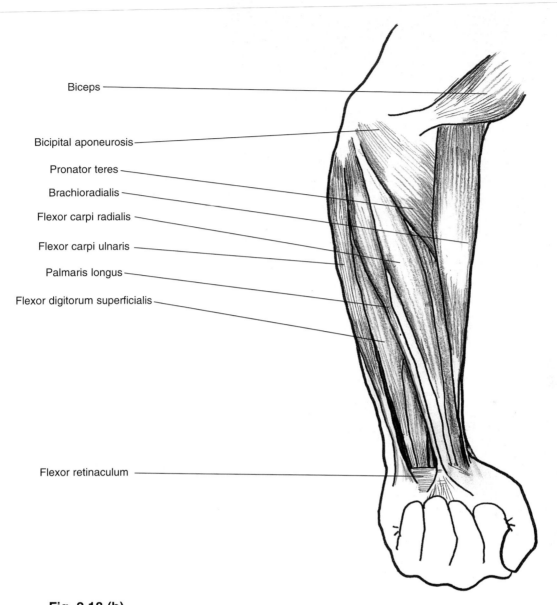

Biceps

Bicipital aponeurosis

Pronator teres

Brachioradialis

Flexor carpi radialis

Flexor carpi ulnaris

Palmaris longus

Flexor digitorum superficialis

Flexor retinaculum

Fig. 2.18 (b)
Muscles of the right forearm
(anterior view)

carpi radialis. Traced distally, the palmaris longus tendon blends with the palmar aponeurosis. Proximally, the narrow belly of palmaris longus can be palpated on the medial side of the previous muscle.

On the anteromedial aspect of the wrist is the stout tendon of flexor carpi ulnaris. Distally it blends with the pisiform bone, while proximally it can be traced almost halfway up the forearm approximately 2 cm anterior to the posterior border of the ulna, being replaced by thick muscle which lies in front of the posterior border of the ulna.

Between the tendons of palmaris longus and flexor carpi ulnaris is a depressed area. If the subject flexes the fingers, particularly the middle and ring

fingers, the tendons of flexor digitorum superficialis can be seen and palpated in that groove. The tendons to the index and little fingers, and those of flexor digitorum profundus, lie deeper and are difficult to differentiate. If the fingers are flexed only at the metacarpophalangeal and proximal interphalangeal joints, flexor digitorum superficialis can be palpated immediately medial to the tendon of palmaris longus. If, however, the fingertips are pressed against the palm of the hand, flexor digitorum profundus can be palpated on the medial side of the forearm, deep to flexor carpi ulnaris. In the palm, the tendons of these muscles are well covered with fascia and are dif-ficult to determine, except for an area just proximal to the metacarpophalangeal joints.

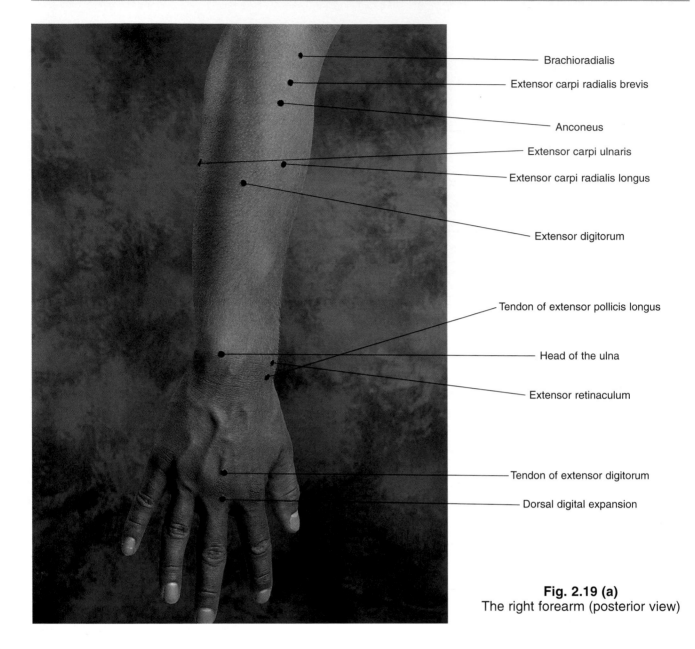

Brachioradialis

Extensor carpi radialis brevis

Anconeus

Extensor carpi ulnaris

Extensor carpi radialis longus

Extensor digitorum

Tendon of extensor pollicis longus

Head of the ulna

Extensor retinaculum

Tendon of extensor digitorum

Dorsal digital expansion

Fig. 2.19 (a)
The right forearm (posterior view)

The posterior aspect of the forearm and wrist

In order to identify muscles in this area, care must be taken to maintain the forearm in the anatomical position, i.e. the arm hanging loosely by the side with the palms facing forwards. Brachioradialis can be palpated most laterally (see page 56). About 1 cm medial to the radial styloid process, two tendons cross the wrist so close to each other that they are often mistaken as one: the lateral is extensor carpi radialis longus which can be traced distally to the base of the second metacarpal; the medial is extensor carpi radialis brevis, attaching to the base of the third metacarpal distally (see Fig. 2.21a). Proximally both muscles can be traced along the medial side of the bulk of brachioradialis to their attachment to, and just above, the lateral epicondyle of the humerus. These become much clearer if the wrist is gently extended.

Passing around the dorsal tubercle of the radius, the tendon of extensor pollicis longus can be palpated, particularly if the thumb is extended. The tendon can be followed to its insertion into the base of the distal phalanx of the thumb. Proximally the tendon is covered almost immediately by superficial muscles (Figs 2.19 and 2.21).

If all the fingers are extended, the tendon of extensor digitorum can be palpated immediately medial to the tendon of extensor pollicis longus (Fig. 2.19). It is broad and flat, dividing into four separate tendons distally. Each tendon can be traced over the back of the hand and along the posterior aspect of each finger, becoming slightly broader over the back of the metacarpophalangeal joint (dorsal digital expansion). Distally, each tendon can be traced to its attachment to the base of the distal phalanx.

Brachioradialis

Extensor carpi radialis brevis

Anconeus

Extensor carpi ulnaris

Extensor carpi radialis longus

Extensor digitorum

Tendon of extensor pollicis longus

Head of the ulna

Extensor retinaculum

Tendon of extensor digitorum

Dorsal digital expansion

Fig. 2.19 (b)
Muscles of the right forearm
(posterior view)

Proximally, the extensor digitorum can be traced up the middle of the forearm medial to the extensor carpi radialis longus and brevis to attach to the lateral epicondyle of the humerus. Often a separate muscle belly can be identified on the lateral side which passes to the index finger only.

Accompanying the extensor digitorum, across the back of the wrist, is the tendon of the extensor indicis, more easily identifiable as it joins the ulnar side of the extensor digitorum tendon to the index finger at the metacarpophalangeal joint.

Passing over the inferior radioulnar joint, the thin tendon of extensor digiti minimi can be traced towards the little finger, joining the tendon of the extensor digitorum at its dorsal digital expan-

sion. The tendon can be traced proximally to a thin fusiform belly which attaches to the lateral epicondyle. The tendon of extensor digiti minimi is much clearer when the little finger is rhythmically extended and relaxed.

Finally, crossing the posteromedial aspect of the wrist, just lateral to the styloid process of the ulna, is the thick tendon of the extensor carpi ulnaris, again becoming much clearer on extension of the wrist. This can be traced distally to the base of the fifth metacarpal and proximally, via its muscle belly, to the lateral epicondyle (Fig. 2.19). In the mid-forearm the muscle belly lies lateral to the posterior border of the ulna.

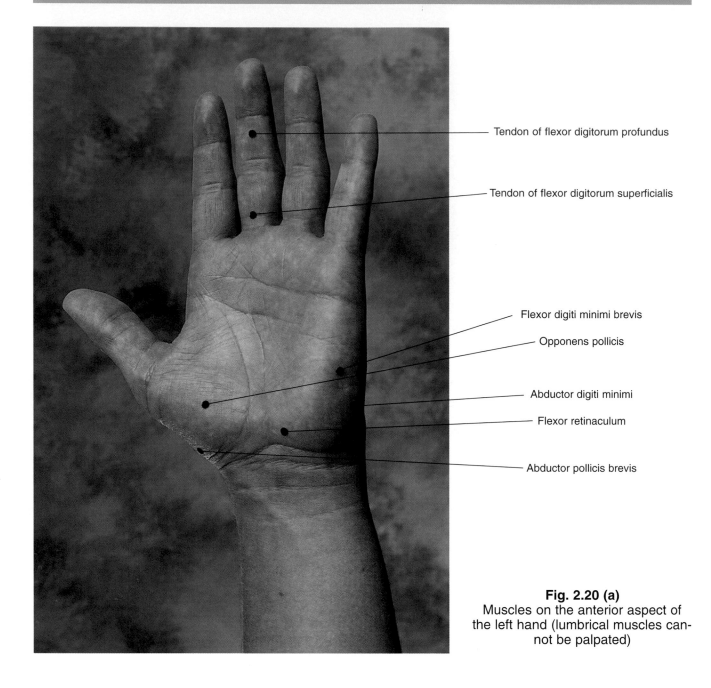

Tendon of flexor digitorum profundus

Tendon of flexor digitorum superficialis

Flexor digiti minimi brevis

Opponens pollicis

Abductor digiti minimi

Flexor retinaculum

Abductor pollicis brevis

Fig. 2.20 (a)
Muscles on the anterior aspect of
the left hand (lumbrical muscles cannot be palpated)

The anterior aspect of the hand

The bones and joints of the hand are moved and controlled by two main groups of muscles: (a) those of the forearm, whose tendons pass over the wrist to attach to particular bony points in the hand and govern the relationships between the forearm and hand (the extrinsic muscles) (see pages 56–59); and (b) those within the hand which change the relationships of the component parts of the hand from within (the intrinsic muscles).

The palm appears to have a flattened central portion with muscular masses on either side which are closer together proximally and diverge distally (Fig. 2.20a). The lateral mass, the thenar eminence, is the larger of the two and consists of muscles responsible for producing movements of the thumb. The medial mass, the hypothenar eminence, consists of muscles responsible for producing movements of the little finger.

It must be remembered that movements of the thumb take place in a plane at right angles to the palm of the hand. Consequently, abduction is movement of the thumb anteriorly away from the index finger, while flexion is movement of the thumb medially across the palm of the hand.

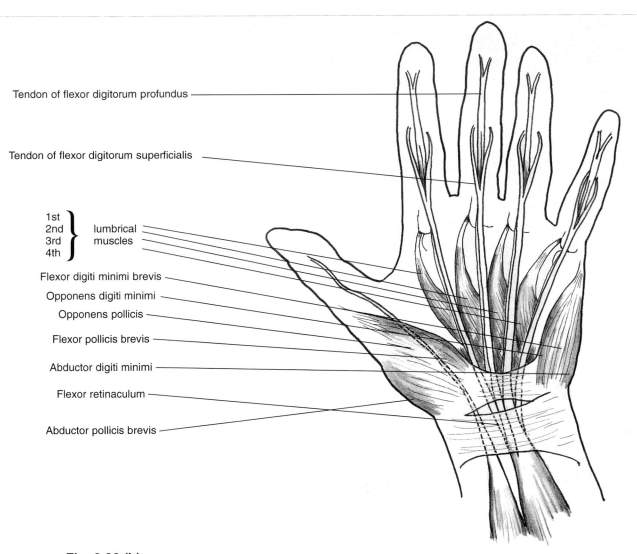

Tendon of flexor digitorum profundus

Tendon of flexor digitorum superficialis

1st
2nd
3rd   } lumbrical
4th   muscles

Flexor digiti minimi brevis

Opponens digiti minimi

Opponens pollicis

Flexor pollicis brevis

Abductor digiti minimi

Flexor retinaculum

Abductor pollicis brevis

Fig. 2.20 (b)
Muscles on the anterior aspect of
the left hand (lumbrical muscles cannot be palpated)

Palpation

If the thumb is abducted, the muscle belly of **abductor pollicis brevis** can be palpated on the lateral side of the thenar eminence, with its tendon passing distally to the lateral side of the proximal phalanx of the thumb (Fig. 2.20). In opposition, i.e. when the pad of the thumb is made to oppose the pad of the fingers, the **opponens pollicis** contracts, causing the whole central section of the thenar eminence to contract and become hard. If the thumb is flexed, against resistance, at the metacarpophalangeal joint, **flexor pollicis brevis**, on the medial aspect of the thenar eminence, will be felt contracting.

On abduction of the little finger, i.e. moving it away from the ring finger, **abductor digiti minimi** can be palpated on the medial side of the hypothenar eminence, which can be traced via a short tendon to the medial side of the base of the

proximal phalanx of the little finger (Fig. 2.20). By opposing the little finger to the thumb, the whole of the hypothenar eminence hardens due to the contraction of **opponens digiti minimi**. With the little finger flexed against resistance, **flexor digiti minimi brevis** can be palpated, with some difficulty, on the lateral side of opponens digiti minimi (Fig. 2.20).

The central section of the palm of the hand is covered by the strong and thick palmar aponeurosis, making palpation of muscles such as adductor pollicis (transverse head), the palmar interossei or the **lumbrical muscles** impossible. The long tendons of the **flexor digitorum superficialis** and **profundus** can be traced, particularly over the fronts of the metacarpophalangeal joints, but again with difficulty. They become more evident if the fingers are flexed against resistance.

Dorsal digital expansion

1st dorsal interosseus

Extensor digitorum tendon to middle finger

Extensor pollicis longus

Extensor retinaculum

Abductor pollicis longus

Extensor carpi radialis longus and brevis

Fig. 2.21 (a)
The posterior aspect of the right
hand (for clarity only the first dorsal
interosseus is identified, but all can
be palpated)

The posterior aspect of the hand [Fig. 2.21a–g]

The skin and fascia on the posterior aspect of the hand are thin and relatively loose, giving easy access for palpation of muscles that are present. As the main function of the hand is to manipulate and hold implements and tools, often with great care and precision, most of the muscles are situated anteriorly. Releasing the grip tends to be left to the long extensor muscles whose muscle bellies lie in the forearm, with their connection to the hand being through long tendons which cross the back of the wrist (see muscles on the posterior aspect of the forearm, page 58–59). Nevertheless, there are a few muscles which can be palpated and are worthy of note.

Palpation

On the lateral side of the thumb the posterior part of abductor pollicis brevis can be palpated (see page 60–61), lying just lateral to the tendon of extensor pollicis longus. Its short tendon can be palpated attaching to the lateral side of the proximal phalanx of the thumb, while its proximal attachment can be traced to the tubercle of the scaphoid. With the thumb abducted and extended, two tendons can be identified crossing the wrist just in front of the radial styloid. These are the abductor pollicis longus and extensor pollicis brevis. The abductor can be traced to the base of the metacarpal and the extensor to the base of the proximal phalanx. Proximal to the radial styloid both tendons wrap posteriorly around the lateral surface of the radius and disappear deep between the other muscles.

In the cleft between the thumb and index finger there is the large muscle mass of the first dorsal interosseus. When the index finger is abducted, i.e. drawn laterally away from the middle finger, contraction of the muscle becomes clear. The muscle belly can be traced from its origin to both the first and second metacarpals, to its tendon which attaches distally to the lateral side of the base of the proximal phalanx of the index finger (Fig. 2.21a). The muscle can easily be demonstrated and identified by placing the fingers on the upper surface of a table with the thumb over the edge running down the vertical section. If the index finger is now abducted, the muscle becomes hard and its belly and tendon easily palpable.

Dorsal digital expansion

2nd, 3rd and 4th dorsal interossei

1st dorsal interosseus

Extensor digitorum tendon to middle finger

Extensor pollicis longus

Abductor pollicis longus

Fig. 2.21 (b)
The posterior aspect of the right
hand

Extensor retinaculum

Synovial membrane

Extensor carpi radialis longus and brevis

When the middle finger is abducted laterally, i.e. towards the index finger, the second dorsal interosseus can be palpated, its fibres bulging between the proximal half of the second and third metacarpals. If the same finger is now abducted medially, i.e. towards the ring finger, the third dorsal interosseus can be palpated between the proximal half of the third and fourth metacarpals (Fig. 2.21d).

Abducting the ring finger, the fourth dorsal interosseus can be palpated between the proximal half of the fourth and fifth metacarpals. In addition, abductor digiti minimi can also be seen and palpated on the medial side of the hand (see page 60–61).

Fig. 2.21 (c)
The posterior aspect of the right
hand

Dorsal digital expansion

Dorsal interossei

Extensor digiti minimi

Extensor pollicis longus

Fig. 2.21 (d)
Muscles and tendons of the right hand (posterior aspect)

Fig. 2.21 (f)
The posterior aspect of the right hand

Extensor indicis

Extensor pollicis longus

Extensor pollicis brevis

Extensor retinaculum

Extensor carpi radialis longus

Extensor carpi radialis brevis

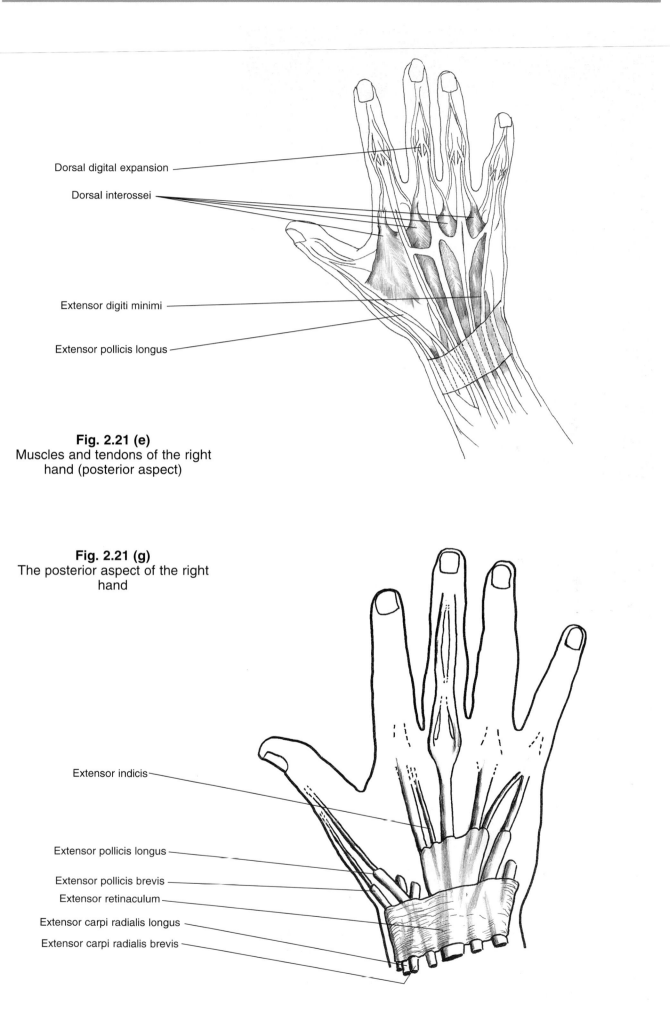

Dorsal digital expansion

Dorsal interossei

Extensor digiti minimi

Extensor pollicis longus

Fig. 2.21 (e)
Muscles and tendons of the right
hand (posterior aspect)

Fig. 2.21 (g)
The posterior aspect of the right
hand

Extensor indicis

Extensor pollicis longus

Extensor pollicis brevis

Extensor retinaculum

Extensor carpi radialis longus

Extensor carpi radialis brevis

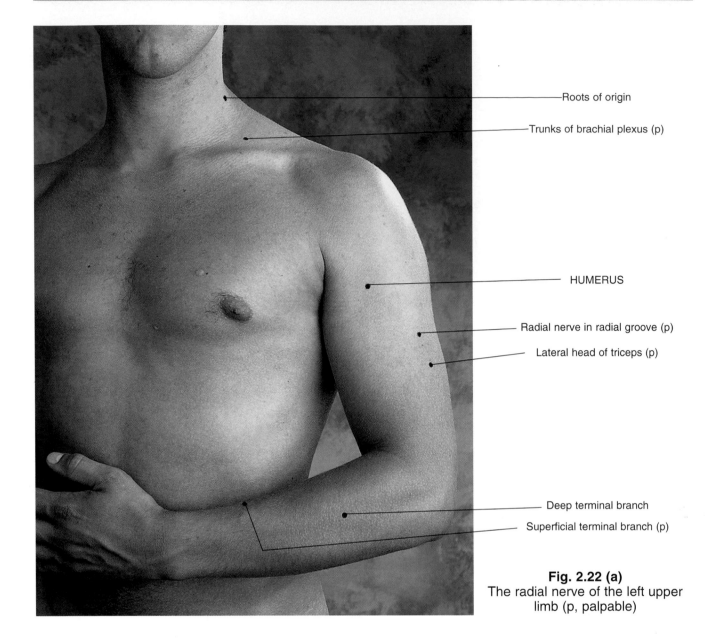

Roots of origin

Trunks of brachial plexus (p)

HUMERUS

Radial nerve in radial groove (p)

Lateral head of triceps (p)

Deep terminal branch

Superficial terminal branch (p)

Fig. 2.22 (a)
The radial nerve of the left upper limb (p, palpable)

NERVES [Figs 2.22 and 2.23]

Most of the upper limb is innervated by nerves via the brachial plexus. The nerve roots contributing to this plexus are C5, 6, 7 and 8 and T1. The root of C5 may receive a contribution from C4 (pre-fixed plexus), while the T1 root may receive a contribution from T2 (post-fixed plexus). The roots combine to form trunks. The upper, middle and lower trunks, each of which divides into anterior and posterior divisions, combine to form the lateral, medial and posterior cords. It is from the cords that the majority of branches arise to be distributed to the whole of the upper limb. For a more detailed description see Palastanga *et al*. (1998).

Palpation

Palpation of nerves must be performed with care. To the palpator, nerves appear as slippery cord-like structures, which only occasionally become superficial, being mostly buried deep to other structures for protection. To the palpated, pressure on a nerve may evoke localized pain, but may also produce a tingling sensation, pain or numbness over the area of its distribution. The accurate location of nerves is important, but over-palpation must be avoided as this may lead to interference, with possible signs and symptoms.

Press the fingers into the depression above the medial end of the clavicle, just lateral to the sternocleidomastoid, and the trunks of the brachial plexus appear as a bundle of tense cords running downwards and laterally. Palpation in this area can be uncomfortable if you apply too much pressure.

Roots of origin

Trunks of brachial plexus (p)

HUMERUS

Radial nerve in radial groove (p)

Lateral head of triceps (p)

Deep terminal branch

Superficial terminal branch (p)

Fig. 2.22 (b)
The radial nerve of the left upper
limb (p, palpable)

The radial nerve

Approximately halfway down the lateral side of the arm, below the insertion of deltoid, a groove can be palpated running downwards and forwards. Again, with careful palpation, particularly just behind the groove, the radial nerve can be rolled against the humerus just anterior to the lateral head of triceps. Anteriorly it enters a muscular groove between brachioradialis and brachialis, passing anterolateral to the elbow joint but too deep to be palpated.

On the lateral side of the radius, at variable points on its lower half, the superficial branch of the radial nerve can be rolled against the bone as it passes from under brachioradialis to its distribution on the back of the lateral side of the hand. Sometimes the nerve is single, whereas in others it splits into five divisions (Fig. 2.22).

With the subject's right forearm in your left hand and the thumb uppermost, glide the radial side of your right thumb up and down the lower end of the radius. The branch(es) of the radial nerve can be felt rolling against the bone. Even though they are lying superficially on the back of the hand, they are still difficult to trace. The subject is likely to experience similar sensations in the distribution of these superficial branches to the posterolateral aspect of the hand and lateral three-and-a-half digits as those experienced on tapping the median nerve on rolling of the superficial branches of the ulnar nerve over the hook of the hamate.

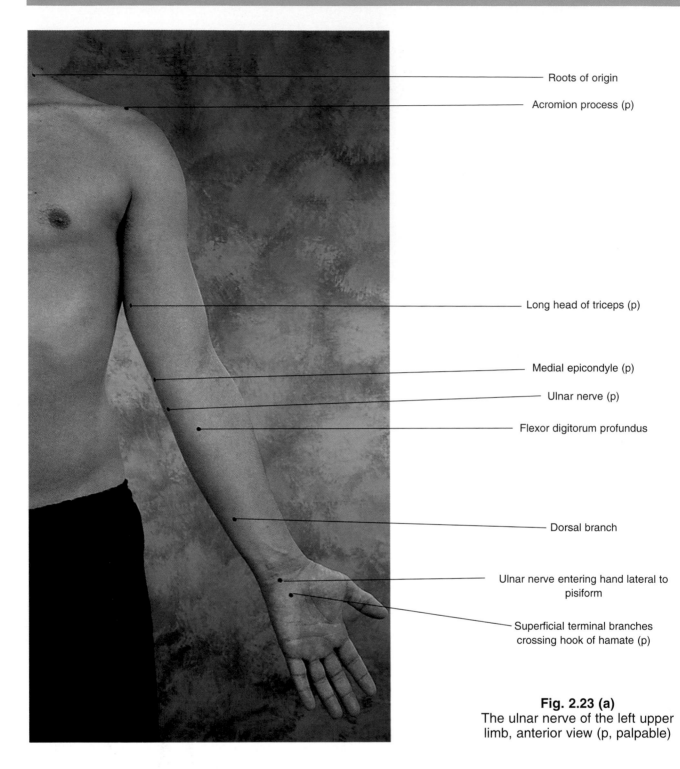

Roots of origin

Acromion process (p)

Long head of triceps (p)

Medial epicondyle (p)

Ulnar nerve (p)

Flexor digitorum profundus

Dorsal branch

Ulnar nerve entering hand lateral to pisiform

Superficial terminal branches crossing hook of hamate (p)

Fig. 2.23 (a)
The ulnar nerve of the left upper limb, anterior view (p, palpable)

Palpation

Press the pads of the fingers against the lateral wall of the axilla (the upper medial surface of the arm), and more cord-like structures can be palpated extending down the medial aspect of the arm. Numerous branches of the brachial plexus, including the ulnar and median nerves, are palpable on the medial side of the arm but they are not easily identifiable. The axillary/brachial artery can, however, be recognized pulsating between them.

The ulnar nerve

Continue down the medial side of the arm until you can palpate the medial supracondylar ridge with the medial epicondyle projecting medially. Move the tips of your fingers to the posterior of this structure. The ulnar nerve can be palpated behind the medial epicondyle as it passes from the medial aspect of the arm, over the medial collateral ligament of the elbow joint, to enter the forearm between the two heads of flexor carpi ulnaris. The whole medial aspect of the arm is tender to palpation, so employ great care here.

Roots of origin

C2
T1
T2

Acromion process (p)

Lateral cord

Median nerve (cut)

Medial cord

Long head of triceps (p)

Medial epicondyle (p)

Ulnar nerve (p)

Flexor digitorum profundus

Dorsal branch

Ulnar nerve entering hand lateral to pisiform

Deep branch of ulnar nerve

Superficial terminal branches crossing hook of hamate (p)

Superficial terminal branches

Fig. 2.23 (b)
The ulnar nerve of the left upper limb, anterior view (p, palpable)

The nerve (Fig. 2.23a,b) can be traced from the groove behind the medial epicondyle down the medial aspect of the elbow joint and medial side of the olecranon until it disappears under the fibrous arch of the flexor carpi ulnaris. It passes down the medial aspect of the forearm deep to this muscle until approximately 7 cm above the wrist, where it appears on the lateral side of the tendon before passing over the flexor retinaculum to enter the medial side of the hand. It can be palpated with some diffi-culty, as it lies lateral to the tendon of flexor carpi ulnaris, often covered with a layer of fascia obs-curing it from palpation. Its two superficial termi-nal branches, however, can be rolled against the hook of the hamate just distal to the pisiform, deep in the hypothenar muscle (see page 67). This proce-dure will give the subject a sensation of tingling over the anterior surface of the medial one-and-a-half digits.

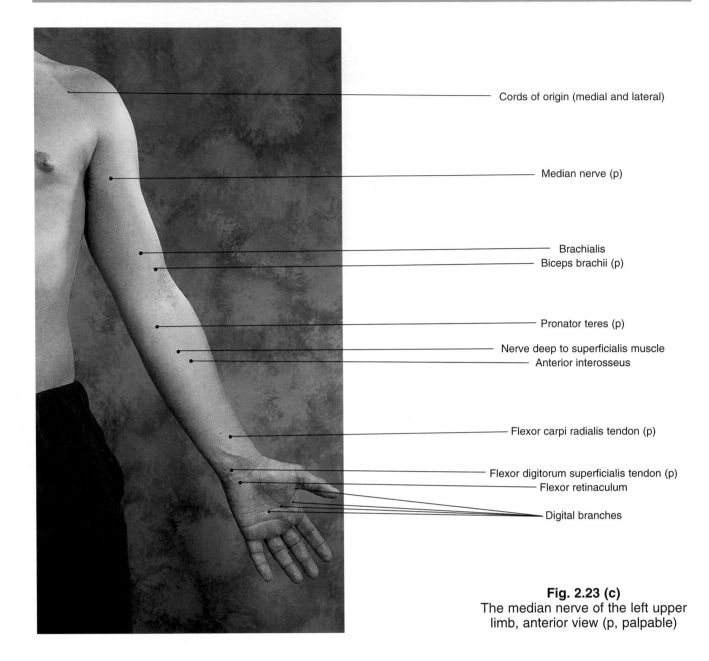

Cords of origin (medial and lateral)

Median nerve (p)

Brachialis
Biceps brachii (p)

Pronator teres (p)

Nerve deep to superficialis muscle
Anterior interosseus

Flexor carpi radialis tendon (p)

Flexor digitorum superficialis tendon (p)
Flexor retinaculum

Digital branches

Fig. 2.23 (c)
The median nerve of the left upper
limb, anterior view (p, palpable)

The median nerve [Fig. 2.23c and d]

The median nerve derives its fibres from the anterior primary rami of the fifth, sixth, seventh and eighth cervical and the first thoracic roots. The nerve is formed in front of the axillary artery after passing through all three trunks and the lateral and medial cords. It passes down the medial side of the arm accompanying the brachial artery, passing across the elbow joint superficial to the brachialis, but deep to biceps. It passes into the forearm between the two heads of pronator teres and passes down towards the front of the wrist under the flexor digitorum superficialis. It crosses the wrist joint under the flexor retinaculum on the radial side between the tendons of flexor carpi radialis and flexor digitorum superficialis, with which it shares a tunnel under the flexor retinaculum. For its distribution throughout the upper limb the reader should refer to *Anatomy and Human Movement* (Palastanga *et al.*, 1998).

Palpation

Although the cord-like structures of nerves can be palpated around the pulsating brachial artery on the medial side of the arm, identification of any particular nerve is virtually impossible. The only place that the median nerve can be palpated in the arm is on the medial side of the biceps just before it forms its tendon. The nerve then passes under the biceps tendon and retinaculum to enter the forearm. It is too well covered by the flexor digitorum superficialis to be palpated in the upper forearm, but becomes superficial as it emerges from the lateral side of the

Cords of origin (medial and lateral)
Latissimus dorsi

Median nerve (p)

Brachialis
Biceps brachii (p)
(cut)

Pronator teres (p)

Nerve deep to superficialis muscle
Anterior interosseus

Flexor carpi radialis tendon (p)

Flexor digitorum superficialis tendon (p)
Flexor retinaculum

Digital branches

Fig. 2.23 (d)
The median nerve of the left upper
limb, anterior view (p, palpable)

muscle, to cross the wrist. Here it can be palpated as a cord-like structure between the tendons of the above muscle and the flexor carpi radialis. It then disappears into the thenar muscles on the lateral side of the hand.

Because the median nerve passes through the same compartment as the tendons of flexor digitorum superficialis and profundus it can become compressed. This is commonly due to tightening of the flexor retinaculum or swelling of the synovial sheath surrounding the flexor tendons. This condi-

tion is referred to as 'carpal tunnel syndrome' and may be tested by tapping the nerve as it passes through the tunnel, which causes a tingling sensation over its distribution in the hand.

Sometimes the patient can suffer severe pain over the distribution of the nerve in the hand and may even lose the ability to use the muscles of the thenar eminence. Permanent dysfunction could occur if the pressure on the nerve is not quickly released. This is normally achieved by an operative procedure.

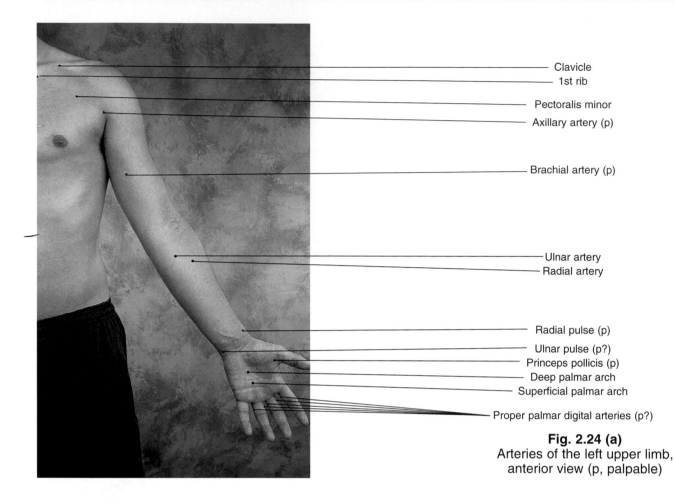

Clavicle
1st rib
Pectoralis minor
Axillary artery (p)

Brachial artery (p)

Ulnar artery
Radial artery

Radial pulse (p)
Ulnar pulse (p?)
Princeps pollicis (p)
Deep palmar arch
Superficial palmar arch
Proper palmar digital arteries (p?)

Fig. 2.24 (a)
Arteries of the left upper limb,
anterior view (p, palpable)

ARTERIES [Fig. 2.24]

A different approach must be made to the palpation of arteries. As stated earlier, when the tissue to be palpated is moving, the fingers should remain stationary. When palpating arteries, the fingertips should be used, never the thumb, as the palpator could be misled by the pulse in his or her own thumb. This is due to the presence of the relatively large artery (princeps pollicis) which supplies its pulp. Although the index finger is commonly used, all the fingertips are extremely sensitive. Sometimes the fingers are placed along the line of the artery, as it may be concealed for a short distance by another structure. Very gentle, sensitive touch must be employed because too much pressure may compress the artery and prevent its pulsations.

Palpation

Palpation of arteries throughout the limb varies from individual to individual, being modified by the texture of the skin, the thickness or tightness of fascial coverings, the bulk of muscles, the quantity of subcutaneous fat, etc. It is also dependent on the size of the artery and the patency of its walls. This varies enormously and may be affected by age and disease, *particularly* of the cardiovascular system.

The blood supply to the upper limbs is via the left subclavian artery, directly from the arch of the aorta, and the right subclavian, via the brachiocephalic trunk. All of these arteries are too deep to palpate, except where the subclavian passes over the first rib. With careful palpation just posterior to the midpoint of the clavicle, behind the insertion of scalenus anterior to the first rib, the pulsations of the subclavian artery can be felt. The artery, now named the axillary artery, then passes into the axilla and can be palpated behind the anterior and against the lateral wall by pressing gently upwards and laterally with the fingers. This may prove uncomfortable for the subject as the cords of the brachial plexus may intervene.

With careful palpation, the pulsations of the brachial artery can be traced down the medial side of the arm lying in a furrow anterior to coracobrachialis, in the upper part, and on the medial side of biceps and its tendon, in the lower part. The whole length of the artery is uncomfortable if too much pressure is applied, as the ulnar nerve lies superficial to it in the upper half, and the median nerve in the lower half of its course. It becomes easier to palpate just prior to passing under the bicipital aponeurosis in front of the elbow joint, but even here it can remain quite elusive. It is here that the pulsation of the brachial artery is auscultated with a stethoscope when taking blood pressure.

Subclavian artery

Clavicle (cut)
1st rib

Pectoralis minor
Axillary artery (p)
Profunda brachii

Brachial artery (p)

Elbow joint

Ulnar artery
Radial artery

Radial pulse (p)
Ulnar pulse (p?)
Princeps pollicis (p)
Deep palmar arch
Superficial palmar arch

Proper palmar digital arteries (p?)

Fig. 2.24 (b)
Arteries of the left upper limb,
anterior view (p, palpable)

The brachial artery divides into the radial and ulnar arteries just below the line of the elbow joint. These are both well covered by muscle and difficult to palpate until they emerge from between the tendons proximal to the wrist.

The radial artery is by far the easier to palpate, lying in a groove between flexor carpi radialis and the anterior border of the radius. This is best approached by wrapping your hand around the back of the subject's wrist with the fingertips resting on the lower end of the anterior border and styloid process of the radius. The fingers are then allowed to move gently medially some 0.5 cm where the pulsation of the radial artery becomes clear. This should be practised regularly, as it is the most common pulse that is checked in the human body. The artery can again be palpated on the lateral side of the scaphoid deep in the 'anatomical snuff box', between the tendons of extensor pollicis longus medially, and extensor pollicis brevis and abductor pollicis longus laterally. This area is, however, quite tender if too much pressure is applied.

The ulnar artery is much more difficult to palpate in the region of the wrist and hand as it is covered by the palmar aponeurosis. Nevertheless, its pulsations are recognizable just lateral to the pisiform bone. It then passes deeply into the palm as the superficial palmar arch, too deep to be palpated.

Throughout the hand, small branches of the radial and ulnar arteries can be palpated by an experienced practitioner beyond the superficial and deep palmar and carpal arches. The posterior metacarpal arteries are palpable between the metacarpal bones, especially at their bases. On each side of the palmar aspect of each finger, the pulsation of the very slender proper palmar digital arteries can be felt. These become clearer beyond the cleft of the fingers. The dorsal digital arteries on either side of the dorsum of each finger are less obvious. In the cleft between the thumb and index finger, the pulsations of the princeps pollicis, a comparatively large artery, can be traced up the anteromedial side of the thumb, particularly opposite the proximal phalanx. On the lateral side of the metacarpal of the index finger, the radialis indicis artery is palpable running up the dorsolateral side of the finger. If the thumb is gently rested against a firm surface, the pulsations of the princeps pollicis can readily be felt by the subject. This is why it is important to use only the fingertips to palpate a pulse.

Sometimes, on a subject with good strong pulsations and thin fascia, the posterior carpal arch arteries can be palpated crossing the posterior aspect of the carpus just below the level of the wrist joint.

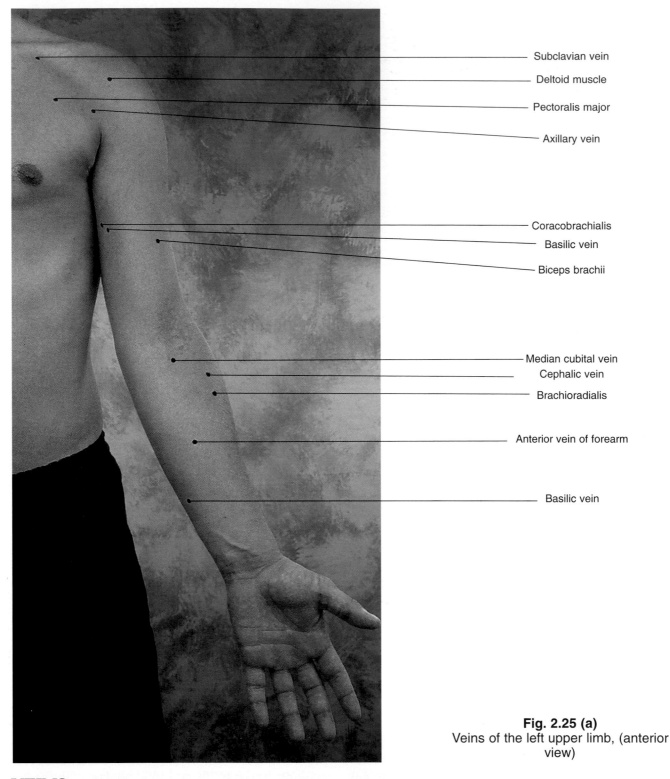

Subclavian vein

Deltoid muscle

Pectoralis major

Axillary vein

Coracobrachialis

Basilic vein

Biceps brachii

Median cubital vein

Cephalic vein

Brachioradialis

Anterior vein of forearm

Basilic vein

Fig. 2.25 (a)
Veins of the left upper limb, (anterior view)

VEINS

The veins of the upper limb are, for convenience of description, divided into two groups, deep and superficial. The deep veins tend to follow the arteries deep within the limb, whereas the superficial veins lie within the superficial fascia forming a variable network. All veins in the upper limb possess valves, more numerous in the deep than in the superficial veins, the function of which is to facilitate venous return to the heart.

Palpation

The superficial veins are extremely difficult to palpate as they are normally thin-walled, variable in position, concealed within the superficial fascia and possess low internal pressure. Thus, only a few of the superficial veins are palpable in the normal limb, the deep veins being impossible to palpate.

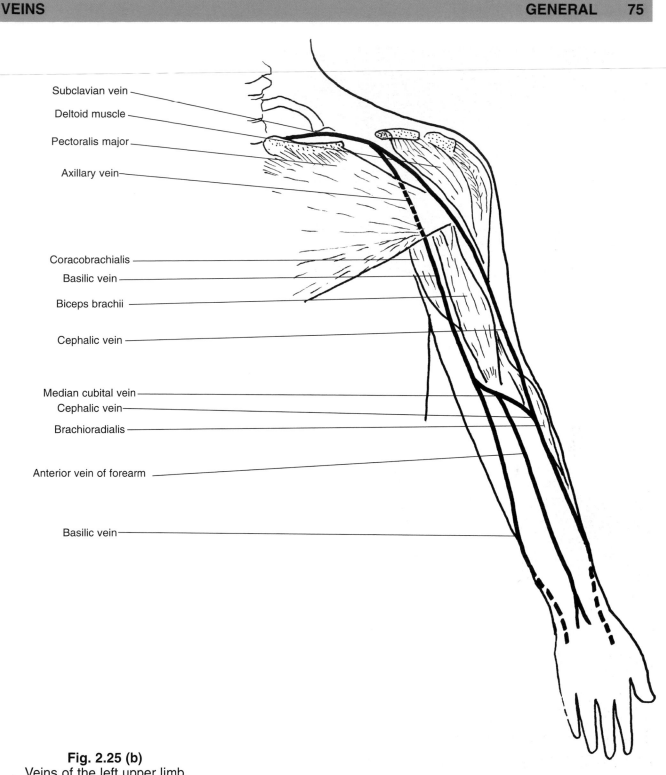

Fig. 2.25 (b)
Veins of the left upper limb
in relation to muscles, (anterior view)

Gentle brushing of the skin surface may be all that is required to indicate the course of superficial veins to the examiner. Some veins merely show as a bluish line just below the skin, while others are accompanied by raised areas. The appearance of the veins in individuals varies considerably, being dependent on factors such as sex, obesity and age. In males the veins are usually more prominent, whereas in the obese they are more difficult to find. Veins tend to show more clearly in the elderly, as the fascia becomes thinner and the veins themselves become tortuous and distended.

The venous network on the dorsum of the hand is palpable in most subjects, particularly if the arm hangs by the side and firm pressure is applied to the inner aspect of the arm anterior to the brachial artery (see page 72).

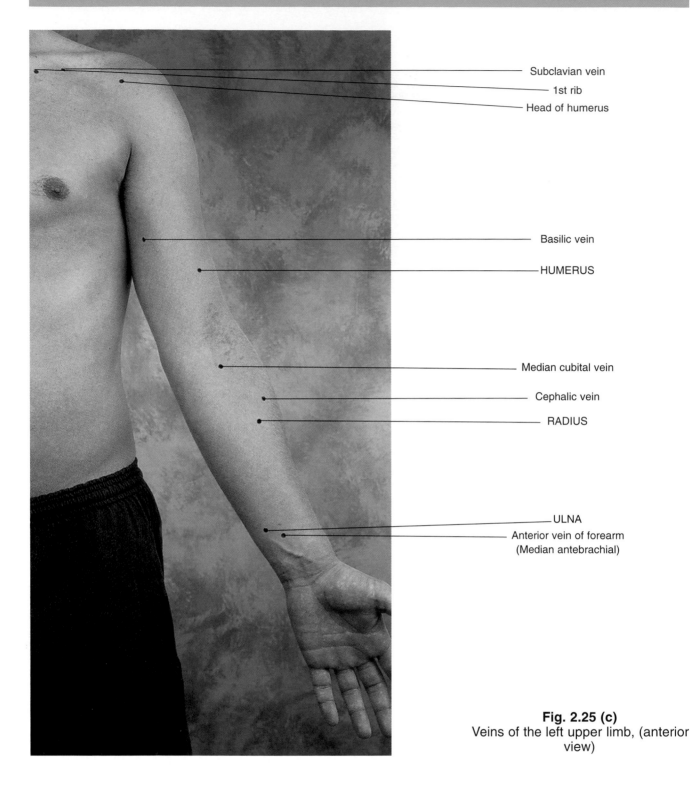

Subclavian vein
1st rib
Head of humerus

Basilic vein
HUMERUS

Median cubital vein
Cephalic vein
RADIUS

ULNA
Anterior vein of forearm
(Median antebrachial)

Fig. 2.25 (c)
Veins of the left upper limb, (anterior view)

Superficial drainage

The cephalic vein [Fig. 2.25]

The origin of the cephalic vein can be traced from the posterolateral aspect of the dorsal venous network, passing upwards around the lateral border of the forearm anterior to the head of the radius. It then ascends on the lateral side of biceps brachii to the groove between deltoid and pectoralis major (Fig. 2.25a,b) to end in the infraclavicular fossa, where it pierces the clavipectoral fascia to join the axillary vein. Proximal to the head of the radius the vein is more difficult to identify.

The basilic vein [Fig. 2.25]

The basilic vein begins on the medial side of the dorsal venous network and passes up the medial aspect of the forearm, coming to lie anterior to the medial condyle of the humerus. It continues up the medial side of the arm, piercing the deep fascia, near the insertion of coracobrachialis, to accompany the brachial vessels before becoming the axillary vein. The distal half of the vein can usually be palpated, whereas proximally it may only appear as a bluish line.

Subclavian vein

1st rib

Head of humerus

Basilic vein

HUMERUS

Cephalic vein

Median cubital vein

Cephalic vein

RADIUS

Basilic vein

ULNA

Anterior vein of forearm
(Median antebrachial)

Fig. 2.25 (d)
Veins of the left upper limb in
relation to bones, (anterior view)

On the front of the forearm there is normally a midline vein, the median antebrachial, which commonly joins with the median cubital vein. The median cubital vein itself passes across the cubital fossa, uniting the cephalic and basilic veins. All of these veins are normally palpable when pressure is applied to the inner aspect of the arm. However, they vary considerably in their position and size between individuals. Compression of these superficial veins is easily achieved by applying light pressure with a finger or thumb. This will emphasize the vein distal to the point of compression, and may, on larger veins, indicate the position of the valves.

3

The lower limb

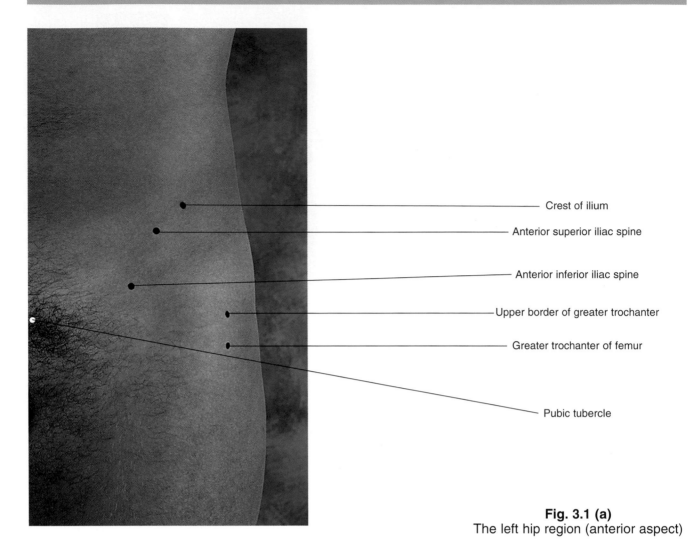

Crest of ilium

Anterior superior iliac spine

Anterior inferior iliac spine

Upper border of greater trochanter

Greater trochanter of femur

Pubic tubercle

Fig. 3.1 (a)
The left hip region (anterior aspect)

BONES

The hip region

The two hip bones on either side and the sacrum, posteriorly, form the pelvic girdle. In its lower section it forms a complete ring (the true pelvis) with the two pubic bones joined at the pubic symphysis, whereas in its upper part (the false pelvis) the two blades of the ilium leave a large space anteriorly.

The hip or innominate bone (*os innominatum* (L) = bone without a name), comprises the ilium, the ischium and the pubis. They are united at the acetabulum, a deep rounded hollow situated on the lateral side of the bone on the constricted area between two blades. That above and posterior is the ilium and that below and anterior is the pubis and ischium. The ilium has an inner and outer surface with a broad crest above a narrow border at the front and back and the upper part of the sciatic notch inferiorly just posterior to its junction with the ischium. The lower blade presents a large foramen, medial to which is the flattened bone of the body of the pubis with a superior ramus above and an inferior ramus passing downwards and laterally. The ischium is situated below the acetabulum and forms the lateral part of the obturator foramen with its ramus passing

from below upwards to join the inferior ramus of the pubis.

The upper end of the femur comprises the head, neck, greater and lesser trochanter. The head lies medially and articulates in the acetabulum, the greater trochanter lies at the lateral end of the neck and the lesser trochanter projects medially and backwards from just below the junction of the neck with the shaft.

Palpation

Owing to the size and thickness of muscle and fascia, this region is much more difficult to investigate than the shoulder. It is often covered by a layer of fat, particularly in women, and this also adds to the difficulty in observation and palpation.

Face the subject, who is standing, and place both hands around the waist. On sliding the hands downwards a bony ridge, the iliac [*ilium* (L) = the flank] crest, is encountered on either side. Each can be traced forwards to end in a well-defined projection, the anterior superior iliac spines (ASIS) (Fig. 3.1). In lean subjects the iliac crest is easily palpated

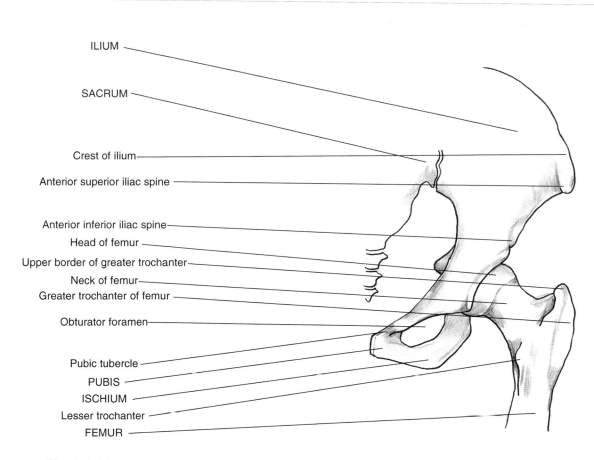

ILIUM

SACRUM

Crest of ilium

Anterior superior iliac spine

Anterior inferior iliac spine

Head of femur

Upper border of greater trochanter

Neck of femur

Greater trochanter of femur

Obturator foramen

Pubic tubercle

PUBIS

ISCHIUM

Lesser trochanter

FEMUR

Fig. 3.1 (b)
Bones of the left hip region (anterior
aspect)

from the ASIS to the posterior superior iliac spine (PSIS). In its anterior two-thirds it is convex laterally, broad and rounded, with inner and outer lips. Five to seven centimetres posterior to the ASIS, on its lateral lip, the tubercle of the crest is easily palpable, giving attachment to the upper end of the iliotibial tract. In its posterior third the iliac crest is concave laterally, less well defined and a little sharper on its superior border. The ASISs are set approximately 30 cm apart, a little more in the female, the abdomen usually protruding forwards between the two. From the ASIS, the sharp concave anterior border of the ilium can be traced downwards to another, less well-defined anterior projection, the anterior inferior iliac spine (AIIS), which lies approximately 2 cm above the rim of the acetablum (Fig. 3.1).

Now place the palm of your hand on the lower abdomen, moving it gently downwards; another ridge of bone can be palpated approximately 4 cm above the genitalia (Fig. 3.1). This is the anterior brim of the true pelvis. This ridge is depressed centrally where the two pubic bones join

(the pubic [*pubes* (L) = the growth of hair in the region in adulthood] symphysis) and is marked superiorly on either side by the pubic tubercles. These are both palpable, approximately 1 cm on either side of the midline on the upper border of the pubis. This area is quite tender on palpation and is frequently covered with a fatty pad of tissue which may make positive identification of these tubercles difficult. Laterally, the superior ramus of the pubis can be palpated, gradually becoming hidden by muscle.

If the line of the pubic crest is extended laterally beyond the region of the hip joint to the lateral aspect of the upper thigh, a hard, bony prominence can be palpated; this is the greater trochanter of the femur (Fig. 3.1). It lies approximately 10 cm below the most lateral aspect of the iliac crest. The trochanters are quadrilateral in shape and, although surrounded by muscle, are easy to identify, being the most lateral bony part of the hip region. This tends to be the level around which the measurement of the hip circumference is erroneously taken.

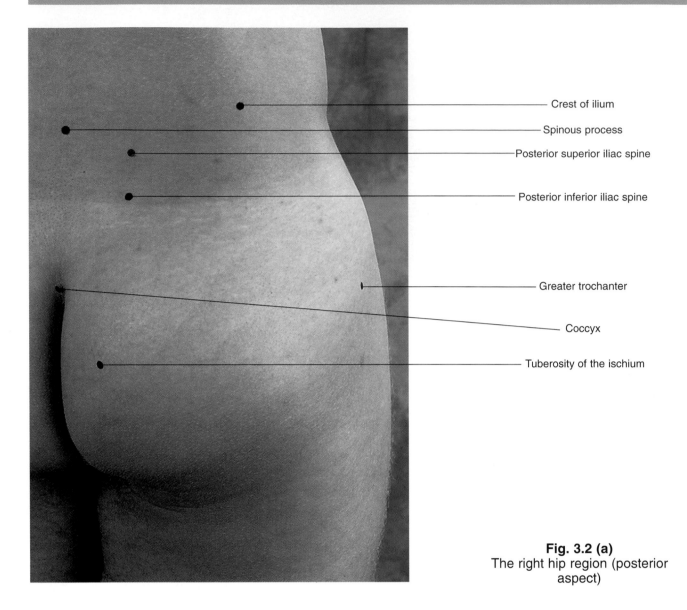

Crest of ilium

Spinous process

Posterior superior iliac spine

Posterior inferior iliac spine

Greater trochanter

Coccyx

Tuberosity of the ischium

Fig. 3.2 (a)
The right hip region (posterior aspect)

From the back, the ease of palpation depends to a large extent on the build of the subject. The region is often covered with a thick layer of fat, particularly in women, rendering precise identification of bony points extremely difficult.

Returning to the iliac crest, it can be traced backwards and medially until the PSIS is reached (Fig. 3.2). This is, however, less easy to identify than the ASIS. In women, it is often located in a small dimple characteristic of this region. From the PSIS the posterior border passes downwards and slightly medially, being concave posteriorly, to terminate approximately 2.5 cm below at the posterior inferior iliac spine (PIIS). From here the posterior border passes forwards, forming the upper boundary of the greater sciatic notch. The notch itself is difficult to identify, except in lean subjects.

The lower lateral border of the sacrum [sacer (L) = sacred; this is believed to be due to it being the only bone to survive a sacrifice] (S4,5) forms the medial component of the sciatic notch. It can easily be identified running downwards and medially to the cleft between the buttocks and terminating at the coccyx, which is often tucked forwards towards the anal canal. The upper part of the sacrum is held between the two ilia posteriorly, its upper border being on a line 2 cm above the level of the PSIS. If you run your hand down the centre of the sacrum posteriorly, a series of up to five tubercles, gradually diminishing in size, can be felt. These lie in line with the spines of the lumbar vertebrae and are termed spinous processes (Fig. 3.2). On either side of these spines, smaller tubercles can be palpated, in line with the articular processes of the vertebrae above. These are therefore known as the articular tubercles. This area is often covered with a fatty pad of tissue which may make positive identification of these tubercles difficult.

The ischial [ischion (Gk) = the socket in which the thigh bone turns] tuberosity is palpable in the standing or prone lying position, being anterolateral to the lateral border of the sacrum and posteromedial to the greater trochanter of the femur (Fig. 3.2). It is much easier, however, to identify these tuberosities if the subject either sits on your hands or is in the prone kneeling position. When sitting, large rounded processes can be felt carrying most of the weight of the trunk to the supporting surface. If the

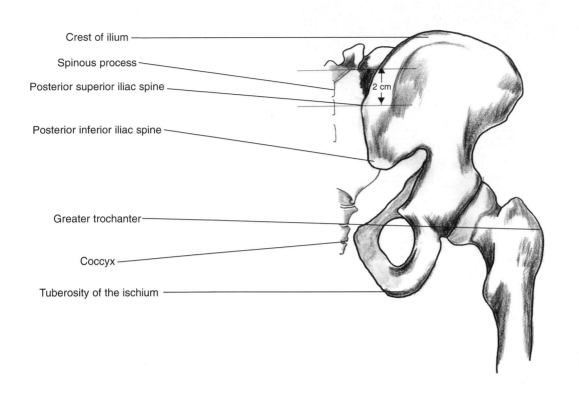

Crest of ilium

Spinous process

Posterior superior iliac spine

2 cm

Posterior inferior iliac spine

Greater trochanter

Coccyx

Tuberosity of the ischium

Fig. 3.2 (b)
Bones of the right hip region
(posterior aspect)

subject is asked to move gently from side to side, the transference of weight from one tuberosity to the other can be observed. In sustained sitting on a hard surface, such as a wooden pew, these tuberosities become very tender and uncomfortable. The pressure is increased if the subject sits upright, preventing his or her sacrum sliding forward to take some of the weight. The tuberosities are covered partially by a bursa posteriorly, and the tendinous attachment of the adductor magnus posteriorly. The bursa may become inflamed after long periods of sitting upright, causing acute pain over the area (bursitis).

Palpation on movement

Once the position and shape of the pelvis has been established by palpation it is useful to know how its position may change during movements. One can normally consider the bony pelvis, i.e. the two hip bones and the sacrum, as one unit which moves as a whole.

Stand on the right side of the standing model and place your right hand on the upper anterior part of the ilium, place your left hand on the sacrum. If the model now drops the lower abdomen forwards by arching the lumbar spine the pelvis will be observed tilting forwards. If the model now pulls in the lower abdomen and flattens the lumbar spine the pelvis will be observed tilting backwards. Both movements occur around a frontal axis running through the heads of both femora.

Now stand facing the model, who is standing on one leg (the right). Place one hand on the crest of both ilia. The model can now draw up the left side of the pelvis by using the left trunk side flexors of the same side and the hip abductors of the standing leg. If these muscles are relaxed the pelvis will drop on the left side. This lateral tilting of the pelvis occurs around a sagittal axis through the right hip joint. Repeat the same procedure using the left leg as the standing leg.

Stand behind the standing model and place your fingers over the two greater trochanters. If the model now flexes and extends one hip rhythmically the trochanter will be observed rotating anticlockwise on flexion and clockwise on extension.

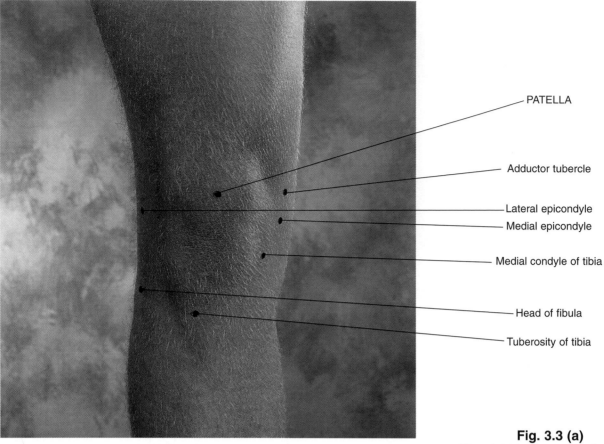

PATELLA

Adductor tubercle

Lateral epicondyle
Medial epicondyle

Medial condyle of tibia

Head of fibula

Tuberosity of tibia

Fig. 3.3 (a)
The right knee region (anterior aspect)

The knee region

There are four bones that can be palpated in this region: the femur, the tibia, the fibula and the patella.

The femur [*femur* (L) = a thigh] is the longest and strongest bone in the human body, taking the weight from the hip and transferring it through the knee joint to the tibia. This beautifully shaped bone narrows in its middle half, becoming more or less cylindrical with a very broad posterior border, the linea aspera. It broadens in its lower half, forming two large condyles at its lower end. These project backwards, being separated from each other by the intercondylar notch. The lateral condyle is stouter than the medial, which is slightly longer from front to back. Both condyles are smooth on their posterior, inferior and anterior surfaces, covered by hyaline cartilage in the living body. The smooth surfaces meet anteriorly at a triangular, patella, surface. The lateral surface of the lateral condyle is roughened and is marked just below its centre by a tubercle termed the lateral epicondyle. The medial condyle is also roughened on its medial side and marked just below its centre by a slightly larger tubercle termed the medial epicondyle. Each condyle has a sharp border above termed the medial and lateral supra-condylar ridges, the medial presenting a tubercle at its lower end, the adductor tubercle

The tibia [*tibia* (L) = a flute] is again a very strong stout bone carrying the body weight to the ankle joint and foot. It is broader above, having two large condyles, both flattened superiorly, being slightly depressed centrally. They are separated by the inter-condylar eminence and a roughened area anteriorly and posteriorly. The shaft narrows as it descends, presenting a large tubercle anteriorly, the tibial tuberosity, just below the level of the knee joint. The sharp anterior border (shin) passes vertically down from this tubercle.

The patella [*patella* (L) = a small plate] is, as its name implies, a small flat bone situated on the front of the knee. It is triangular in shape with the apex downwards and has a roughened anterior surface and a smooth posterior surface divided into two articular facets with the roughened apex below.

The fibula [*fibula* (L) = a pin] is a long, thin bone situated lateral to the tibia, having complex surfaces and a border mainly produced by the muscles attaching to it. It is expanded above and below: the upper expansion, the head, articulates with the under surface of the lateral condyle of the tibia and takes no part in the knee joint. The lower expansion forms the lateral malleolus and takes part in the formation of the ankle joint.

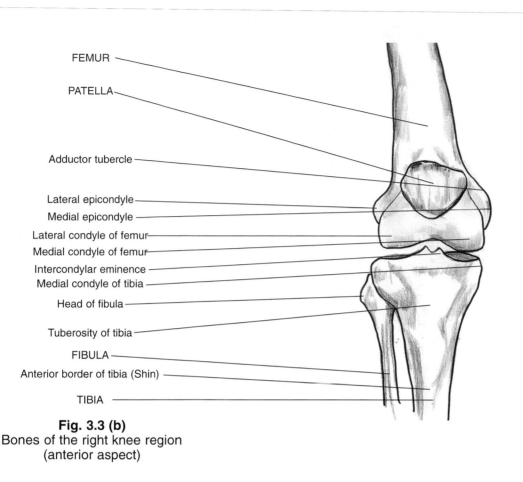

FEMUR

PATELLA

Adductor tubercle

Lateral epicondyle

Medial epicondyle

Lateral condyle of femur

Medial condyle of femur

Intercondylar eminence

Medial condyle of tibia

Head of fibula

Tuberosity of tibia

FIBULA

Anterior border of tibia (Shin)

TIBIA

Fig. 3.3 (b)
Bones of the right knee region
(anterior aspect)

Anterior aspect

Palpation

The obvious bony feature anteriorly is the patella. Place your fingers on its anterior surface and gently move them around, investigating its surfaces and borders. The patella is broader superiorly, narrowing to a rounded point below, where it is continuous with the ligamentum patellae. The borders are rounded, while the anterior surface, although appearing slippery due to the presence of the prepatellar bursa, has rough vertical ridges in line with the fibres of the tendon of quadriceps femoris.

With the knee flexed to 90 degrees, the patella becomes more prominent, situated on the medial and lateral femoral condyles, each of which is clearly palpable either side. Each femoral condyle is convex forwards, and presents a strip either side of the patella. It is narrow superiorly, due to the breadth of the patella, but becomes broader below due to the comparative narrowness of the ligamentum patellae. These condylar surfaces pass posteriorly into the knee joint itself.

The medial and lateral tibial condyles are easily recognisable below the femoral condyles, with their flattened upper surfaces being marked by a sharp circumference separating them from the more vertical surfaces of the shaft.

Below and centrally the large tibial tuberosity is easily identified (Fig. 3.4); the lower part is smooth and slippery, due to the presence of the superficial infrapatellar bursa, while its upper part gives attachment to the ligamentum patellae. The tuberosity is particularly noticeable when the knee is extended. With the knee flexed to 90 degrees place your fingers in the small triangular fossae on either side of the ligamentum patellae. Here the upper surfaces of the tibial condyles can be felt below, the under surface of the femoral condyles above, while between your fingers lies the ligamentum patellae. Directly posteriorly is the cleft of the knee joint, with the medial and lateral menisci between. These are not always palpable, although the anterior edge of the medial meniscus can be observed bulging forwards on medial rotation of the tibia. The anterior edge of the lateral meniscus also becomes palpable, but to a lesser extent, on lateral tibial rotation.

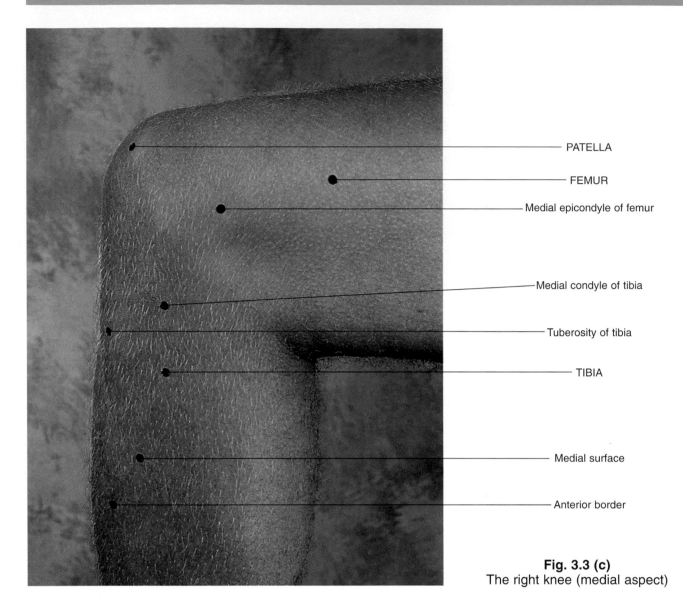

PATELLA

FEMUR

Medial epicondyle of femur

Medial condyle of tibia

Tuberosity of tibia

TIBIA

Medial surface

Anterior border

Fig. 3.3 (c)
The right knee (medial aspect)

Medial aspect

On the medial side of this region the large, elongated medial condyle of the femur sits on top of the flattened plateau of the medial tibial condyle. The centre of the medial surface of the femoral condyle is marked by a tubercle termed the medial epicondyle. Vertically above this is the medial supracondylar line marked at its lower end by the adductor tubercle.

Below the femoral condyle the flattened medial tibial condyle continues downwards as the medial surface of the tibial shaft, bounded in front by its anterior border marked at its upper end by the tibial tuberosity

Palpation

The medial surface of the femoral condyle is readily palpable, with the epicondyle projecting from its mid point (Fig. 3.3). Approximately 2 cm proximal to the medial epicondyle the adductor tubercle is just palpable, being hidden to a certain extent by the attachment of the tendinous part of the adductor magnus. This tubercle represents the most distal part of the medial supracondylar ridge, little of which can be palpated.

The medial tibial condyle (Fig. 3.3c, d) is also easily palpable below the femoral condyle. It appears to be larger than the lateral, and can be traced around the medial side, becoming continuous below with the

PATELLA

FEMUR

Medial epicondyle of femur

Medial condyle of tibia

Head of fibula

Tuberosity of tibia

TIBIA

FIBULA

Medial surface

Anterior border

Fig. 3.3 (d)
Bones of the right knee (medial
aspect)

medial surface of the shaft of the tibia and its anterior border (the shin), the whole of which is subcutaneous and palpable as far as the medial malleolus.

Palpation on movement

With the model standing and the knee extended place the fingers of one hand on the medial condyle of the femur and the fingers of the other hand on the medial border of the patella. If the model now flexes the knee the patella will be observed sliding downwards and backwards on the femoral condyle until it lies inferiorly. Return the knee to the extended position. Now move the fingers from the patella and place them on the upper part of the medial surface of the medial condyle of the tibia, close to the joint line. If the knee is flexed again the tibial condyle will be observed moving backwards and upwards on to the posterior aspect of the femoral condyle. As in the case of the lateral condyles, in this position the anterior part of the tibial condyle appears to part from the femoral condyle due to the smaller articular surface at the posterior part of the femoral condyle.

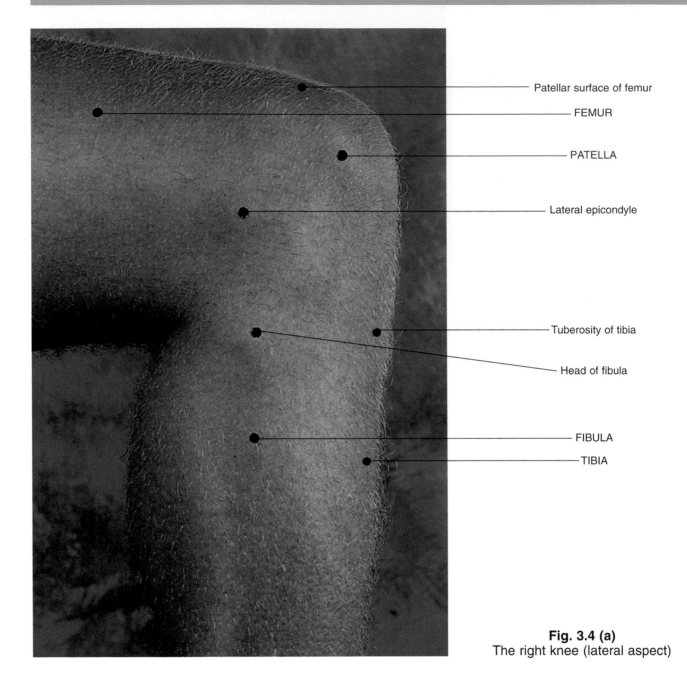

Patellar surface of femur

FEMUR

PATELLA

Lateral epicondyle

Tuberosity of tibia

Head of fibula

FIBULA

TIBIA

Fig. 3.4 (a)
The right knee (lateral aspect)

Lateral aspect

On the lateral side of this region the stout lateral condyle of the femur sits on top of the plateau of the lateral condyle of the tibia. Posteriorly, the two condyles are close together; however anteriorly, they diverge into a small hollow which is bounded at the front by the lower section of the patella and the ligamentum patellae. The head of the fibula lies below and posterior to the knee joint.

Palpation

With the model standing, the flat lateral surface of the lateral femoral condyle can readily be palpated, lying posterior to the lateral border of the patella. It is marked by a tubercle at its centre (the lateral epicondyle). Running your fingers upwards from this lateral epicondyle the lateral supracondylar ridge may be just palpable running vertically upwards. This is difficult to palpate as the iliotibial tract tends to follow the same line.

Approximately 2 cm below the lateral epicondyle the lower border of the lateral femoral condyle and the upper border of the lateral tibial condyle can be palpated running horizontally and diverging anteriorly. Finally, approximately 1 cm below this rim, the head of the fibula can be palpated, with its styloid process projecting upwards, and the narrower neck just below (Fig. 3.4). The remainder of the upper end

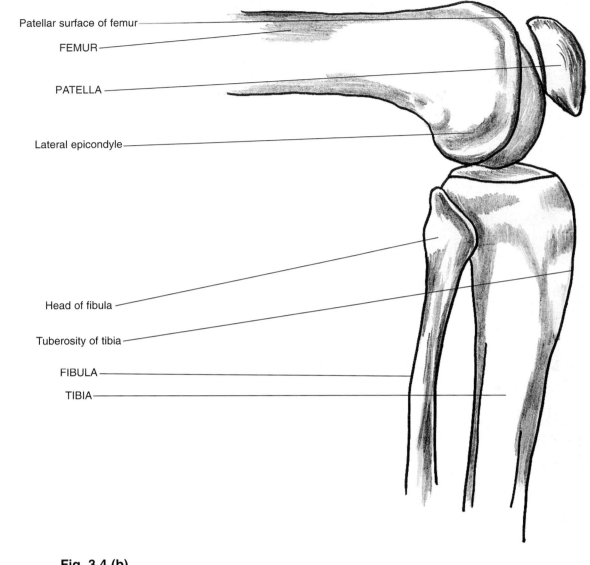

Patellar surface of femur

FEMUR

PATELLA

Lateral epicondyle

Head of fibula

Tuberosity of tibia

FIBULA

TIBIA

Fig. 3.4 (b)
Bones of the right knee (lateral
aspect)

of the shaft of the fibula is surrounded by muscles and is therefore not palpable. The head can easily be located by running the palm of the hand up the lateral aspect of the leg.

Palpation on movement

With the model's knee fully extended, place your fingers of one hand on the lateral side of the patella and the fingers of the other hand on the lateral surface of the femoral condyle. If the model now flexes the knee the patella will be observed sliding downwards and backwards under the condyle, finally ending up inferiorly. Return the knee back to the extended position. Now remove the fingers from the patella and place them on the lateral condyle of the tibia close to the knee joint. If the model flexes the knee again the tibia will be observed gliding backwards and upwards on to the posterior surface of the femoral condyles. At this position the anterior part of the tibial condyle appears to part from the femoral condyle. This is due to the posterior surface of the femoral condyle being smaller than that of the tibia.

The head of the fibula moves with the tibia.

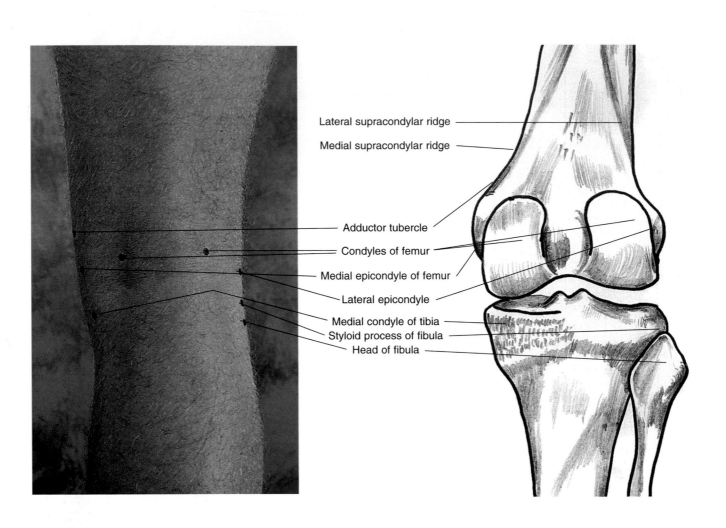

Fig. 3.4 (c), (d)
The right knee region (posterior aspect)

Posterior aspect

Virtually no bony features can be palpated on the posterior aspect of the knee, either when it is flexed or extended. The posterior aspect of the sides of each femoral condyle and the medial surfaces of the tibia soon become hidden by the fascia and muscles at the back of the knee. The head of the fibula (Fig. 3.4), however, can easily be palpated on the lateral side of the popliteal fossa, with the tendon of biceps femoris attaching to its upper section. Palpation from this aspect must be approached with care, as the common peroneal nerve passes down the back of the head of the fibula *en route* to its passage around the lateral side of the neck.

When the knee is extended and the quadriceps femoris is relaxed, the patella can easily be moved from side to side, producing a knocking effect as it crosses either side of the grooved patellar surface of the femur. This manoeuvre, an accessory movement, exposes a strip of the patellar surface of the femur, on the side away from the direction of the movement. If held to one side, the articular surface of the patella on that side can also be palpated for approximately 1 cm on its posterior surface.

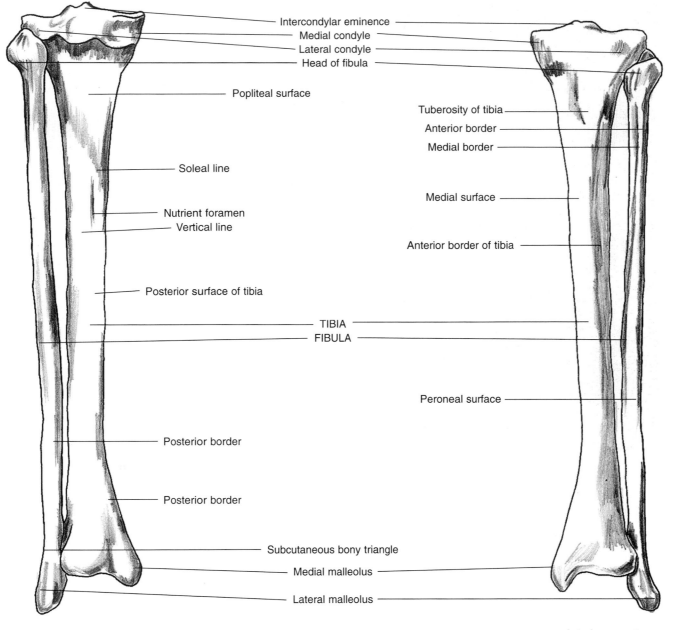

Intercondylar eminence
Medial condyle
Lateral condyle
Head of fibula

Popliteal surface

Tuberosity of tibia
Anterior border
Medial border

Medial surface

Soleal line

Anterior border of tibia

Nutrient foramen
Vertical line

Posterior surface of tibia

TIBIA
FIBULA

Peroneal surface

Posterior border

Posterior border

Subcutaneous bony triangle
Medial malleolus
Lateral malleolus

Posterior aspect

Anterior aspect

Fig. 3.4 (e), (f)
The tibia and fibula

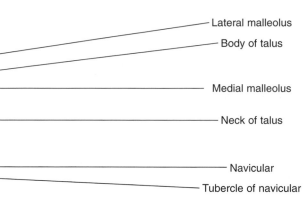

Lateral malleolus
Body of talus
Medial malleolus
Neck of talus
Navicular
Tubercle of navicular

Fig. 3.5 (a)
The right ankle region (anterior aspect)

The ankle region

There are four bones taking part in the formation of this area: the lower ends of the tibia and fibula, the talus and the calcaneus

The lower end of the tibia

From its narrowest cross-section, two-thirds of the way down the shaft, the bone expands to form part of the mortice for the formation of the ankle joint. Its medial side presents a large projection downwards, termed the medial malleolus. On its lateral side there is an elongated triangular area for the attachment of an extremely strong interosseous ligament which binds the two bones together. Its under surface and the lateral side of the malleolus are smooth for articulation with the talus in the ankle joint.

The lower end of the fibula

The slender shaft of the fibula expands below to form the pointed lateral malleolus, which forms the lateral section of the mortice of the ankle joint. It is flattened from side to side, having a smooth articular surface on its medial side and a roughened surface on its lateral, subcutaneous side.

The talus

This bone is formed of a body, a neck and a head. The body is narrower at the back and wider anteriorly. It is pulley-shaped superiorly and slightly concave inferiorly. It has smooth, articular surfaces on its superior, inferior, lateral and the upper part of its medial surfaces.

The neck passes forwards and medially to expand into the head, which articulates with the posterior surface of the navicular.

The calcaneus (see page 94)

At the ankle the muscles of the leg have become tendinous and thus the bones are easier to palpate and identify between and deep to the tendons and retinacula.

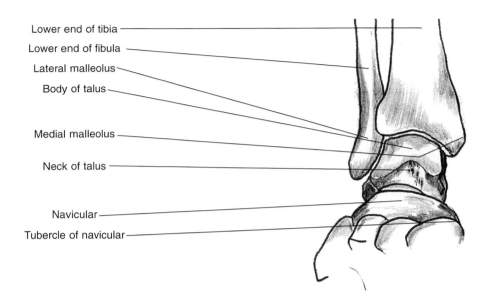

Lower end of tibia
Lower end of fibula
Lateral malleolus
Body of talus
Medial malleolus
Neck of talus
Navicular
Tubercle of navicular

Fig. 3.5 (b)
Bones of the right ankle region
(anterior aspect)

Palpation

Anterior aspect. Placing the hands on the subcutaneous medial surface of the tibia, trace down to the medial malleolus. The anterior border of the tibia (shin) appears to form the anterior part of the malleolus, which is clearly defined (Fig. 3.5a,b). It has an anterior border and tip which can be palpated, and a posterior border which is partially hidden by tendons and the flexor retinaculum. The anterior border of the malleolus [*malleolus* (L) = a small hammer] continues upwards and laterally under the extensor tendons and extensor retinacula, marking the line of the ankle joint.

On the lateral side of the ankle the lateral malleolus of the fibula is the most outstanding feature (Figs 3.4e, f, 3.5). From its tip, which lies at a lower level than that of the medial malleolus, both the anterior and posterior borders can be traced upwards, encompassing the large prominence of the malleolus. Just above the level of the ankle joint, at approximately 2.5 cm, the fibula narrows to a trian-

gular subcutaneous lateral surface. The shaft can be traced upwards for approximately 15 cm, where it becomes hidden by muscle, the peroneus tertius anteriorly and the peroneus brevis and tendon of peroneus longus posteriorly.

With your right hand over the front of the ankle region, place your index finger on the lateral, and your thumb on the medial, malleolus of the subject's left ankle. Draw your finger and thumb forward into a small hollow on either side. Between your thumb and finger you will feel the head of the talus. Immediately anterior you can palpate the narrow gap of the talonavicular joint and posterior part of the navicular with its prominent tubercle, medially. If the foot is plantar flexed, the neck of the talus [*talus* (L) = the ankle bone] can also be palpated, and deep beneath the tip of your index finger, just lateral to the head of the talus, you will feel the anterior section of the upper surface of the calcaneus [*calx* (L) = a heel] and the origin of extensor digitorum brevis.

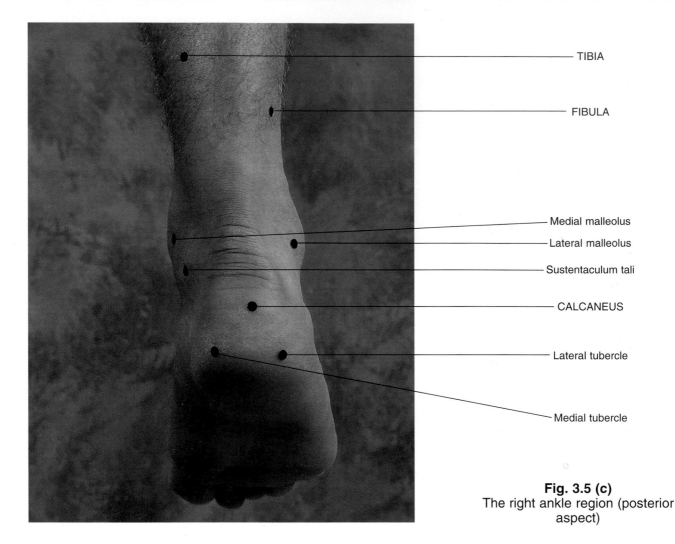

TIBIA

FIBULA

Medial malleolus

Lateral malleolus

Sustentaculum tali

CALCANEUS

Lateral tubercle

Medial tubercle

Fig. 3.5 (c)
The right ankle region (posterior aspect)

Posterior aspect. From the posterior aspect very little of the talus can be seen as the body has narrowed down to just two tubercles and a groove running downwards and medially. The mortice of the ankle joint (see page 92) is formed by the two malleoli and the inferior border of the tibia. Both the malleoli are marked posteriorly by a fossa for the attachment of ligaments.

The calcaneus

This is the largest of the tarsal bones and is situated below the talus and behind the navicular and cuboid. It is oblong in shape, projecting forwards and backwards beyond the talus. The backward projection forms the heel. It has six surfaces: an anterior, which is smooth, a superior, marked by a smooth articular surface centrally, and a medial, which is fairly smooth and converted into a hollow by the projection medially from its upper section by the sustentaculum tali. The lateral surface is roughened, presenting two tubercles, and the posterior surface is rounded and roughened across its centre for the attachment of the tendocalcaneus. Its inferior surface is slightly concave downwards and is roughened for the attachment of muscles and fascia. It

presents three broad, rounded tubercles. The medial and lateral lie posterior, almost on the junction with the posterior surface, and the anterior lies central, approximately 1 cm from its anterior border.

Palpation

Place your hands at the tip of the medial malleolus. Move your fingers 1 cm down from this tip and you will feel the horizontal ridge of the sustentaculum tali. It runs for approximately 2–3 cm and is clearer anteriorly and posteriorly. If the foot is everted the sustentaculum tali becomes more prominent. At the anterior end of this ridge there is a small gap before encountering the tubercle of the navicular. This gap is spanned by the 'spring ligament'.

Because the tendocalcaneus lies almost 2 cm clear of the ankle joint, few bony features can be identified posteriorly. On close examination of the posterior borders of the lateral and medial malleoli, a small depression can be palpated, the malleolar fossa. Tracing superiorly, the posterior border of the lateral malleolus forms the posterior border of the triangular area referred to above. The posterior surface of the medial malleolus is continuous with the posterior border of the medial surface of the tibia (Fig. 3.5c, d).

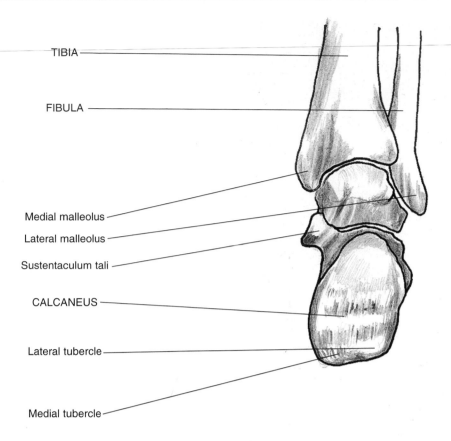

Fig. 3.5 (d)
Bones of the right ankle region
(posterior aspect)

Palpation on movement

Anterior. With the model lying, stand facing the lateral side of the model's right ankle region. With your left hand grip the two malleoli with your fingers on the medial and your thumb on the lateral. With your right hand grip the anterior part of the body and neck of the talus with your fingers in the hollow just anterior to the medial malleolus and your thumb in the hollow just anterior to the lateral malleolus. Both sets of fingers and both sets of thumbs should be close to each other.

Starting from the fully plantarflexed position, if the model now dorsiflexes the foot you will feel the anterior part of the body disappearing into the gap between the two malleoli. In fact, the fingers of your right hand will now be gripping the neck and head of the talus. At this point the ankle is in its close-packed position and no side-to-side movement is possible. When the model fully plantarflexes from the dorsiflexed position the head and neck of the talus will move forwards and downwards and the anterior section of the body will reappear from within the mortice. At this point the head and neck of the talus can be rocked from side to side. This is an accessory movement.

Medial. With the ankle returned to the mid position, adopt the same position with your hands but now move the fingers of your right hand to just below the tip of the medial malleolus. Here you will find the horizontal rim of the sustentaculum tali. If the model now rhythmically plantar- and dorsiflexes the ankle, you will feel the sustentaculum tali moving forwards and backwards, describing a shallow arc around the medial malleolus.

Lateral. Similarly, if the left hand remains in its original position and your right thumb is placed on the two tubercles below the lateral malleolus, movement forwards and backwards around the malleolus can be observed when plantar- and dorsiflexion is performed.

Posterior. With the model and yourself in the same position, keep your left hand gripping the two malleoli, place your right hand under the heel with the fingers resting on the posterior aspect of the calcaneus either side of the tendocalcaneus. As the model moves into dorsi- and plantarflexion, the calcaneus will be observed moving forwards and backwards away and towards the posterior part of the tibia. It is worth noting that when it passes downwards it is nearly impossible to move from side to side. This is due to the anterior part of the talus moving into the mortice of the ankle joint.

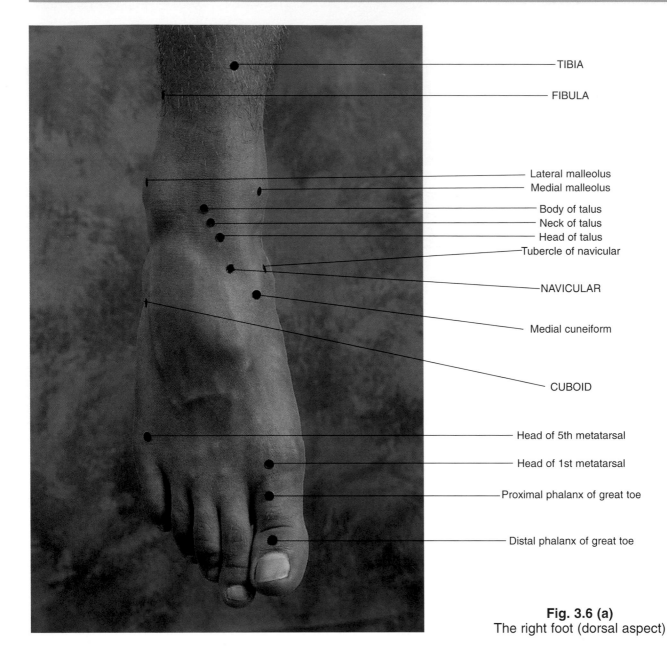

TIBIA

FIBULA

Lateral malleolus
Medial malleolus

Body of talus
Neck of talus
Head of talus
Tubercle of navicular

NAVICULAR

Medial cuneiform

CUBOID

Head of 5th metatarsal

Head of 1st metatarsal

Proximal phalanx of great toe

Distal phalanx of great toe

Fig. 3.6 (a)
The right foot (dorsal aspect)

The foot

There are three main groups of bones forming the skeleton of the foot. Posteriorly is the tarsus, comprising large irregular bones, while anteriorly are the phalanges, miniature long bones forming the toes. Between these two groups are the metatarsals, which are also miniature long bones, linking them together (Fig. 3.6).

The calcaneus forms the heel and is the largest and most posterior of the group of tarsal bones. In front and to the lateral side is the cuboid [*kubgides* (Gk) = cube shape]. Sitting on the middle section of the upper surface of the calcaneus is the body of the talus, with its neck and head passing forwards and medially, superomedially to the cuboid. The navicular lies in front of the head of the talus with the three cuneiform [*cuneus* (L) = a wedge] bones interposed between the anterior surface of the

navicular and the three medial metatarsal bones. The two lateral metatarsals lie anterior to the cuboid.

Dorsal aspect

From the medial and lateral malleoli run your index finger and thumb forwards, as before, until the head of the talus is gripped between them. The upper part of the talocalcaneonavicular joint can be palpated. The roughened dorsal surface of the navicular can be traced medially to its large tuberosity which projects downwards and medially, being approximately 2.5 cm downwards and forwards from the tip of the medial malleolus (Figs 3.5a, b, 3.6). Immediately distal to the navicular the medial cuneiform can also be palpated, projecting downwards. The dorsal surfaces of the middle and lateral cuneiforms can be

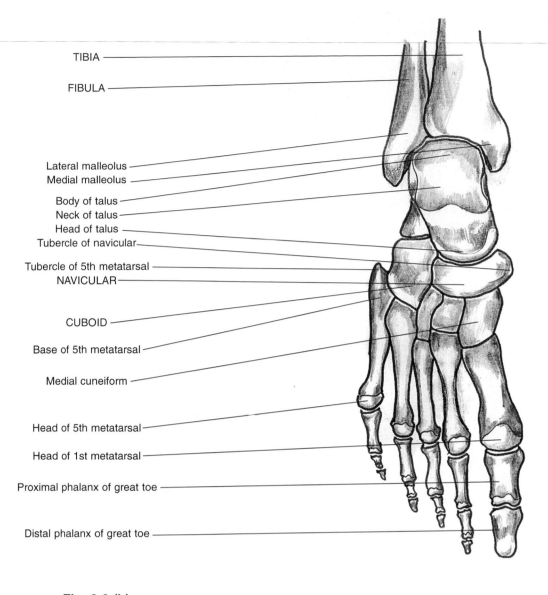

TIBIA

FIBULA

Lateral malleolus
Medial malleolus
Body of talus
Neck of talus
Head of talus
Tubercle of navicular
Tubercle of 5th metatarsal
NAVICULAR

CUBOID

Base of 5th metatarsal

Medial cuneiform

Head of 5th metatarsal

Head of 1st metatarsal

Proximal phalanx of great toe

Distal phalanx of great toe

Fig. 3.6 (b)
Bones of the right foot (dorsal
aspect)

identified on the dorsum of the foot, lying lateral to the medial cuneiform. The base, shaft and head of the first metatarsal are clearly identifiable, being much stouter than those of the other four. In some individuals the head projects medially, carrying the base of the toe with it. This causes inflammation of the bursa on its medial side, often accompanied by pain and swelling. Such medial deviation of the metatarsal head commonly progresses to a condition termed 'hallux valgus'.

Carefully running the pads of your fingers over the dorsum of the foot, the base, shaft and head of each of the remaining metatarsals can be palpated. The base of the second metatarsal is traced further proximally than the others to the middle cuneiform, the third to the lateral cuneiform and the fourth and fifth to the cuboid (Fig. 3.6). The base of the fifth metatarsal is more expanded than the rest and has,

projecting proximally, a tubercle or styloid process on its lateral side. The base is easily located by tracing backwards along the shaft of the fifth metatarsal. The large lateral projection is elongated proximally and overlies the lateral side of the cuboid.

The lateral side of the calcaneus is marked by the peroneal tubercle 1 cm below and just anterior to the tip of the lateral malleolus. This tubercle is elongated downwards and forwards and if the foot is everted, two tendons appear to pull clear. The one above the tubercle is peroneus brevis, the one below is peroneus longus. This tubercle must not be confused with that of the calcaneofibular ligament which can be found with careful palpation just below and posterior to the tip of the lateral malleolus.

- Lateral tubercle
- Medial tubercule
- CALCANEUS
- Sustentaculum tali
- Tubercle of navicular
- Medial cuneiform
- Base of 5th metatarsal
- Base of 1st metatarsal
- Head of 5th metatarsal
- Head of 1st metatarsal

Fig. 3.7 (a)
The right foot (plantar aspect)

Plantar aspect

As in the palm of the hand, very few bony points are palpable in this region due to the presence of over-lying muscles, as well as a dense and thick layer of plantar fascia, termed the 'plantar aponeurosis'.

The heel is the most posterior and inferior aspect of the **calcaneus**, on either side of which are two large broad **tubercles** (**medial** and **lateral**) which give attachment to the more superficial of the plantar muscles. On the posterior aspect of the heel there is often a horizontal raised area to which the tendo-calcaneus attaches. The tendon and its attachment are usually quite clear (see Fig. 3.22b). Below this the posterior surface of the calcaneus is covered with a pad of tough fibrous tissue and fat.

Below and in front of the tip of the lateral malleo-lus, the calcaneus is marked by an elongated tub-ercle (the peroneal tubercle), which has the tendons of peroneus brevis above and peroneus longus below.

Immediately below the tip of the medial malleo-lus, a horizontal ridge can be felt – the sustenta-culum tali – which is slightly hidden by the tendon of flexor digitorum longus. The inferior surface of

the navicular tuberosity can be palpated on the medial side of the foot 3 cm anteroinferior to the tip of the medial malleolus. On the lateral side of the foot, the base of the fifth metatarsal and its tubercle are covered by the plantar fascia and muscles. The **heads** of the metatarsals are relatively easy to find (Fig. 3.7). Those of the **first** and **fifth metatarsals** lie deep to a pad of harder skin at the broadest part of the foot on the medial and lateral side, respectively. The heads of the second, third and fourth meta-tarsals are less easy to palpate, lying on a well-formed anterior metatarsal arch; normally they can be palpated with little difficulty when the arch is flat. If the toe is grasped between the finger and thumb of one hand and passively extended, the metatarsal head can readily be felt on the plantar surface proximal to the base of the toe. If, however, the toe is flexed at the metatarsophalangeal joint, the metatarsal head appears on the dorsum of the foot, as the knuckles would in the hand.

The base of the proximal phalanx can be identi-fied just beyond the corresponding metatarsal head. The heads of the proximal phalanges, particularly

Lateral tubercle
Medial tubercule
CALCANEUS
Sustentaculum tali
Head of talus
Tubercle of navicular
Medial cuneiform
Base of 5th metatarsal
Base of 1st metatarsal
Head of 5th metatarsal
Head of 1st metatarsal

Fig. 3.7 (b)
Bones of the right foot (plantar
aspect)

those of the second, third and fourth, are often flexed and project forwards on their dorsum, being covered by hard skin and a bursa which often swells and becomes inflamed and may lead, if not corrected, to a condition known as 'hammer toes'. If the toes are extended at the proximal interphalangeal joint, the small bicondylar head can be identified (Fig. 3.7).

Palpation on movement

Take up the same position and the same hand holds as for palpation on movement, anterior aspect (page 95). If the model now plantarflexes the ankle and then moves the foot into adduction and abduction, the head of the talus can be observed moving from side to side. Remember, this will not occur in dorsiflexion due to the close-packed nature of the ankle joint.

Now move your hands down so that the head of the talus is gripped in the left hand and the right

fingers come into contact with the tubercle of the navicular and the thumb grips around the base of the fifth metatarsal. As the model everts the foot, the tubercle will descend and the metatarsal rises. As the model inverts the foot, the tubercle will rise and the metatarsal will descend. The navicular is rotating around an axis running through the neck and head of the talus.

If the hands are now moved down to the base of the great toe and the left hand grips the first metatarsal just proximal to the head and the right hand grips the proximal phalanx, when the model extends the toe, the head becomes quite clear with the phalanx moving towards the dorsum of the head. When the toe is flexed, the phalanx can be palpated moving downwards around the head. This movement can be observed in all the metatarsophalangeal joints, but to a lesser extent.

A similar movement can be felt in the interphalangeal joints with the head of the phalanx becoming quite palpable when the toes are flexed.

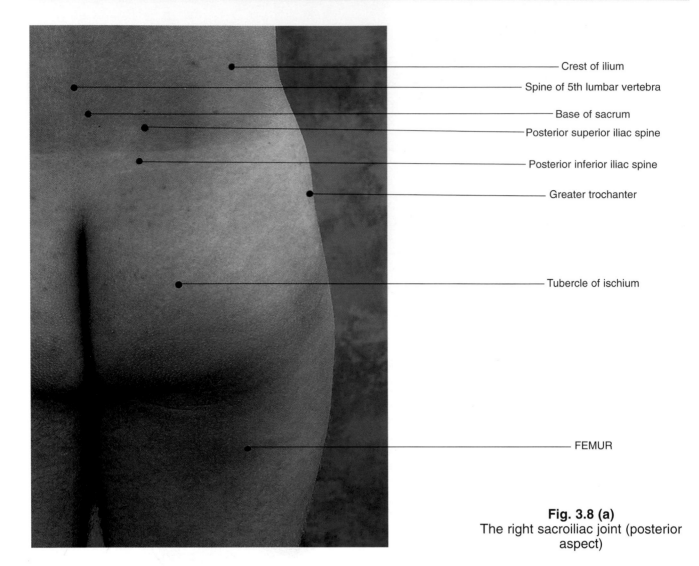

Fig. 3.8 (a)
The right sacroiliac joint (posterior aspect)

Labels:
- Crest of ilium
- Spine of 5th lumbar vertebra
- Base of sacrum
- Posterior superior iliac spine
- Posterior inferior iliac spine
- Greater trochanter
- Tubercle of ischium
- FEMUR

JOINTS

Although the joints of the lower limb are structurally similar to their counterparts in the upper limb, they tend to be more stable. Movement at the lower limb joints is more limited, with the weight transmitted across them being considerably more than in the upper limb. The sacroiliac joint and the pubic symphysis are really associated with the pelvis, but as this is the region from which the lower limb functions, they are included in this section.

The sacroiliac joint

Structure

This joint is situated deeply in the back of the pelvis and is formed by the auricular surface on the lateral side of the sacrum and the sacropelvic surface of the hip bone. It is a synovial joint surrounded by a capsule and lined with synovial membrane. The capsule is supported by anterior, posterior and interosseous ligaments and the joint is further supported by two accessory ligaments, the sacrotuberous and the sacrospinous.

Palpation and surface marking

This joint is set deeply at the back of the pelvis and is thus difficult to palpate. Nevertheless, certain landmarks can be identified, giving an accurate indication of its position (Fig. 3.8).

Find the posterior superior and inferior iliac spines, as outlined above (pages 82–83). The line of the joint can be marked by an oblique line passing downwards and medially at an angle of approximately 25° from a point 5 cm lateral to the spine of the fifth lumbar vertebra to a point just lateral to the posterior inferior iliac spine. The joint is, however, in a plane running forwards and laterally under the posterior part of the ilium, reaching as far forward as the apex of the greater sciatic notch (Fig. 3.9b).

Accessory movements

There is much controversy concerning the movements that may occur at this joint. The fact that it is a synovial joint with plane, although irregular, articular surfaces suggests that it is designed for

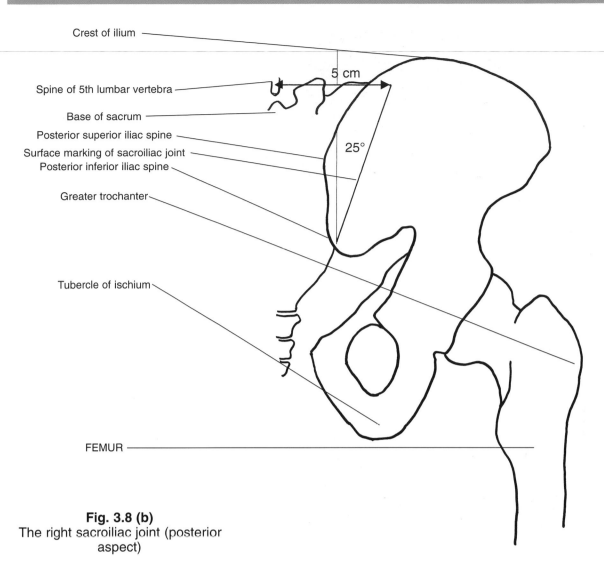

Crest of ilium

Spine of 5th lumbar vertebra

Base of sacrum

Posterior superior iliac spine

Surface marking of sacroiliac joint

Posterior inferior iliac spine

Greater trochanter

Tubercle of ischium

FEMUR

5 cm

25°

Fig. 3.8 (b)
The right sacroiliac joint (posterior aspect)

movement. However, the irregularity of the articular surface, together with the presence of extremely strong, short interosseous ligaments, means that in reality little movement is possible. In the young female, movement is often considerable, whereas in the elderly male, little or no movement is possible. The two joints on either side of the **sacrum** and the symphysis pubis anteriorly allow slight rotation and gapping movements to occur, which reduces the stresses imparted on the pelvis from the trunk and lower limbs.

Slight rotation of the sacrum forwards and backwards around a frontal axis running through its interosseous ligament may be regarded as normal physiological movement. It can, however, be aided by pressure placed alternately on the upper and lower aspects of its posterior surface, with the subject in prone lying, thereby rocking the sacrum between the ilia.

Rotation of the ilium can be enhanced by using the **femur** as a lever and localizing the movement of the joint with the other hand. With the subject lying on one side, stand behind the hip region and take the upper femur into extension; the other hand should be placed on the posterior aspect of the **iliac crest**. Considerable fixation of the rest of the pelvis can be achieved if the subject holds the alternate knee up to the chest. Flexion of the femur on the pelvis produces a backward rotation of the ilium on the sacrum, which can be enhanced by pressure applied from the front on the anterior superior iliac spine, and fixation by the subject extending the alternate lower limb.

With the subject supine, slight gapping of the posterior part of the sacroiliac joint can be achieved by rotating the pelvis and flexed lower limb to the side and applying a downward and inward pressure on the femur, towards the hip. During these movements, associated gapping and twisting occur at the pubic symphysis. For additional information consult the manipulation literature.

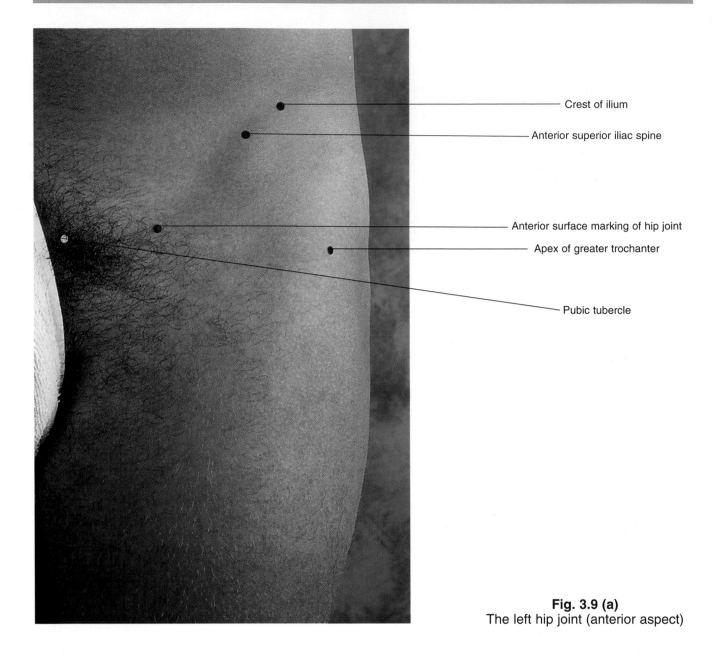

Crest of ilium

Anterior superior iliac spine

Anterior surface marking of hip joint

Apex of greater trochanter

Pubic tubercle

Fig. 3.9 (a)
The left hip joint (anterior aspect)

The hip joint [Fig. 3.9]

This is a large synovial ball-and-socket joint between the head of the femur and the acetabulum of the hip bone. It lies on the anterolateral aspect of the pelvis and affords a considerable amount of mobility to the lower limb. It is surrounded by a capsule which encloses a large part of the femoral neck, both lined with synovial membrane. The capsule is supported, externally, by the very powerful iliofemoral, ischiofemoral and pubofemoral ligaments. In addition further support is afforded internally by the ligament of the head deep inside the joint and the acetabular labrum, which attaches to the rim of the acetabulum and transverse ligament, thus surrounding the head.

Surface marking

The joint lies in the groin some 1.5 cm below the mid point of the inguinal ligament, i.e. halfway between the anterior superior iliac spine and the pubic tubercle (pages 80–81). The acetabulum extends 4 cm vertically below this point deep to the head of the femur. Midway between the upper and lower limits, i.e. at the mid point of the joint, the acetabulum extends 2 cm either side of this vertical line (Fig. 3.9).

An alternative method of establishing the centre of the hip joint can be by tracing a line horizontally and medially from the upper border of the greater trochanter to a point below the mid point of the inguinal ligament. When viewed posteriorly, the hip joint centre lies 5 cm above and 3 cm lateral to the ischial tuberosity.

Palpation

Palpation of the joint from any aspect is, however, virtually impossible as it is covered by thick muscle crossing the joint, particularly posteriorly and laterally. Only if the hip is fully extended can movement

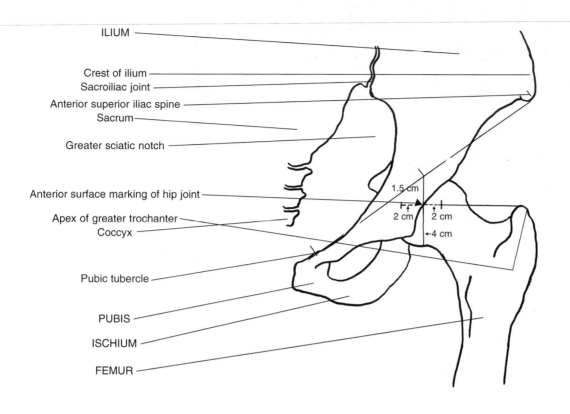

ILIUM

Crest of ilium
Sacroiliac joint
Anterior superior iliac spine
Sacrum
Greater sciatic notch

Anterior surface marking of hip joint
Apex of greater trochanter
Coccyx

Pubic tubercle

PUBIS

ISCHIUM

FEMUR

1.5 cm
2 cm   2 cm
←4 cm

Fig. 3.9 (b)
Bones of the left hip joint (anterior
aspect)

be detected and then only anteriorly. If the fingers are placed on the anterior surface marking of the joint, with the subject standing, and the limb is then taken into approximately 15° of extension, the head of the femur can be palpated projecting forwards under the anterior covering of muscles (iliopsoas and pectineus).

Accessory movements

There is very little accessory movement at this joint. With the subject lying supine and the hip flexed approximately 30°, slight parting of the articular surfaces is possible. This is produced by applying strong traction to the femur.

Movements of flexion, extension and rotation of the hip, however, with the hands carefully controlling the movement from the lower end of the femur,

can be a source of important information for the palpator. Quality and range of movement can be assessed and areas of 'grinding' and limitation can be located. Linked with the patient's symptoms and reactions, a much clearer picture of the problems involved can be visualized.

Combining the three components of movement, i.e. flexion/extension, abduction/adduction and medial/lateral rotation, can test the joint movement and function to extremes. Testing in these confined movements is often referred to as the 'quadrants' and for further information concerning these manoeuvres the manipulation and mobilization literature should be consulted (Maitland, 1991). Fixation of proximal and distal joints in testing of the hip joint is essential, as compensatory movement is common in this area and can lead to incorrect diagnosis.

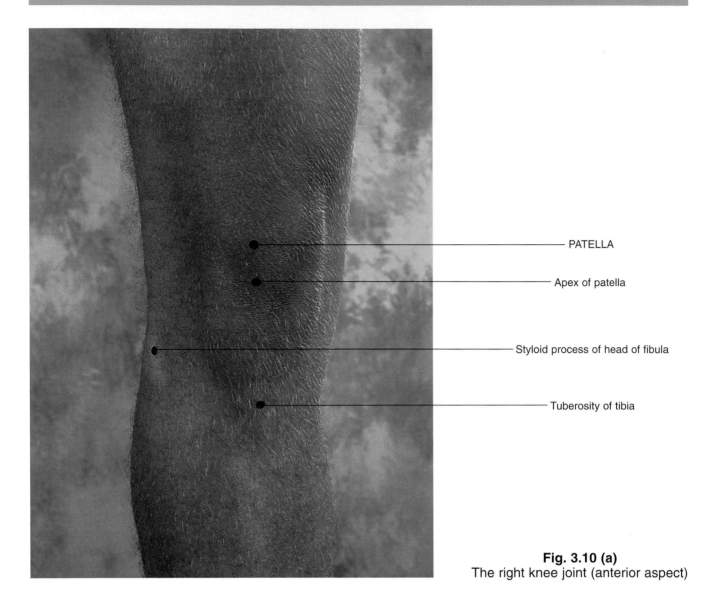

PATELLA

Apex of patella

Styloid process of head of fibula

Tuberosity of tibia

Fig. 3.10 (a)
The right knee joint (anterior aspect)

The knee joint [Fig. 3.10]

The knee joint is a synovial composite joint comprising the bicondylar section between the condyles of femur and tibia and the plane joint between the patella and the patellar surface of the femur. The joint functions as a modified hinge, with the main movements being flexion and extension. Rotation can be produced in the semiflexed position and in the final few degrees of full extension.

It is the largest joint in the human body and perhaps the most complex (see *Anatomy and Human Movement*, Palastanga *et al.*, 1998).

The articular surfaces are covered with articular cartilage, but are not congruent. Those on the femur cover the superior, posterior, inferior and anterior surfaces of the large condyles, coming together anteriorly to form a triangular surface which is narrow at the top and is called the patellar surface. The articular surfaces of the tibia only cover the central section of the upper surface; its outer sections are covered by two crescentic-shaped menisci.

The joint is supported on its posterior, lateral and medial side by a fibrous capsule. Anteriorly the capsule is formed by the lower section of the quadriceps femoris, the patella and the ligamentum patellae. The joint is lined by an extensive and complex synovial membrane and is supported by numerous ligaments, including the oblique popliteal, the tibial collateral, the fibula collateral externally and the anterior and posterior cruciate ligaments internally. It also relies heavily on the powerful surrounding muscles for its stability.

Anterior to the condylar section is the patellofemoral joint between the posterior surface of the patella and the patellar surface of the femur. This is a synovial plane joint, separate from the knee although it shares the same joint space and synovial membrane.

The knee joint appears at first sight to be a very unstable joint with the two rounded condyles of the femur sitting on top of the two flattened surfaces of the tibia. This, however, is not so. This joint rarely dislocates and even then only under extreme force, such as a car or aeroplane crash. It is, however, subject to many stresses and strains, particularly in sport.

Fig. 3.10 (b)
The right knee joint (anterior aspect)

Surface marking

The joint lies on a line which bisects the ligamentum patellae horizontally (Fig. 3.10b,d), halfway between the lower tip of the patella and the tibial tuberosity. An alternative method of marking the joint is by drawing a line horizontally 1 cm above the tip of the styloid process of the fibula.

Palpation

With the fingers either side of the ligamentum patellae, two triangular depressions can be felt. These are bounded by the tibia below, the femur above and the ligamentum patellae centrally. At the apex of the depression, running horizontally, is the knee joint space; your fingers are now resting against the ante-

rior aspect of the medial and lateral menisci. These can be observed moving forwards during rotation at the joint, the lateral meniscus on lateral rotation and the medial on medial rotation. Tracing the joint posteriorly, the space becomes narrower until just behind the mid point it becomes hidden by the medial collateral ligament medially and the lateral part of the joint capsule laterally. Posteriorly the joint is impossible to palpate due to the presence of muscle, tendon and fascial coverings, although the joint can be represented by a horizontal line drawn across the back of the popliteal fossa 1 cm above the tip of the styloid process of the head of the fibula (Fig. 3.10f).

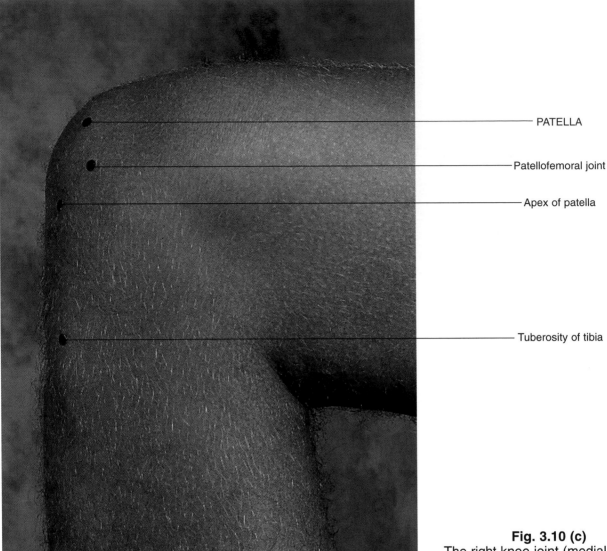

PATELLA

Patellofemoral joint

Apex of patella

Tuberosity of tibia

Fig. 3.10 (c)
The right knee joint (medial aspect)

Accessory movements

The knee joint becomes 'close packed' on full extension; therefore, accessory movements should only be performed avoiding the extreme of extension. With the subject lying supine, the knee flexed to 90° and the foot firmly fixed on the supporting surface (often achieved by the investigator sitting on the foot), the tibial condyles can be drawn forwards (anterior draw test), and pushed backwards, producing a gliding of the tibial condyles against the femoral condyles. There should be only a slight movement in either direction, forward movement of the tibia being limited by the anterior cruciate ligament and posterior movement being limited by the posterior cruciate ligament.

With the subject again lying supine with the knee flexed 15°, stabilize the under surface of the thigh with one hand and grasp the lower end of the leg just above the ankle with the other. A side-to-side movement can be produced. Distraction of the joint can also be achieved by pulling on the leg in the mid position, with the subject seated on a high plinth with the foot clear of the floor.

The **patellofemoral joint** lies deep to the **patella**, between it and the patellar surface of the femur, 1 cm deep to its anterior surface (Fig. 3.10c, d), sharing the same joint space as the bicondylar articulation. It is easily marked by tracing around the perimeter of bone. When the knee is in an extended and relaxed position, the patella can be moved from side to side across the patellar surface of the femur, resulting in a knocking effect. It can also be moved up and down as a gliding movement along the vertical groove of the femoral surface.

With the patella moved laterally, the medial edge of the patellar surface of the femur can be palpated, marked by a sharp ridge. In this position, the under surface of the lateral edge of the patella can also be palpated. Conversely, if the patella is moved medially, the lateral edge of the patellar surface of the femur and the medial under surface of the patella also become palpable.

PATELLA

Patellofemoral joint

Apex of patella

Line of knee joint

Equidistant

Tuberosity of tibia

1 cm

Fig. 3.10 (d)
The right knee joint (medial aspect)

Functional anatomy

Little stress is applied to the structural components of the knee joint, on which it relies for its stability during normal activities, such as walking, running, jumping, swimming, etc. However, enormous tension is applied to these components during sporting activities where the lower limbs are used for varied directional propulsion and kicking. Lateral or medial forces applied to the knee, particularly when the knee is in its extended 'close-packed' position may cause strains, partial tears or even complete ruptures to medial or lateral ligaments. Violent over-extension of the knee may rupture the anterior cruciate ligament, and the posterior cruciate ligament may rupture when enormous force is applied to the anterior aspect of the proximal end of the tibia. When the knee is over-rotated in a flexed position the menisci, especially the medial, sometimes get trapped between the rolling condyle of the femur on the tibia, producing a tear in the meniscus.

In addition to all the ligamentous problems, the very powerful muscle surrounding the joint, on which stability is also dependent, may be partially torn or even completely ruptured. On a violent extension force such as kicking a stationary object, or falling from a height on to the feet, the quadriceps femoris tendon may rupture causing complete dysfunction of the joint.

When one considers all the fractures that may occur through direct or indirect violence to the bones of the joint and the degeneration due to age and all the stresses applied by virtually the whole body weight being transferred through the joint during movement, it is hardly surprising that the knee joints are a source of much pain and suffering, for many, in their senior years.

(For detailed study of structure, stability, function, dysfunction, remedies, etc., see *Anatomy and Human Movement*, Palastanga *et al.*, 1998.)

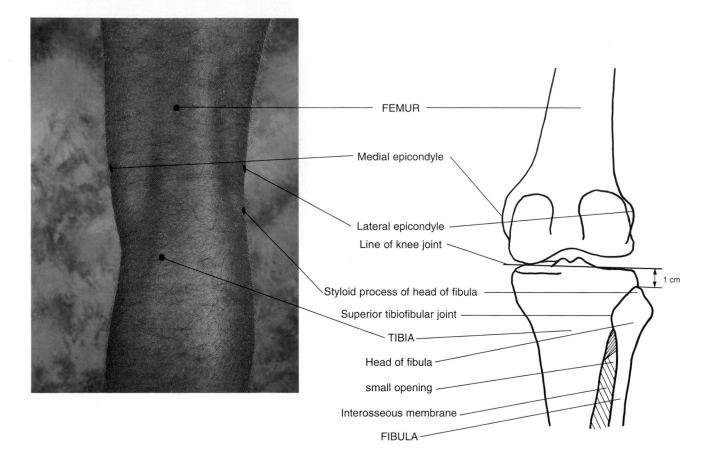

Fig. 3.10 (e), (f)
The right knee joint (posterior aspect)

The tibiofibular union

The tibia and fibula are joined together by two joints, the superior tibiofibular joint and the inferior tibiofibular joint, and an interosseous membrane. They unite the bones so tightly that very little movement occurs between the two. The interosseous membrane is composed of strong fibrous tissue with its fibres passing downwards and laterally. There is a small opening above (see Fig. 3.10f), with an additional group of fibres passing in the opposite direction just below the superior tibiofibular joint.

The superior tibiofibular joint

This is a synovial joint, with its surfaces covered with articular cartilage and it is surrounded by a capsule lined with synovial membrane. The capsule is supported by the anterior and posterior tibiofibular ligaments.

Surface marking

This joint can be represented, both anteriorly and posteriorly, by a line 1.5 cm in length running downwards and slightly medially just medial to the head of the fibula (Fig. 3.11a,b).

Palpation

With the model in supine lying and the knee straight, stand on the right side just below the level of the knee. Place the index finger of your left hand on the styloid process of the head of the fibula. From that point your thumb can trace downwards and medially along the anterior aspect of the joint. Your middle finger is just behind the joint, and similarly to the thumb, can trace downwards and medially along the posterior joint line. This is a little more difficult to palpate as it is covered by the lateral head of gastrocnemius.

Accessory movements

Although the head of the fibula can be felt gliding up and down during dorsiflexion and plantar flexion of the ankle joint, accessory movement between the two bones is virtually impossible. With the subject lying supine and the ankle joint plantar flexed, direct pressure, applied by the thumb, on the head of the fibula can produce a slight backward gliding. Forward gliding can be achieved using the same technique but with the subject lying prone. Extreme care must be taken, when performing this procedure, to avoid the common peroneal nerve as it winds around the neck of the fibula.

Medial condyle of tibia
Intercondylar eminence
Lateral condyle of tibia
Head of fibula
1.5 cm
Superior tibiofibular joint
Interosseous membrane
FIBULA
TIBIA
Inferior tibiofibular joint
2.5 cm
Medial malleolus
Lateral malleolus

Anterior view | Posterior view

Fig. 3.11 (a), (b)
The superior and inferior tibiofibular joints and union of the left side

The inferior tibiofibular joint

This joint is a fibrous syndesmosis [*syndesmos* (Gk) = a band] between the lower lateral rough triangular surface on the tibia and a similar surface on the lower medial side of the fibula. The surfaces are bound together by a very strong interosseous ligament which is a continuation downwards of the interosseous membrane. The joint is further supported by an anterior, posterior and transverse tibiofibular ligament, the latter forming part of the socket of the ankle joint.

Surface marking

This joint can be represented by a vertical line 2.5 cm long running superiorly from the line of the ankle joint (see page 110) on the medial side of the lateral malleolus

Palpation

Again it is difficult to palpate, except for its upper edge, as it is mostly covered by the superior extensor retinaculum and extensor digitorum longus tendons. Posteriorly, little can be palpated owing to the presence of the tendocalcaneus.

Accessory movements

Accessory movement of the inferior tibiofibular joint is not possible, except when diastasis (a parting of the inferior tibiofibular joint) has occurred. It is unwise to increase the unwanted movement in this injury, as this leads to even further instability of the ankle joint.

The fibrous interosseous ligament between the two bones holds the two bones together and is referred to by some as a fibrous syndesmosis.

Lateral malleolus

Tip of lateral malleolus
Tip of medial malleolus

Neck of talus

Head of talus

Fig. 3.12 (a)
The right ankle joint (anterior aspect)

The ankle joint [Fig. 3.12]

The ankle joint is a synovial hinge joint involving the distal ends of the **tibia** and **fibula** proximally and the **body of the talus** distally. The weight-bearing surfaces are the trochlear surfaces of the tibia and talus. The stabilizing surfaces are those of the **medial** and **lateral malleoli**, which grip the body of the talus. The articular surfaces are composed of, above, the inferior surface of the tibia, the medial surface of the lateral malleolus and lateral surface of the medial malleolus, and, below, the superior, lateral and upper part of the medial surface of the talus. The surfaces are covered with articular cartilage. The joint is surrounded by a capsule lined with synovial membrane and is supported by very powerful lateral and medial (deltoid) ligaments. These two ligaments are delta-shaped, being narrower above and broader below. Above they are attached to the anterior and posterior borders, tip and fossae of each

malleolus. Below, the medial attaches to the navicular, calcaneonavicular 'spring' ligament, sustentaculum tali and medial tubercle of talus, with a deep section attaching to the medial surface of the talus. The lateral has three portions, the anterior and posterior attaching to the talus and the middle portion to the calcaneus. The transverse tibiofibular ligament which passes across the posterior of the ankle joint, forming part of its socket, attaches to both malleoli and the lower border of the tibia.

A horizontal line drawn across the anterior surface of the ankle 2 cm above the tip of the medial and 3 cm above that of the lateral malleolus marks the superior limit of the joint. It is continued down the medial side of the lateral malleolus and the lateral side of the medial malleolus to their tips which completes the joint line (Fig. 3.12b, d, f).

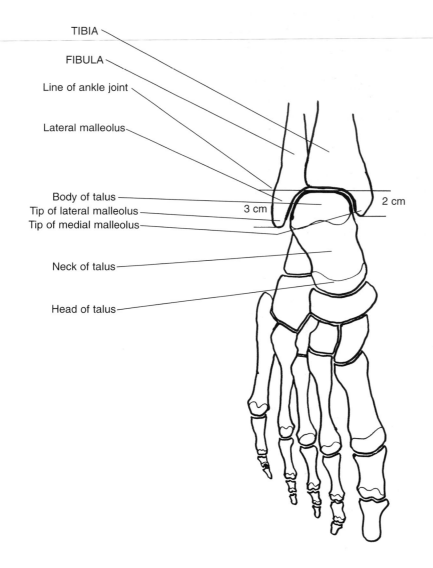

TIBIA

FIBULA

Line of ankle joint

Lateral malleolus

Body of talus

Tip of lateral malleolus

Tip of medial malleolus

3 cm   2 cm

Neck of talus

Head of talus

Fig. 3.12 (b)
The right ankle joint (anterior aspect)

Palpation

Careful palpation between the extensor tendons in the region of the horizontal part of the joint line reveals the lower border of the tibia. Medially the joint line can be traced on to the anterior border of the medial malleolus and down to the tip. It can be traced up the posterior border of the medial malleolus, above the malleolar fossa where the joint line is hidden by tissue which lies between the tendo calcaneus and the joint. Laterally the joint line can be palpated between the talus and lateral malleolus anteriorly, and can be traced down to the tip of the malleolus. As on the medial side, its posterior border can be traced upwards above the malleolar fossa until it too is lost under similar fascia. With the ankle plantarflexed, the body of the talus, i.e. its upper, lateral and medial surfaces, can be felt gliding forwards (Fig. 3.12c, d). Posteriorly the joint is hidden by tendons and fascia.

Accessory movements

The ankle joint allows the movements of dorsiflexion and plantarflexion. Side-to-side movement is limited by the presence of the two malleoli, there being no movement possible when the joint is dorsiflexed and 'close packed' as the body is gripped between the two malleoli. However, when the joint is plantarflexed, by gripping the foot with one hand and stabilizing the leg with the other, the narrower part of the body of the talus can be moved from side to side, as well as forwards and backwards.

Commonly the lateral (and less frequently the medial) malleolus is fractured by a lateromedial or mediolateral force. Unless the malleolus is replaced exactly, the talus is able to move sideways and the joint becomes less stable. The same mechanical problem will occur if the two bones are parted at the inferior tibiofibular joint (diastasis – see page 109).

Fig. 3.12 (c)
The right ankle joint (medial aspect)

TIBIA

Tip of medial malleolus

Head of talus

Tubercle of navicular

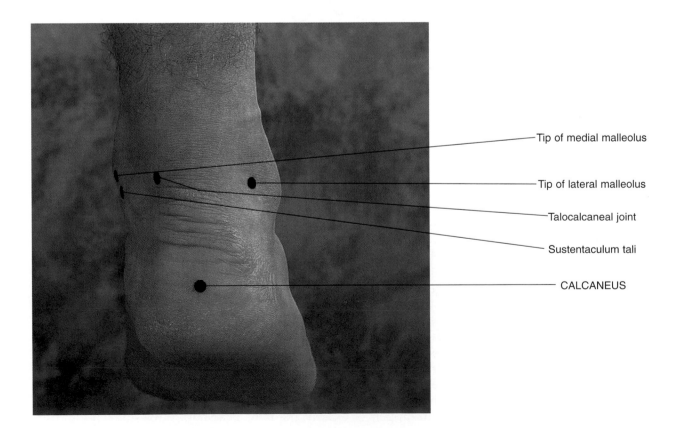

Fig. 3.12 (e)
The right ankle joint (posterior aspect)

Tip of medial malleolus

Tip of lateral malleolus

Talocalcaneal joint

Sustentaculum tali

CALCANEUS

TIBIA

Line of ankle joint
Tip of medial malleolus

2 cm

Head of talus

Tubercle of navicular

Medial cuneiform

1st metatarsal

CALCANEUS

Fig. 3.12 (d)
The right ankle joint (medial aspect)

FIBULA

TIBIA

TALUS

Line of ankle joint

Tip of medial malleolus

Tip of lateral malleolus

2 cm

3 cm

Talocalcaneal joint

Sustentaculum tali

CALCANEUS

Fig. 3.12 (f)
The right ankle joint (posterior aspect)

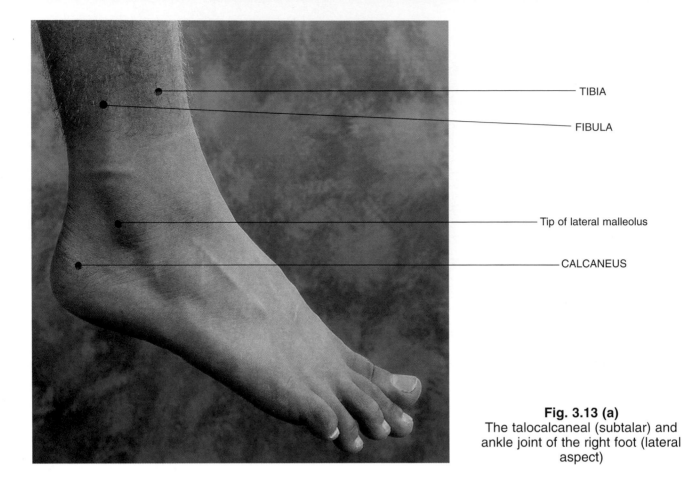

TIBIA

FIBULA

Tip of lateral malleolus

CALCANEUS

Fig. 3.13 (a)
The talocalcaneal (subtalar) and
ankle joint of the right foot (lateral
aspect)

The foot

The joints of the foot are divided into those between the tarsal bones (the intertarsal joints) and the tarsal and metatarsal bones (the tarsometatarsal joints); between the metatarsal bases (the intermetatarsal joints); between the metatarsals and phalanges (the metatarsophalangeal joints) and those between the phalanges (the interphalangeal joints). Most of the joints are readily identifiable on the dorsum of the foot as they are only covered by thin fascia and the tendons of the long extensor muscles, whereas the plantar aspect of the foot is covered by numerous intrinsic muscles, in four layers, and very thick layers (up to 80) of plantar fascia.

The talocalcaneal (subtalar) joint [Fig. 3.13]

The talocalcaneal joint lies below the talus and is often referred to as the subtalar joint. The joint surfaces taking part in this joint are the inferior surface of the talus and the middle section of the superior surface of the calcaneus. Both surfaces are covered with articular cartilage and the joint is surrounded by a fibrous capsule lined with synovial membrane. The capsule is supported by medial, posterior, lateral and interosseous ligament. The interosseous ligament lies anterior to the joint and separates it from the talocalcaneonavicular joint. There is also a short ligament which joins the neck of the talus to the sustentaculum tali at the lateral end of the sinus tarsi.

Surface marking

The joint is marked by a line running horizontally 1 cm below the tip of the lateral malleolus on the

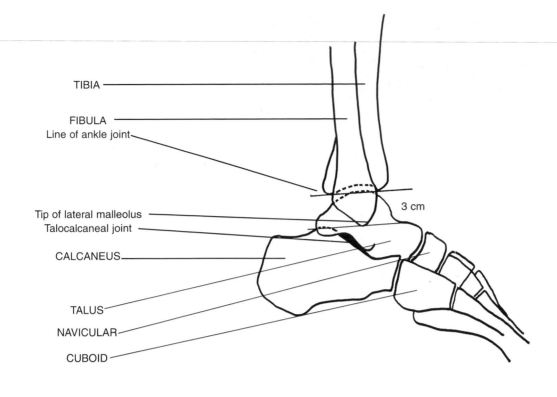

Fig. 3.13 (b)
The talocalcaneal (subtalar) and
ankle joint of the right foot (lateral
aspect)

lateral side to a point 1.5 cm below the tip of the
medial malleolus on the medial side (Fig. 3.13b).

Palpation

This is a very difficult joint to palpate due to the fact
that the medial and lateral malleoli and the powerful ligaments tend to hide the joint. Find the tip of
the lateral malleolus and move forward into the hollow. Below your finger you will feel the sharp edge
of the upper border of the **calcaneus**. This is the
anterior part of the lateral side of the joint.

On the medial side find the tip of the **medial
malleolus**. Move down 2 cm and you will be able to
palpate a horizontal ridge. This is the medial edge of
the **sustentaculum tali** and its upper border is the
lower boundary of the subtalar joint.

Accessory movement

With the model in supine lying, stand to the lateral
side of the right foot (similar to the position adopted
for accessory movements of the ankle joint). With
your left hand grip the neck of the talus with your
finger on the medial side and thumb laterally. With
your right hand fit the model's heel into your palm
with your fingers wrapping around the back of the
calcaneus. The calcaneus can now be made to glide
very slightly backwards and forwards. The calcaneus can also be rocked from side to side producing a slight gapping of the lateral and medial side of
the joint alternately.

Tip of medial malleolus

Talocalcaneal joint

Sustentaculum tali

Head of talus

Tubercle of navicular

Fig. 3.13 (c)
The right talocalcaneal (subtalar)
joint (medial aspect)

TIBIA

FIBULA

Medial malleolus

TALUS

Talocalcaneal joint

Sustentaculum tali

CALCANEUS

3 cm

1 cm

Fig. 3.13 (e), (f)
The talocalcaneal (subtalar) joint (posterior aspect)

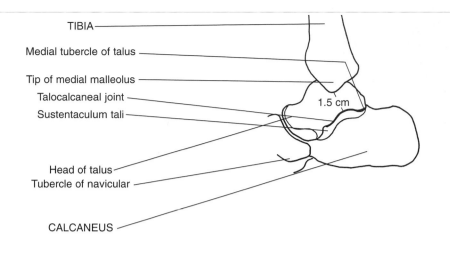

TIBIA
Medial tubercle of talus
Tip of medial malleolus
Talocalcaneal joint
Sustentaculum tali
1.5 cm
Head of talus
Tubercle of navicular
CALCANEUS

Fig. 3.13 (d)
The right talocalcaneal (subtalar)
joint (medial aspect)

TIBIA
FIBULA
Tip of lateral malleolus
Head of talus
CALCANEUS
Talocalcaneal
(subtalar joint)

Fig. 3.13 (g), (h)
The talocalcaneal (subtalar) joint of the right foot (lateral aspect)

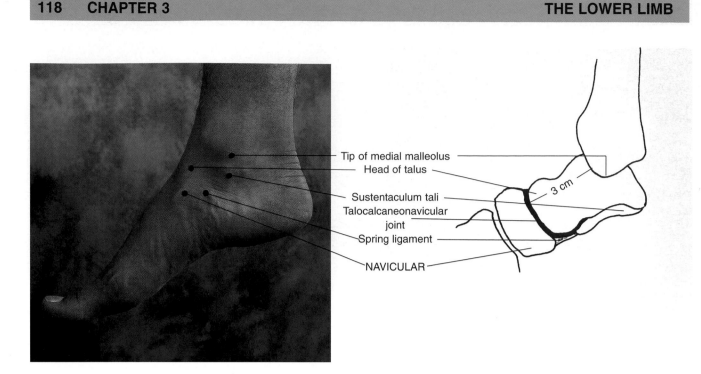

Fig. 3.14 (a), (b)
The talocalcaneonavicular joint of right foot (medial aspect)

The talocalcaneonavicular joint [Fig. 3.14a–d]

This is a synovial, modified ball-and-socket joint between the **head of the talus** and a socket comprising the posterior surface of **navicular**, the superior surface of the **sustentaculum tali** of the calcaneus and the 'spring' ligament which joins the two (Fig. 3.14). It is surrounded by a capsule lined with synovial membrane and is supported by the talonavicular ligament dorsally, the medial band of the bifurcate ('Y'-shaped) ligament laterally, the tibionavicular part of the deltoid ligament medially and posteroinferiorly, under the neck, by the anterior section of the interosseous ligament in the sinus tarsi. The plantar calcaneonavicular (spring) ligament is a fibroelastic ligament forming part of the socket and lies below the head of the talus, having articular cartilage on its superior surface.

Surface marking

The surface marking of the joint can be represented by a line, convex distally, drawn transversely across the medial half of the dorsum of the foot at the level of the tubercle of the navicular.

As with nearly all the joints in the foot, palpation and identification is only possible on the dorsum. The plantar aspect is hidden deep to many layers of the plantar fascia, many short but powerful muscles and strong, dense ligaments.

— Tip of lateral malleolus
— Head of talus
—Talocalcaneonavicular joint
— NAVICULAR
— Calcaneocuboid joint
— CUBOID

2 cm

Fig. 3.14 (c), (d)
The talocalcaneonavicular and calcaneocuboid joints of right foot (lateral aspect)

Palpation

The tubercle of the navicular is situated 2.5 cm anteroinferior to the tip of the medial malleolus and is clearly palpable. As it projects slightly backwards, it is in line with the joint. The head of the talus can be traced down the proximal side of the tubercle to a small gap underneath, housing the 'spring' ligament. Posterior to the gap, the anterior section of the sustentaculum tali is palpable. If the foot is held in slight plantarflexion and the muscles relaxed, the joint can be traced across the dorsum of the foot almost to the mid point where the head of the talus and the navicular dip towards the bifurcate ligament. The tendons of tibialis anterior and extensor hallucis longus may have to be moved to the side to follow the line clearly.

Accessory movements

Stand lateral to the foot. With your proximal hand, stabilize the talus from the medial side with your fingers on the plantar and thumb on the dorsal aspect. With your distal hand, grasp the forefoot as far backwards as the navicular, again with your fingers on the plantar and thumb on the dorsal aspect. Slight up-and-down gliding can be obtained of the navicular on the head of the talus. Rotation of the forefoot on the head of the talus is also possible, but this is of course movement normally occurring during inversion and eversion.

Fig. 3.14 (e), (f)
The talocalcaneonavicular and calcaneocuboid joint of right foot (plantar aspect)

The calcaneocuboid joint

This is a synovial, plane joint between the quadrilateral anterior surface of the calcaneus and the posterior surface of the cuboid. Both surfaces are covered with articular cartilage and the joint is surrounded by a capsule, lined with synovial membrane and supported by the lateral portion of the bifurcate ligament medially, by the dorsal calcaneocuboid ligament and by the plantar calcaneocuboid and long plantar ligaments.

Surface marking

The line of the joint is just proximal to the tubercle of the fifth metatarsal bone on the lateral and dorsal aspect of the base of the foot. It is slightly concave forwards.

Palpation

This joint is difficult to identify, although certain landmarks can be palpated. From the tip of the tubercle of the fifth metatarsal move dorsally 2 cm. Just proximal to your finger you will feel the ant-erior border of the superior surface of the calcaneus. This is 2 cm anterior to the tip of the lateral malleolus. The border can be traced medially until it dips towards the bifurcate ligament, and laterally to the anterior border of the lateral surface almost down to the tubercle.

Accessory movement

This plane synovial joint allows slight upward movement during eversion and slight downward movement during inversion accompanying the rotation of the navicular on the head of the talus. This movement is physiological and its loss would severely interfere with the functional movement of the foot. With the model in supine lying, stand to the right of the right foot. Stabilize the talus and calcaneus by gripping below the two malleoli with the fingers on the inside. With the right hand, grasp the cuboid with the thumb on the dorsum and the index and middle fingers underneath. Now move the cuboid up and down. Note, only slight movement will be present.

Ankle joint

Medial malleolus

Tip of lateral malleolus

CALCANEUS

Line of calcaneocuboid joint

Talocalcaneonavicular joint

Tubercle of navicular

Cuboideonavicular joint

Styloid process of 5th metatarsal

1 cm

Fig. 3.14 (g), (h)
The midtarsal joint of the right foot (dorsal aspect)

The cuboideonavicular joint [Fig. 3.14h]

This joint between the navicular and the cuboid is normally a syndesmosis. The articular surfaces are joined entirely by a strong fibrous interosseous ligament and this is further supported by dorsal and plantar ligaments. Sometimes it is replaced by a small synovial joint which is surrounded by a capsule, lined by synovial membrane and supported by dorsal and plantar ligaments.

Surface marking

The joint is marked by a line 1 cm long running from back to front, 1 cm forward and 1 cm lateral to the lateral side of the head of the talus.

Palpation

The joint is impossible to palpate.

Accessory movements

As in all syndesmoses, there is usually a very minimal amount of movement, and as this restriction of movement is its function there is little point in trying to move the joint.

The midtarsal joint [Fig. 3.14g and h]

This is a composite articulation of the talocalcaneonavicular joint medially and the calcaneocuboid joint laterally. The two proximal bones are firmly united by the interosseous ligament in the sinus tarsi and the two distal bones are firmly united by the cuboideonavicular syndesmosis. The two joints are therefore considered to move as one unit, particularly in inversion and eversion of the foot.

Surface marking

The joint line can be marked across the dorsum of the foot by a line from just proximal to the tuberosity of the navicular medially to a point 1 cm proximal to the tip of the tubercle of the fifth metatarsal laterally (Fig. 3.14g, h).

Palpation

As in the separate joints above.

Accessory movements

As in the separate joints above.

Fig. 3.14 (i), (j)
The cuneonavicular and cuneometatarsal joints of right foot (medial aspect)

The cuneonavicular and intercuneiform joints [Figs 3.14i,j and 3.15c,d]

The three cuneiform bones articulate proximally with the distal surface of the navicular by plane synovial joints. They are surrounded by a common capsule which is lined by synovial membrane and is supported by relatively weak dorsal and stronger plantar ligaments. The cuneiform bones are also bound together distally by interosseous ligaments.

Palpation

The cunceonavicular joint can be palpated on its medial and dorsal aspects just distal to the navicular tuberosity and, with care, can be traced across the foot between the extensor tendons, being slightly concave proximally (Fig. 3.14i, j).

The joints between the cuneiforms themselves, and between the lateral cuneiform and the cuboid, are extremely difficult to palpate, although the joint lines can be determined by following proximally from the first, second and third metatarsal bones (Fig. 3.15a, b).

Accessory movements

The joints between the navicular and the cuneiforms, as well as those between the cuneiforms themselves, are all plane synovial joints but as they also possess interosseous ligaments which bind the adjacent surfaces together, they possess very little movement. They can be moved passively by stabilizing the most proximal component with the fingers and thumb of one hand and gliding the distal component up and down with the other hand, the grip being similar to that used on the talocalcaneonavicular joint. Although only slight gliding is present at these joints, loss of this movement can lead to complete dysfunction of the foot.

The cuneocuboid joint is synovial but is also tightly bound together by an interosseous ligament, becoming, in part, a syndesmosis. Consequently, passive accessory movement between the two bones is virtually impossible.

Fig. 3.15 (a), (b)
The cuneonavicular and cuneometatarsal joints of the right foot (lateral aspect)

The tarsometatarsal joints

The **tarsometatarsal joints** exist between the bases of the metatarsals and the cuneiform and cuboid bones. The first metatarsal articulates with the medial cuneiform bone, the second fits in between the medial and lateral cuneiforms with its base articulating with the middle, shorter, cuneiform, and the third metatarsal articulates with the lateral cuneiform. The fourth and fifth articulate with the cuboid. They are all plane synovial joints surrounded by a capsule which is lined with synovial membrane and supported by dorsal and plantar tarsometatarsal ligaments. There are also two or possibly three interosseous ligaments, two to the base of the second metatarsal as it fits into this mortice and the other between the lateral cuneiform to the fourth metatarsal.

Palpation and surface marking

The joint between the first metatarsal and the medial cuneiform can be palpated 2 cm distal to the navicular tuberosity. It can also be identified by following the first metatarsal proximally to where its base is marked by an expanded area. This line can be traced on to the dorsum of the foot, being crossed here by the tendon of extensor hallucis longus (Fig. 3.14i, j).

The joint between the second metatarsal and the middle cuneiform is extremely difficult to palpate as it is set more proximally between the medial and lateral cuneiforms. That between the third metatarsal and the lateral cuneiform, however, can be identified by following the line of the metatarsal to its base, which is slightly raised.

The same procedure will enable the joints between the fourth and fifth metatarsals and the cuboid to be identified. Its surface is marked by a line running laterally and proximally towards the tip of the tubercle on the fifth metatarsal (Figs 3.15a, b and 3.17a, b).

Accessory movements

With the model in supine lying, stand to the right of the right foot. With the cleft between your thumb and fingers of your left hand gripping the cuneiform bones and your right hand gripping the first metatarsal, movements up and down and even a little rotation can be obtained. There is a little movement obtained at these joints when the metatarsals are moved on each other (see Intermetatarsal joints, page 124).

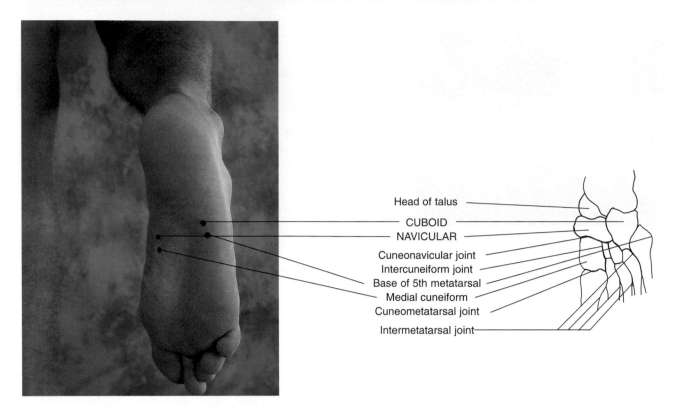

Head of talus
CUBOID
NAVICULAR
Cuneonavicular joint
Intercuneiform joint
Base of 5th metatarsal
Medial cuneiform
Cuneometatarsal joint
Intermetatarsal joint

Fig. 3.15 (c), (d)
Joints of cuneiform bones and metatarsals of right foot, plantar aspect (not palpable)

The intermetatarsal joints [Fig. 3.15c–f]

These are four small synovial joints between the adjacent sides of the bases of the second to fifth metatarsal. They are surrounded by a capsule lined with synovial membrane and their joint space is continuous with that of the tarsometatarsal joints. The capsule is supported by a dorsal and plantar ligament and an interosseous ligament at its distal end. The base of the first metatarsal is connected to the base of the second by an interosseous ligament only.

Surface marking

From a line drawn across the dorsum of the foot from the base of the first metatarsal to the tubercle on the base of the fifth, the joints pass distally for 0.5 cm in line with the spaces between the second to fifth metatarsal.

Palpation

If a finger is placed between the metatarsals on the dorsum of the foot and drawn proximally, the space between them gradually narrows, with the bones eventually coming into contact with each other. These small plane joints run anteroposteriorly for approximately 0.5 cm, as far proximally as the line drawn across the dorsum of the foot from the base of the first metatarsal and the tubercle on the lateral side of the base of the fifth. That between the second and third metatarsals is slightly smaller due to the arrangement of the cuneiforms (Fig. 3.15e, f).

The interosseous ligament between the first and second metatarsals can be marked in a similar fashion.

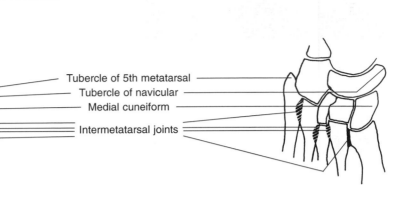

Tubercle of 5th metatarsal
Tubercle of navicular
Medial cuneiform
Intermetatarsal joints

Fig. 3.15 (e), (f)
The intermetatarsal joints of right foot (dorsal aspect)

Accessory movements

Movement between the metatarsal bases and either the cuneiforms or the cuboid is virtually non-existent. Only slight movements can be produced, even when the metatarsals are used as levers. Obviously this also results in a slight gliding movement at the intermetatarsal joints. With the subject lying supine, grip one metatarsal head between the fingers and thumb of one hand and the adjacent head with the other hand, both thumbs being on the dorsum of the foot. Downward pressure on one metatarsal head, and upward pressure on the other, results in a small degree of movement. This small movement between the heads creates an even smaller, but definite, movement between the bases. If the lateral metatarsal head is taken in one hand and the metatarsal of the great toe is taken in the other, a considerable forward and backward movement is achieved due to combined movement of all metatarsal bases.

Although there is no contact between the two metatarsal heads, they are joined to each other by the powerful deep transverse metatarsal ligament. Occasionally this may become shortened; movement of one metatarsal head against its neighbour will help to mobilize this region.

Fig. 3.16 (a), (b)
The metatarsophalangeal and interphalangeal joints of the right foot (dorsal aspect)

The metatarsophalangeal joints [Figs 3.16 and 3.17]

These joints exist between the smooth, rounded heads of the metatarsal bones and the shallow cavity on the base of the proximal phalange. They are synovial condyloid joints, surrounded by a fairly loose capsule which is lined with synovial membrane. The articular surface on the head of the metatarsal extends onto its dorsal, distal and particularly plantar surfaces. The capsule is supported by cord-like collateral and strong plantar ligaments. A deep transverse metatarsal ligament links all the plantar ligaments together, forming a strong link between the heads of the metatarsals while allowing some up-and-down movement to occur between them.

Surface marking

The metatarsophalangeal joints lie on a line drawn from just distal to the head of the first metatarsal to just distal to the head of the fifth metatarsal. The line is slightly convex forward at its centre.

Palpation

Grip the **head of the first metatarsal** between your fingers and thumb. Let them slide slightly forwards. The joint space can easily be identified on the medial and dorsal aspect just distal to the head. Although the under surface of the head is masked by a thick pad of fascia, the line of the joint can be traced with some difficulty.

If the lesser toes are strongly flexed, the heads of the metatarsals protrude on the dorsum of the foot. The joints can be palpated, with care, just beyond these heads. The tendons of extensor digitorum longus and brevis may have to be moved to the side. The joint of the fifth metatarsal can easily be palpated on its lateral side just beyond the head.

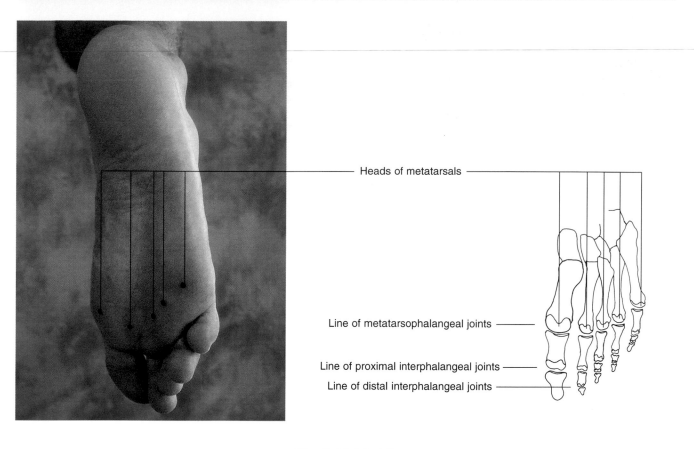

Fig. 3.16 (c), (d)
The metatarsophalangeal and interphalangeal joints of the right foot (plantar aspect)

With all the toes strongly extended, the joints can be identified from their plantar aspect but again they are partially masked by the thick fascia which covers them.

If the toes are rhythmically flexed and extended the proximal phalanges can be observed gliding over the heads of the metatarsals.

Accessory movements

Movement at the metatarsophalangeal joints is similar to that at the metacarpophalangeal joints of the hand, although a little more difficult to perform. These movements include rotation and a gliding of the proximal phalanx on the corresponding metatarsal head.

Grip the whole toe to be moved between the fingers and thumb of one hand, while stabilizing the remainder of the foot with the other. The toe can now be rotated about its long axis, and moved upwards, downwards and from side to side against the metatarsal head.

As in the case of many of the synovial joints with comparatively loose capsules, these joints can also be distracted, although not as much as the metacarpophalangeal joints of the hand and certainly not enough to cause the 'popping' sound that can be produced sometimes in the hand.

Stabilize the whole foot with one hand and grip the appropriate phalange with the fingers and thumb of the other. Now just apply a traction force on the phalange.

Although abduction and adduction is an active movement at these joints, it is often quite difficult to perform. This movement is easily obtainable, however, using the same technique as above and moving the phalange from side to side.

Fig. 3.17 (a), (b)
The metatarsophalangeal and interphalangeal joints of the right foot (lateral aspect)

The interphalangeal joints [Figs 3.16 and 3.17]

These joints exit between the proximal and middle, and middle and distal phalanges of each of the lesser toes. As there are only two phalanges in the great toe, there is only one interphalangeal joint. These joints are synovial hinge joints surrounded by a capsule which is lined with synovial membrane and supported by strong collateral and thick plantar ligaments. The plantar ligaments are composed of fibrocartilage and form part of the joint capsule.

At the distal end of each distal phalange the joint surface is replaced with the nail bed.

Palpation

On the second to fifth toes, the proximal interphalangeal joints are usually flexed so that the head of the proximal phalanx is easy to palpate. In many subjects it is marked by a small bursa on its dorsal aspect. These joints can be palpated as a faint, horizontal line just beyond this bicondylar head, particularly if the middle phalanx is gripped between the finger and thumb and gently moved forwards and backwards. The joint is difficult to palpate on its plantar aspect. The distal interphalangeal joint is usually hyperextended and, although the joint itself is difficult to feel, the movement available clearly marks its line, particularly when palpated from the plantar aspect (Figs 3.16c, d and 3.17).

The interphalangeal joint of the great toe can be palpated just beyond the head of the proximal phalanx, particularly when the toe is flexed, and again can be emphasized by moving the distal phalanx forwards and backwards in a similar fashion to the lesser toes (Fig. 3.16c, d).

Accessory movements

The interphalangeal joints are hinge joints. However, with the joint in slight flexion some side-to-side rocking of the joint can be produced.

Fig. 3.17 (c), (d)
The metatarsophalangeal and interphalangeal joints of the right foot (medial aspect)

Grasp the proximal of the two phalanges between finger and thumb of one hand and the more distal in a similar grip with the other hand. The distal phalanx can now be moved from side to side.

The joints of the foot are generally more difficult to mark and palpate. They are, however, all important in the functions of the foot, especially locomotion. Stiffness of just one small joint may lead to severe pain and dysfunction. It is therefore important to be able to locate and mobilize all joints, noting the direction of their articular surfaces and the resultant shape of the part as a whole.

Most feet react favourably to fairly strong manipulative techniques being performed on them, and these combined with the correct strengthening and mobilizing exercises can improve function dramatically.

All the joints of the foot, including the ankle, contribute to the overall position and shape of the foot. This will vary considerably according to its function at the time, i.e. weight-bearing or non-weight-bearing, mobile or stationary. It is therefore important to examine the structure in as many varying positions as possible.

In the standing position, weight transference through the foot is worthy of close examination. Body weight is transmitted through the tibia to the talus and then via the longitudinal and transverse arches to the ground. The shape and position of the foot depend on where this downward force is applied to the arches and how the weight is distributed through the fore- and hind-foot to the ground. If the weight is applied too far to the medial side, the medial longitudinal arch becomes flattened, whereas if the weight is applied to the lateral side, the lateral longitudinal arch becomes flattened and the medial arch raised.

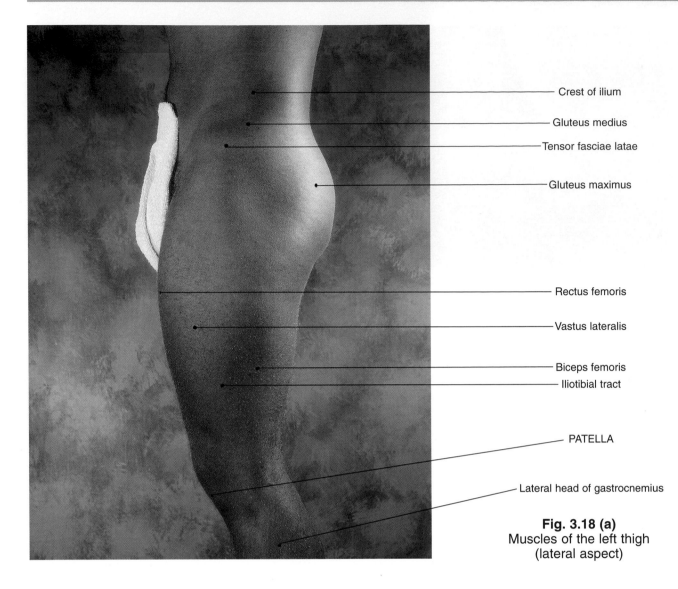

Crest of ilium

Gluteus medius

Tensor fasciae latae

Gluteus maximus

Rectus femoris

Vastus lateralis

Biceps femoris

Iliotibial tract

PATELLA

Lateral head of gastrocnemius

Fig. 3.18 (a)
Muscles of the left thigh
(lateral aspect)

MUSCLES

The lateral and anterior aspect of the hip

Gluteus medius, *gluteus minimus and tensor fasciae latae*

On the lateral aspect of the ilium, just anterior and deep to gluteus maximus, between the most lateral part of the iliac crest and the greater trochanter of the femur, gluteus medius can be located (Fig. 3.18a and b). It is covered by strong, thick fascia, but can, nevertheless, be felt contracting and relaxing when either, in standing, the weight is transferred from one leg to the other, the muscle preventing the pelvis dropping to the opposite side, or, in side lying, when the limb is raised and lowered. Anterior to gluteus medius, the bulk of gluteus minimus, covered by the tensor fasciae latae (Fig. 3.18a, b), is readily palpable between the anterior section of the iliac crest and the greater trochanter. The contraction of these two muscles is produced in lying or standing when the foot is medially rotated, as in the weight-bearing phase of walking when the lower limb is moving

into extension and medial rotation, just before the thrust phase produced by the gastrocnemius.

It is important to practise the palpation of these muscles, gluteus maximus, medius, minimus and tensor fasciae latae, in the subject or patient during ambulation. Much information can be gained from this region regarding the relationships of the bony structures and the power and timing of muscle contraction. As noted above, the gluteus medius should contract on the weight-bearing limb to prevent the pelvis dropping to the other side when the foot is raised from the ground. Therefore, the distance between the iliac crest and the greater trochanter of the femur, on the weight-bearing limb, should remain the same or even decrease slightly.

It is also worth noting, through palpation of these muscles, that as the weight-bearing limb moves

Crest of ilium

Gluteus medius

Tensor fasciae latae

Gluteus maximus

Greater trochanter of femur

Rectus femoris

Vastus lateralis

Biceps femoris

Iliotibial tract

PATELLA

Lateral head of gastrocnemius

Fig. 3.18 (b)
Muscles of the left thigh
(lateral aspect)

from the flexed to the extended position, the muscles appear to contract in sequence from posterior to anterior. As the heel comes in contact with the ground, the limb is in lateral rotation and the posterior section of gluteus medius and possibly gluteus maximus are contracted. As the hip moves forwards over the foot, the middle of gluteus medius can be felt contracting, and as the limb moves into extension and medial rotation, the anterior section of gluteus medius, gluteus minimus and tensor fasciae latae are contracted. During this sequence, the pelvis will rotate around the weight-bearing hip joint towards the weight-bearing side. Finally, it is worth noting that immediately the limb is weight-bearing, the gluteus medius contracts.

Dysfunction of the hip joint may upset the precise *firing off* of these muscles.

Iliopsoas and pectineus

The front of the hip joint is crossed by iliopsoas and pectineus, the former being a broad tendon and the latter a quadrilateral muscle. Because they are both covered by several layers of fascia, as well as the femoral sheath and its contents, they are difficult to palpate (see Fig. 3.20a, b).

Palpation

With the subject lying supine and both the hip and knee supported and flexed to 90°, place your fingers on the anterior aspect of the hip joint 3.5 cm below the centre of the inguinal ligament. If the subject now gently flexes and extends the hip joint, the contraction of both iliopsoas laterally and pectineus medially can be palpated.

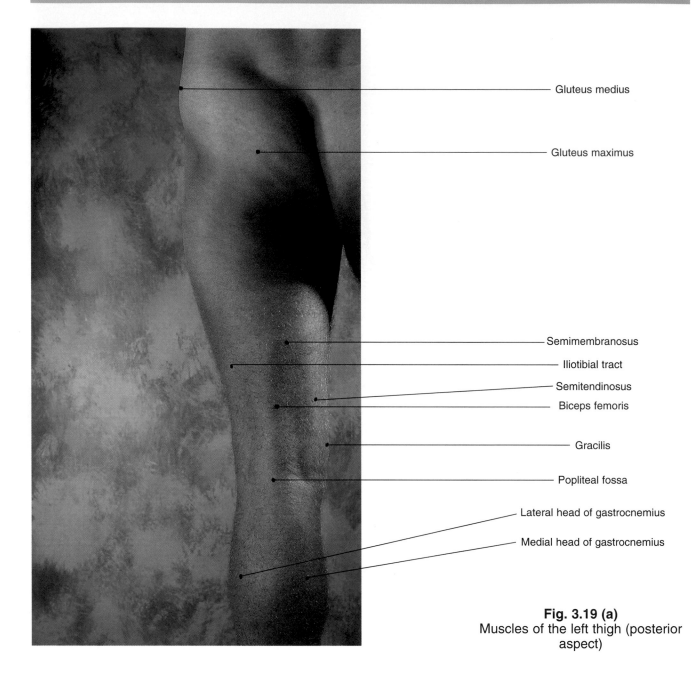

- Gluteus medius
- Gluteus maximus
- Semimembranosus
- Iliotibial tract
- Semitendinosus
- Biceps femoris
- Gracilis
- Popliteal fossa
- Lateral head of gastrocnemius
- Medial head of gastrocnemius

Fig. 3.19 (a)
Muscles of the left thigh (posterior aspect)

The posterior aspect of the hip and thigh

Gluteus maximus

The extremely well-developed muscles around the hip joint are the gluteal muscles, especially the gluteus maximus, which is important in maintaining the upright posture. It is a large and powerful muscle, giving the gluteal region its rounded shape.

Gluteus maximus (Figs 3.18 and 3.19) lies between the posterior part of the iliac crest superiorly, the anal cleft medially and the gluteal fold inferiorly. With care, its coarse fibres can be traced running downwards and laterally towards the greater trochanter of the femur. It is often possible, especially with the hip extended, to trace the more superficial fibres to their attachment into the fascia lata (iliotibial tract). The extent of the muscle is made clearer if the subject extends the hip when lying prone.

The hamstrings

Below the gluteal fold the hamstrings are evident. These powerful muscles cover the whole of the back of the thigh. Semitendinosus and semimembranosus pass downwards and medially, with the biceps crossing to lie laterally as it passes down to the knee. The muscle bellies of the hamstrings separate approximately two-thirds of the way down the thigh, giving rise to their tendons – semitendinosus and semimembranosus medially and biceps femoris laterally (Fig. 3.19).

Gluteus medius

Gluteus maximus

Semimembranosus

Iliotibial tract

Semitendinosus

Biceps femoris

Gracilis

Popliteal fossa

Lateral head of gastrocnemius

Medial head of gastrocnemius

Fig. 3.19 (b)
Muscles of the left thigh (posterior
aspect)

Palpation

With the subject lying prone and flexing the knee against resistance, the tendon of biceps femoris stands clear on the posterolateral side of the knee, and can be traced to its insertion to the head of the fibula. Proximally the superficial fusiform muscle belly can be followed towards the ischial tuberosity (Fig 3.2). The deeper fibres of biceps femoris can be palpated on the medial side of the tendon in the upper part of the popliteal fossa. The tendon of semitendinosus can be observed, and palpated, on the posteromedial side of the knee joint as it passes downwards to its attachment on the medial surface of the tibial condyle and shaft. Proximally, its fusiform muscle belly joins that of biceps femoris near the gluteal fold. A slightly thinner tendon, lying anteromedial, can be identified. This is the tendon of

gracilis whose muscle belly can be traced up the medial side of the thigh as far as the body of the pubis, particularly when the knee is flexed against resistance. Semimembranosus lies deep to semitendinosus just above the knee. It is difficult to palpate, even at its distal end, because it attaches, via a broad aponeurosis, to the postero-medial aspect of the medial condyle of the tibia.

With the knee supported in approximately 60° of flexion, press your fingertips and thumb into the space on either side of the semitendinosus tendon approximately 5 cm above the level of the knee joint. As the subject gently flexes and extends the knee, the muscle below can be felt contracting and then relaxing.

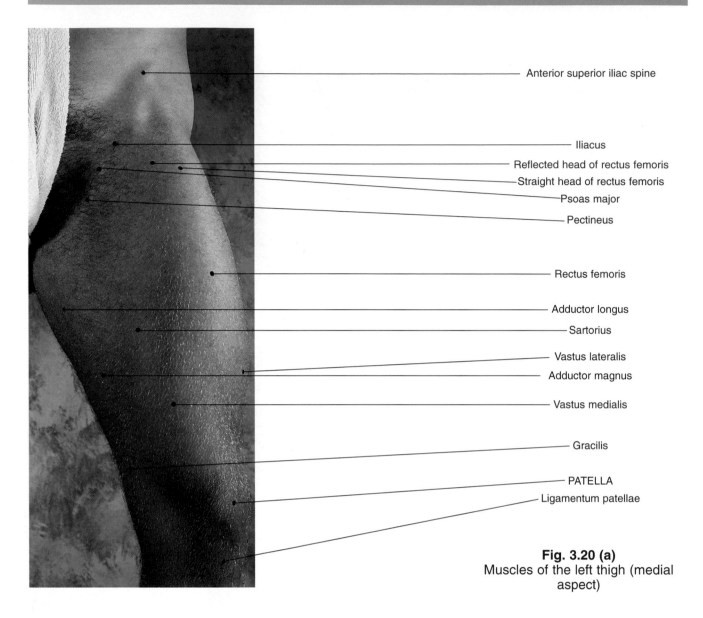

Anterior superior iliac spine

Iliacus

Reflected head of rectus femoris

Straight head of rectus femoris

Psoas major

Pectineus

Rectus femoris

Adductor longus

Sartorius

Vastus lateralis

Adductor magnus

Vastus medialis

Gracilis

PATELLA

Ligamentum patellae

Fig. 3.20 (a)
Muscles of the left thigh (medial aspect)

The anterior and medial aspects of the thigh

The adductors and quadriceps femoris

If the thigh is now adducted, the adductor group of muscles comes into action. The following can be palpated: the tendinous part of **adductor magnus** running down the medial aspect of the thigh from the ischial tuberosity to the adductor tubercle, **adductor longus** lying anteriorly and laterally with adductor brevis and the aponeurotic part of adductor magnus lying more posteriorly. However, it is difficult to identify the adductor muscles separately.

The great bulk of muscle on the front of the thigh is the quadriceps femoris, consisting of **vastus medialis**, **vastus intermedius**, **vastus lateralis** and **rectus femoris**. It extends from the anterior inferior iliac spine and above the acetabulum (the attachment of the rectus femoris) via the **patella** to the **tibial tuberosity** (Fig. 3.20).

Palpation

Three of the four bellies of quadriceps femoris can readily be palpated when the knee is extended against resistance. The belly of the vastus intermedius lies deep to the other three and is difficult to identify separately.

Rectus femoris passes straight down the front of the thigh from the anterior inferior iliac spine to the base of the patella. Its proximal and distal tendons can clearly be identified. Its belly appears as a fusiform shape on the front of the thigh.

The belly of **vastus lateralis** can be identified halfway down the lateral surface of the thigh, being flattened posteriorly by the fascia lata iliotibial tract (Fig. 3.18).

Vastus medialis can be identified on the medial side of the thigh just above the level of the patella. It varies considerably in size according to its use and is the first part of the quadriceps to show signs of weakness. Its lowest fibres can be traced running almost horizontally and laterally to attach to the medial border of the patella.

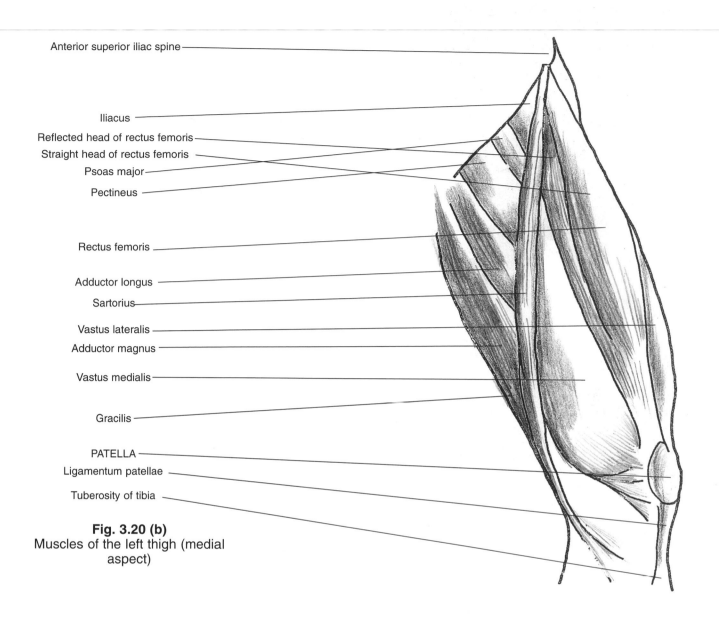

Anterior superior iliac spine

Iliacus

Reflected head of rectus femoris

Straight head of rectus femoris

Psoas major

Pectineus

Rectus femoris

Adductor longus

Sartorius

Vastus lateralis

Adductor magnus

Vastus medialis

Gracilis

PATELLA

Ligamentum patellae

Tuberosity of tibia

Fig. 3.20 (b)
Muscles of the left thigh (medial aspect)

The tendon of the quadriceps, particularly of rectus femoris and vastus intermedius, can be identified attaching to the upper border of the patella. There are often small depressions on its medial and lateral edges where it joins the expansion of vastus lateralis and vastus medialis. The patella is a sesamoid bone and lies within the tendon of quadriceps femoris, the ligamentum patellae being a continuation of the quadriceps tendon (Fig. 3.20). The ligamentum patellae joins the apex of the patella to the upper part of the tibial tuberosity. It is approximately 5 cm long and 2 cm wide, with its central point level with the knee joint (see pages 105 and 107). When the knee is fully extended, a strong tendon-like structure can be palpated lying lateral to the patella and running down to attach to the lateral tibial condyle (Fig. 3.21a,b). This is the lower part of the iliotibial tract, and can be traced superiorly along the lateral side of the thigh to the ilium.

Sartorius

With the subject lying supine, resist the movement of flexion, lateral rotation, abduction of the hip and flexion of the knee by applying resistance to the heel. The long strap-like sartorius muscle can be observed and palpated, crossing the thigh from the anterior superior iliac spine above to the medial condyle of the tibia below (Fig. 3.20). Its upper third appears to stand away from the groin region. With the subject sitting with the knees extended, contraction of both muscles simultaneously produces the 'tailor sitting' position. Sartorius [*sartor* (L) = tailor] can be observed and palpated during this action.

Vastus lateralis
Biceps femoris
Iliotibial tract

PATELLA

Gastrocnemius (lateral head)
Tibialis anterior
Soleus
Peroneus longus
Extensor digitorum longus

Peroneus brevis

Superior extensor retinaculum
Tendo calcaneus
Inferior extensor retinaculum
Extensor digitorum brevis
CALCANEUS

Fig. 3.21 (a), (b)
Muscles of the right leg (lateral aspect)

The anterior and lateral aspect of the leg and foot

The muscles in the anterior compartment of the leg are somewhat easier to identify than those in the corresponding aspect of the forearm. Even so, differentiation is easiest where the tendons pass over the front of the ankle joint. Consequently, palpation should begin here.

Tibialis anterior

With the subject lying supine and the foot dorsiflexed, find the most medial tendon, that of tib-ialis anterior (Fig. 3.21). Although it lies deep to the superior and inferior extensor retinacula, it is clear to see and feel. Distally it can be traced to its insertion on the medial cuneiform and base of the first metatarsal. Proximally, the strong tendon gives way to a firm but narrow muscle which fills the space lateral to the anterior border of the tibia. The muscle is contained within strong fascia and becomes particularly hard on contraction. There is often a narrow space between the muscle and the tibia anteriorly.

Extensor hallucis longus

The tendon lying lateral to tibialis anterior at the ankle joint is that of extensor hallucis longus (Fig. 3.21c, d). It also stands clear of the joint and can be traced across the medial side of the foot to the great toe where, if the toe is extended, it can be followed to its insertion into the base of the distal phalanx. Proximally, the tendon is soon lost between the other muscles; however, if the line of the tendon is continued to the middle of the fibula, the muscle can be felt contracting deep to extensor digi-torum longus.

Extensor digitorum longus

Lateral to the tendon of extensor hallucis longus lies the tendon of extensor digitorum longus (Fig. 3.21a–d). Immediately distal to the ankle it can be seen dividing into four separate tendons, which can be traced to the dorsal surface of the lateral four toes. Occasionally, when the toes are flexed at the metatarsophalangeal joint, the tendons can be felt and seen to 'bowstring' across the joint. Proximally, the tendon soon becomes muscular, extending supe-riorly as far as the superior tibiofibular joint, lying

Extensor hallucis longus
Superior extensor retinaculum
Tibialis anterior
Medial malleolus
Lateral malleolus
Inferior extensor retinaculum
Peroneus tertius
Tendon of extensor digitorum longus
Extensor digitorum brevis
Tendon of extensor hallucis longus

Fig. 3.21 (c), (d)
Tendons and muscles of the left foot (dorsal aspect)

between tibialis anterior medially and the fibula laterally.

Peroneus tertius

Although this small muscle is named as one of the peroneal muscles, peroneus tertius is considered to be part of the extensor digitorum longus, in fact its fifth tendon. This may be borne out as it does arise from the lower third of the fibula in line with, and does pass under, the superior extensor retinaculum and through the loop of the inferior retinaculum, with, and lateral to, the extensor digitorum longus. However, unlike the extensor digitorum longus, it does not insert into the digits but into the medial side of the dorsal surface of the base of the fifth metatarsal. In a small percentage of subjects the muscle is absent.

The tendon of the peroneus tertius is difficult to find, but is best located as it crosses the lateral part of the dorsum of the foot on its way to attach to the medial side of the base of the fifth metatarsal (Fig. 3.21c, d).

Palpation

From the base of the fifth metatarsal, draw a line from its medial side towards the lower quarter of the shaft of the fibula. It is along this line that the tendon is most likely to be palpated, particularly when the foot is everted.

Extensor digitorum brevis

Extensor digitorum brevis presents as a large swelling some 2 cm anterior to the lateral malleolus on the dorsolateral aspect of the foot (Fig. 3.21). Four narrow tendons can be palpated, leaving its distal aspect passing towards the medial four toes. In the second, third and fourth toes the tendons join those of extensor digitorum longus, while in the great toe the tendon passes to the lateral side of the proximal phalanx.

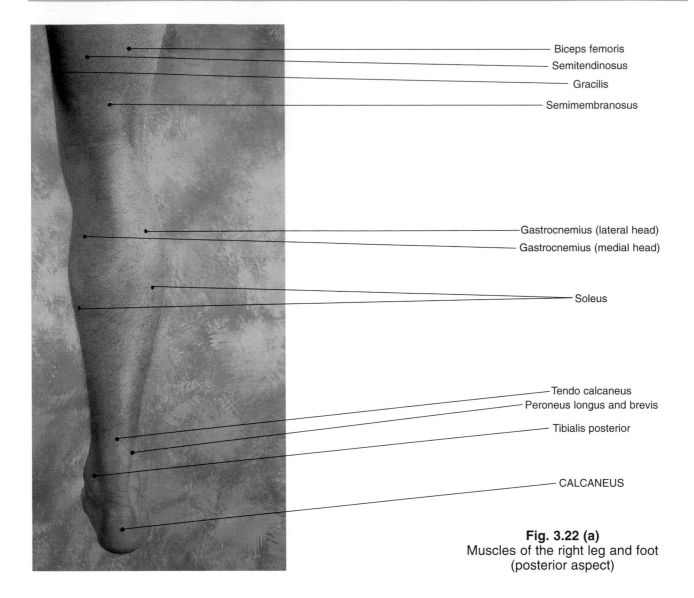

Biceps femoris
Semitendinosus
Gracilis
Semimembranosus

Gastrocnemius (lateral head)
Gastrocnemius (medial head)

Soleus

Tendo calcaneus
Peroneus longus and brevis
Tibialis posterior

CALCANEUS

Fig. 3.22 (a)
Muscles of the right leg and foot
(posterior aspect)

The posterior and plantar aspects of the leg and foot

Popliteus

Popliteus lies deep within the popliteal fossa high up on the posterolateral aspect of the knee joint. Its tendon, however, can be palpated as it passes below the lateral epicondyle of the femur. With the subject sitting and the knee flexed 90°, place the tips of your fingers on the lateral surface of the femoral condyle just below and in front of the lateral epicondyle. If medial rotation of the leg at the knee joint is now performed, the tendon of popliteus can be palpated as it runs forwards, in a groove, towards its femoral attachment.

Triceps surae (calf)

The posterior aspect of the leg is dominated by the beautifully shaped calf muscles gastrocnemius and soleus, the former being more superficial and the latter deep. Together they are attached distally by the tendo calcaneus to the posterior surface of the calcaneus. The two muscles, however, arise from different bones. The gastrocnemius from the femur, its medial head from the upper part of the medial condyle and the lateral head from just above the lateral epicondyle. The soleus, which is believed to derive its name from a flat fish, the sole, arises below the knee joint from the posterior surfaces of the tibia, fibula and interosseous membrane.

Plantaris, when present, passes lateral to medial, from the upper part of the lateral condyle of the femur downwards, between gastrocnemius and soleus to attach adjacent to the tendo calcaneus.

Biceps femoris
Semitendinosus
Gracilis
Semimembranosus

Popliteal fossa

Gastrocnemius (lateral head)
Gastrocnemius (medial head)

Soleus

Tendo calcaneus
Peroneus longus and brevis

Tibialis posterior

CALCANEUS

Fig. 3.22 (b)
Muscles of the right leg and foot
(posterior aspect)

Palpation

With the subject standing, begin at the posterior aspect of the heel, where the broad tendo calcaneus can easily be identified attaching to the calcaneus. Follow the tendon upwards for some 8 cm as it narrows to a width of approximately 1 cm, after which it rapidly widens into an aponeurosis about 8 cm wide. Here the muscle fibres of gastrocnemius can be palpated attaching to the superficial surface of the aponeurosis. Two large bellies, the medial and longer belly, stretch to the medial femoral condyle, and the lateral belly to the lateral femoral condyle (Fig. 3.22). The two bellies are separated by a faint vertical line which is easily palpable in a well-developed calf.

Soleus lies deep to gastrocnemius, its fibres contributing to the deep surface of the tendo calcaneus Its upper attachment is to the posterior aspect of the tibia (soleal line) and to the head and shaft of the fibula. The muscle belly is broad and thick. As soleus is primarily a postural muscle, preventing the tibia from tilting forwards in the standing position, it is easier to palpate when the subject is standing.

First locate the broad aponeurosis of the tendo calcaneus where it joins the muscle fibres of gastrocnemius, and run your fingers to the outer borders. Immediately adjacent is the muscle belly of soleus bulging either side and deep to the aponeurosis (Fig. 3.22). If the subject gently raises the heel, the muscle fibres of gastrocnemius can be felt contracting.

If the subject then fully flexes the knee and plantarflexes the foot, soleus can be felt contracting while gastrocnemius remains relaxed. This is because the upper (femoral) and lower (calcaneal) attachments of gastrocnemius are brought closer together, shortening the muscle and essentially preventing it from contracting. This is known as 'muscle insufficiency'.

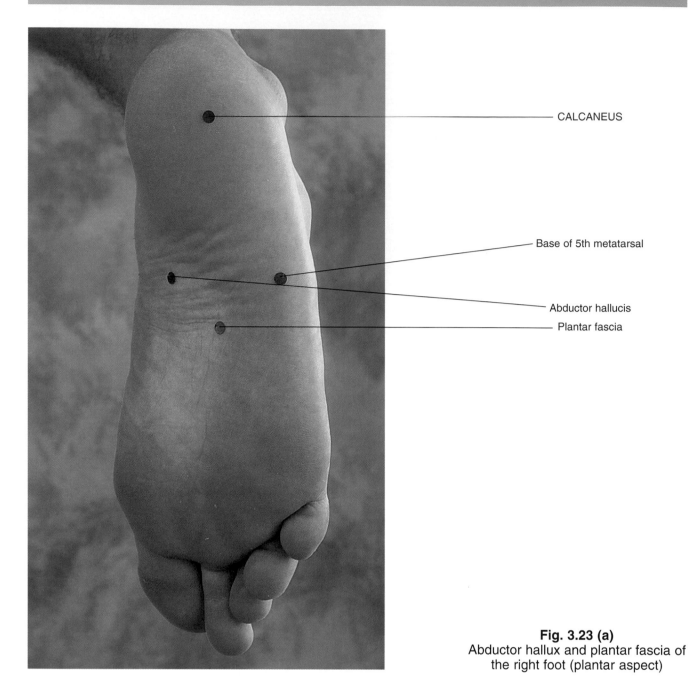

CALCANEUS

Base of 5th metatarsal

Abductor hallucis

Plantar fascia

Fig. 3.23 (a)
Abductor hallux and plantar fascia of
the right foot (plantar aspect)

Plantar muscles

The plantar surface of the foot is covered centrally by a thick dense layer of fascia known as the plantar aponeurosis. This is triangular in shape, being narrower posteriorly, where it attaches to the calcaneus, and broader anteriorly, where it splits to attach either side of the proximal phalanx of each toe. It gives the central portion of the plantar aspect a pale appearance, the heel, lateral border and under the metatarsal heads being darker and covered with harder skin for weight-bearing.

The plantar muscles are arranged in four layers deep to the plantar fascia, and are relatively easily recognized on dissection. The deepest muscles are the shortest, whereas those just deep to the plantar aponeurosis are the longest. All of these muscles except abductor hallucis are difficult to palpate due to the thickness and tension of the fascia.

Palpation

Only abductor hallucis is easily recognizable on the medial side of the foot. Some subjects may be able to abduct their great toe, in which case the belly of abductor hallucis can be palpated along the medial border of the foot. The broad fusiform-shaped muscle belly passes forwards from the medial tubercle of the calcaneus, continuing as a tendon to the medial side of the proximal phalange of the great toe.

If the subject is unable to abduct the great toe (really more of a party trick than anything else), shortening the foot while weight-bearing produces a powerful contraction of the muscle. This is most probably the muscle's main functional activity. The bulk of the muscle is palpated in the posterior section of the muscle, with the relatively thick tendon

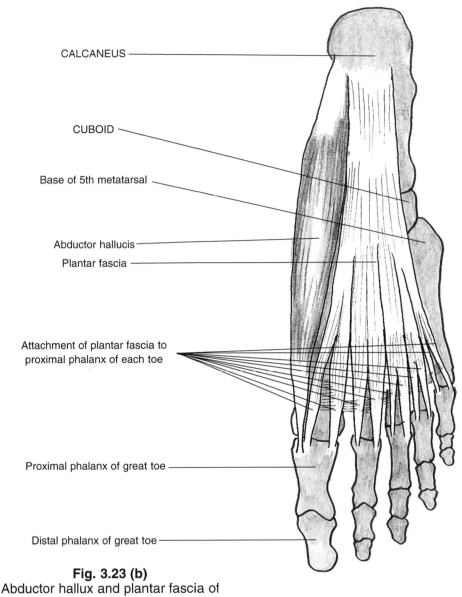

CALCANEUS

CUBOID

Base of 5th metatarsal

Abductor hallucis

Plantar fascia

Attachment of plantar fascia to
proximal phalanx of each toe

Proximal phalanx of great toe

Distal phalanx of great toe

Fig. 3.23 (b)
Abductor hallux and plantar fascia of
the right foot (plantar aspect)

distinct in its anterior half inserting into the medial side of the base of the proximal phalanx of the great toe. If the toe is extended, the medial edge of the plantar fascia can be palpated as it is being stretched.

The use and type of footwear, if any, habitually worn, together with the activities and weight of the subject, will influence the structure and appearance of the foot. There is usually a thickening of the fascia and hardening of the skin over weight-bearing areas, these normally being over the heel, lateral border of the foot and heads of the metatarsals, particularly the first and fifth.

The amount of the sole of the foot which is in contact with the supporting surface is inversely proportional to the height of the plantar arches. The medial side of the foot is rarely in contact with the ground, except in subjects with extremely flat feet. Anteriorly, the metatarsal heads are normally in contact with the ground and may show a downward convexity, producing areas of hardened skin (callus), under the second, third and fourth metatarsal heads.

Sciatic nerve anterior to piriformis

Sciatic nerve deep to gluteus maximus

Biceps femoris (cut)

Sciatic nerve deep to biceps femoris

Common peroneal nerve medial to biceps tendon

Tibial nerve in popliteal fossa

Tibial nerve deep to gastrocnemius and soleus

Tendo calcaneus (cut)

Medial plantar nerve

Lateral plantar nerve

Fig. 3.24 (a), (b)
The sciatic nerve and branches in the left lower
limb (posterior view)

NERVES

The nerves of the lower limb are normally deep within the tissues and thus extremely difficult to palpate. Nevertheless, it is important to be aware of their location and to be able to palpate those that venture close to the surface.

The whole of the lower limb is supplied from the lumbar, sacral and coccygeal plexi. The lumbar plexus derives its fibres from T12, L1, L2, L3 and L4 roots. The sacral (lumbosacral) plexus derives its fibres from L4, L5, S1, S2, S3 and S4. The coccygeal (sacral) plexus derives its fibres from S4 and S5. These form a complex arrangement of nerves, most of which are not palpable, but nevertheless remain essential knowledge for the anatomist. The reader should refer to *Anatomy and Human Movement* (Palastanga *et al.*, 1998) for further study.

Surface marking

The **sciatic nerve** derives its fibres from the anterior primary rami of L4 and L5 through the lumbosacral trunk, and S1, S2 and S3. It is formed **in front of piriformis** in the posterior part of the pelvis and emerges from the pelvis through the sciatic notch below piriformis and **deep to the gluteus maximus** It is the largest peripheral nerve in the body. It runs vertically down the back of the thigh, deep to **biceps femoris**, having emerged from below piriformis approximately halfway between the greater trochanter of the femur and the ischial tuberosity. About two-thirds of the way down the thigh, it splits into its terminal branches – the **tibial** and **common peroneal nerves** (Fig. 3.24a–d). Although it is difficult to palpate the nerve directly, pressure applied over the area of its course can cause considerable discomfort to the subject.

The tibial nerve (Fig. 3.24a, b) continues through the popliteal fossa to enter the calf **deep to gastrocnemius** and **soleus**, to lie between superficial and deep groups of muscles. It is again difficult to palpate in this region, although an unpleasant sensation can be produced if excessive pressure is applied. In the lower third of the leg the tibial nerve becomes medial to the **tendo calcaneus**, and continues to the space behind the **medial malleolus** where it is palpable. It can be traced proximally into

Fig. 3.24 (c), (d)
Branches of the common peroneal nerve of the right leg (anterior aspect) (p, palpable)

the leg, and distally into the foot, where it almost immediately divides into the **medial and lateral plantar nerves**. These terminal branches soon become too deep to be palpated.

The common peroneal nerve, the lateral terminal branch of the sciatic nerve, enters the popliteal fossa. It passes down the medial side of the **tendon of biceps femoris** where it can be palpated passing behind the head of the fibula to the neck (Fig. 3.24). It then winds anteriorly around the neck of the fibula, immediately splitting into superficial and deep branches.

Palpation

With the knee semiflexed, locate the tendon of biceps femoris as it passes down to the head of the fibula, posterolateral to the knee. Below the level of the knee joint the common peroneal nerve will be found just medial and deep to this tendon, passing behind the head of the fibula and winding forwards around the neck of the fibula (Fig. 3.24). It is easier to

palpate posteriorly but more difficult anteriorly as it becomes covered by peroneus longus and tibialis anterior.

The deep peroneal nerve lies deep within the anterior compartment of the leg and is impossible to palpate until it crosses the anterior aspect of the ankle joint between the tendons of extensor hallucis longus and **extensor digitorum longus**.

First find the anterior tibial pulse on the front of the ankle joint between extensor hallucis longus and extensor digitorum longus. The nerve runs just lateral to this, but it is difficult to find as it lies deep to the **superior extensor retinaculum**.

The **superficial peroneal nerve** can be palpated passing over the anterolateral aspect of the ankle, just medial to the anterior border of the lateral malleolus. It can be traced proximally for approximately 5 cm to where it emerges from between peroneus brevis and extensor digitorum longus. Distally it can be traced on to the lateral side of the dorsum of the foot, dividing into fine terminal cutaneous branches (Fig. 3.24c, d).

Fig. 3.25 (a), (b)
The arteries of the right lower limb (anterior aspect) (p, palpable)

ARTERIES

As in the upper limb, most of the large arteries are located deep within the tissues and are normally difficult to palpate.

The pulsation of the femoral artery can be palpated in the groin just below the mid point (halfway between the anterior superior iliac spines and the pubic tubercle) of the inguinal ligament directly anterior to the head of the femur at the hip joint. Above, the vessel lies within the abdomen and below it is hidden by fascia as it lies in the femoral triangle on the proximal anteromedial aspect of the thigh. Just above the knee the femoral artery passes through the opening in adductor magnus (adductor hiatus) lying deep to the sartorius muscle in the adductor (subsartorial) canal to enter the popliteal fossa, becoming the popliteal artery. This can be

palpated with deep, sensitive pressure as it crosses the back of the knee joint. Its identification is facilitated if tension of the superficial tissues is reduced by bending the knee to about 45°. Success in palpation is largely dependent on the amount of fat within the fossa and, in reality, it is extremely difficult to find. This is, therefore, a good region in which to practise the careful use of the fingers in palpation of pulses.

As the popliteal artery enters the calf, it divides into the anterior and posterior tibial arteries. The anterior tibial artery passes over the main section of the interosseous membrane and below the most superior fibres (see pages 108, 109), into the anterior compartment of the leg, deep to the anterior tibial muscles. The posterior tibial artery passes down the

Superior extensor retinaculum

Tibialis anterior tendon

Extensor digitorum longus tendon

Anterior tibial artery

Inferior extensor retinaculum

Extensor hallucis longus tendon

Dorsalis pedis artery (p)

Arcuate artery (p)

Dorsal metatarsal arteries (p)

Dorsal digital arteries (p?)

Fig. 3.25 (c), (d)
The arteries of the right foot (dorsal aspect) (p, palpable)

back of the leg deep to the gastrocnemius, soleus and plantaris (triceps surae).

The **anterior tibial artery** can be palpated as it crosses the anteromedial aspect of the ankle joint between the tendons of **extensor hallucis longus** and **extensor digitorum longus** where it lies medial to the deep branch of the common peroneal nerve. With careful palpation it can be traced down to the space between the first and second metatarsals where it passes into the plantar aspect of the foot between the two bones. Beyond the **extensor retinaculum** the artery is called the **dorsalis pedis** (Fig. 3.25a–d), and is commonly the point at which the arterial supply is checked. Care must be taken not to palpate too distally, as the artery will

have already passed through to the plantar aspect of the foot. In subjects with a good blood supply to the foot, the **arcuate artery**, a continuation of the dorsalis pedis on the dorsum of the metacarpals, can be palpated.

The posterior tibial artery crosses the ankle joint **behind the medial malleolus** between the tendons of flexor digitorum longus and flexor hallucis longus, medial to the posterior tibial nerve (Fig. 3.25a, b). Although it is quite clear as it crosses the ankle joint, it is difficult to trace into the medial side of the foot and the lower part of the leg.

It is important to practise finding these arterial pulses, as they give a good indication of the competence of the blood supply to the lower limb.

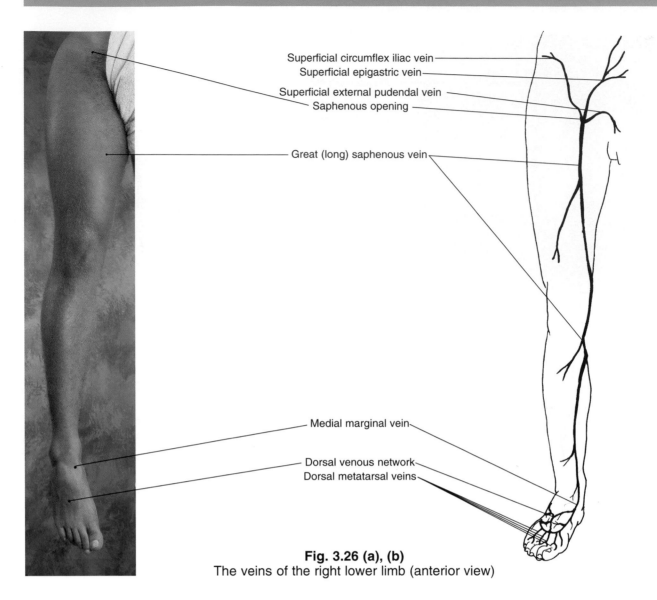

Superficial circumflex iliac vein
Superficial epigastric vein
Superficial external pudendal vein
Saphenous opening

Great (long) saphenous vein

Medial marginal vein

Dorsal venous network
Dorsal metatarsal veins

Fig. 3.26 (a), (b)
The veins of the right lower limb (anterior view)

VEINS

The arrangement of veins in the lower limb is similar to that in the upper limb (see pages 74 and 75), there being two main systems – deep, accompanying the arteries, and superficial, contained within the superficial fascia. All veins of the lower limb possess valves, which facilitate central venous return. The valves in the communicating vessels normally only permit blood to flow from the superficial to the deep system.

The deep veins

The smaller arteries are normally accompanied by two small veins (venae comitantes), one either side of the artery. The larger arteries are usually accompanied by a single large vein of approximately the same diameter as the artery. None of the deep veins can be palpated.

The superficial veins

In normal subjects most veins are difficult to see or palpate, except in the distal part of the leg and on the dorsum of the foot.

With the subject standing, the network of vessels on the dorsum of the foot appear blue and raised. They can be palpated with little difficulty. One vein on either side of the network appears to be slightly larger than the rest; these are termed marginal veins.

The great (long) saphenous vein

The great or long saphenous vein (Fig. 3.26a, b) begins on the medial side of the dorsal venous network as a continuation of the medial marginal vein It passes proximally in front of the medial malleolus, along the medial side of the calf and crosses the knee joint just posterior to the medial condyles of both the tibia and femur. The vein then ascends on the medial side of the thigh to join the deep system (femoral vein) after passing through the saphenous opening which lies below the mid point of the inguinal ligament immediately medial to the pulsations of the femoral artery (see Fig. 3.25a, b).

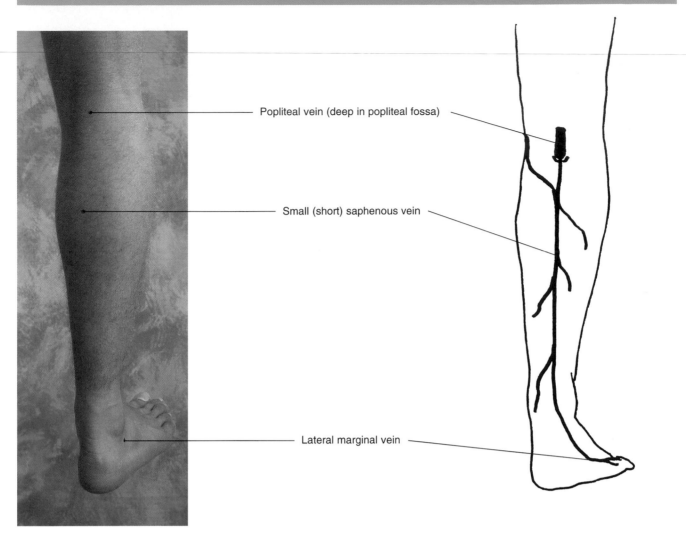

Fig. 3.26 (c), (d)
The veins of the right leg (posterior view)

Palpation

Only the lower part of the vein can normally be palpated as it lies deep within the superficial fascia. With the subject standing, find the medial marginal vein (the major vessel on the medial aspect of the dorsum of the foot). Brushing the skin surface with the fingertips, move up to the medial malleolus. Above this level the vein can be felt passing up the medial aspect of the calf. It can often be traced posteromedial to the knee, but soon disappears as it enters the thigh. In some individuals it can be seen in the thigh as a bluish line running upwards towards the mid point of the groin.

The small (short) saphenous vein

Beginning on the lateral side of the dorsal venous network as a continuation of the lateral marginal vein, the small or short saphenous vein passes behind the lateral malleolus and up the lateral side of the tendo calcaneus to the posterior aspect of the calf. It pierces the deep fascia in the lower part of the popliteal fossa to join the deep popliteal vein (Fig. 3.26c, d).

Palpation

The lateral marginal vein is a little more difficult to recognize than the medial. It can be traced along the lateral side of the dorsum of the foot, but its continuation is difficult to palpate behind the lateral malleolus. That part between the lateral malleolus and the popliteal fossa is variable in its palpability; however, after a long period of standing it usually becomes quite visible and therefore easily palpable.

In some individuals, particularly the elderly, a network of vessels can be palpated on the medial side of the leg and thigh, which roughly follow the course of the great saphenous vein. Most of these join with the great saphenous vein along its length.

4

The head and neck

Frontal bone

Coronal suture

Bregma

Parietal bone

Sagittal suture

Lambda

Lambdoid suture

Occipital bone

Fig. 4.1 (a)
The skull (superior aspect)

BONES

The skull

Superior aspect [Fig. 4.1a]

The skull, viewed from above, is shaped like a flattened egg. It is broader across the posterior dimension and narrower across the anterior dimension. Its length, from front to back, is normally almost twice its breadth from side to side.

It comprises the frontal, two parietal [*paries* (L) = a wall] and part of the occipital [*occipitum* (L) = the back of the head) bones. Viewed from above, the frontal bone makes up the anterior section, forming approximately one-third. The two parietal bones form most of the posterior two-thirds. The occipital bone fits into just the central posterior part of the skull.

The frontal bone joins the anterior borders of the two parietal bones at the coronal [*corona* (L) = crown] suture which runs transversely across the skull. The intersection of all three bones is known as 'bregma' [*brechein* (Gk) = to moisten, the most humid and delicate part of the infant's brain]. The two parietal bones join at the sagittal [*sagitta* (L) = an arrow, the direction in which an arrow would pass through the body) suture, which runs anteroposteriorly along the centre of the skull. The posterior borders of both parietal bones meet the anterior border of the squamous part of the occipital bone at the lambdoid [*lambda* = the Greek letter 'L'] sutures. The point at which all three bones meet is termed 'lambda'.

Palpation

The skull is covered, superiorly, by a fibromuscular sheet (aponeurosis) from the eyebrows anteriorly to the external occipital protuberance and the superior nuchal lines posteriorly. This is thick and adherent to the skin covering the skull but only attached to the pericranium by areola tissue. This gives it a certain amount of freedom to move over the skull. It is continuous laterally with the temporal and zygomatic fascia.

Due to this arrangement and the fact that there is normally a covering of hair, palpation of the bones, sutures and landmarks of the skull requires a slightly different technique if exact location is required. Use all the fingertips of both hands to locate and mark the structures, using a gentle forward and backward motion, moving the aponeurosis on the underlying bone.

Place your fingers anterior and posterior to the vertex of the skull. On pressing the tips in and moving them from side to side, the sagittal suture can be palpated, particularly posteriorly. Halfway between the vertex and the external occipital protuberance a hollow can be felt with two sutures running downwards and laterally in front of the occipital bone. This is the point 'lambda'. Moving approximately 5 cm forwards from the vertex there is another palpable slight hollow with the coronal suture running laterally to either side. This point is termed 'bregma'. In front of the coronal suture one can feel the frontal bone (forehead), sometimes with a central raised line where the two bones have fused.

Either side of the sagittal suture, behind the frontal bones and in front of the occipital bone, are the two large plates of the parietal bones.

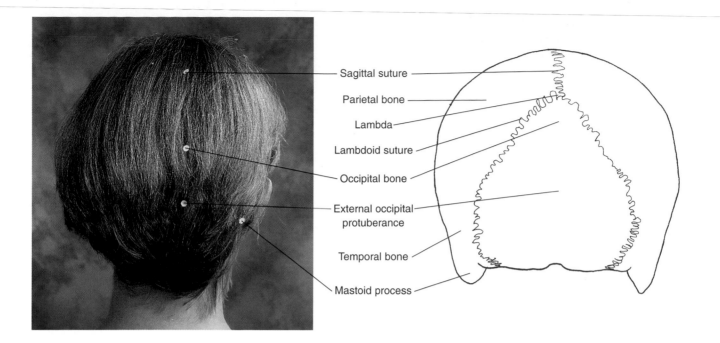

Sagittal suture

Parietal bone

Lambda

Lambdoid suture

Occipital bone

External occipital protuberance

Temporal bone

Mastoid process

Fig. 4.1 (b), (c)
The skull (posterior aspect)

Posterior aspect [Fig. 4.1b and c]

The posteroinferior part of the skull consists mainly of the occipital bone. On either side it joins the temporal bones, each of which has a large downward-projecting prominence termed the mastoid [*mastos* (Gk) = a breast, *oeides* (Gk) = shape] process. Superiorly it joins the two parietal bones forming the vault of the skull. Its anterior portion forms the base of the skull, surrounding the foramen magnum and projecting forward as the basilar section.

Posteriorly, at its apex, the occipital bone fits between the two parietal bones at the point lambda (see previous page). Running downwards and laterally from this point, the two lambdoid sutures divide the occiput from the two parietal bones. The bone presents a large tuberosity, about 5 cm below the point lambda, termed the external occipital protuberance, with superior, middle and inferior nuchal lines radiating laterally. The external occipital protuberance varies considerably in its size, being very prominent in some and almost non-existent in others.

Palpation

The most prominent bony feature of the posterior aspect of the skull is the external occipital protuberance situated just below its centre. It varies in size and shape between individuals, being large and prominent in some and difficult to find in others. Radiating laterally and upwards from the external occipital protuberance are the two superior nuchal (believed to come from Arabic '*nugraph*' = the back of the neck) lines. These are palpable in their central section on most subjects, but are difficult to trace more than a few centimetres laterally. Approximately 5 cm above the external occipital protuberance the sagittal suture meets two occipitoparietal sutures. In the young child this is the region of the posterior fontanelle [*fons* (L) = small fountain or spring) which in the adult becomes the lambda. Inferiorly the occipital bone can be traced forwards under the skull, but is soon lost in the deep hollow at the level of the tubercle of the first cervical vertebra. Moving to either side, just behind the pinna of each ear, the mastoid process of the temporal bone can be palpated. It is pointed at its inferior aspect where sternocleidomastoid attaches.

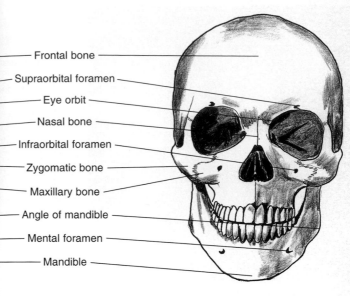

Frontal bone
Supraorbital foramen
Eye orbit
Nasal bone
Infraorbital foramen
Zygomatic bone
Maxillary bone
Angle of mandible
Mental foramen
Mandible

Fig. 4.2 (a), (b)   The skull (anterior aspect)

Anterior aspect [Fig. 4.2a and b]

Each **eye orbit** is formed superiorly by the **frontal bone** (which forms the forehead), laterally by the **zygomatic bone**, medially by the **nasal bone** and inferiorly by the **maxilla**. The upper teeth are associated with the maxilla, while the lower teeth are located in the superior border of the **mandible**.

Palpation

Deep to the eyebrow the upper rim of the eye orbit can be palpated, being slightly notched at its centre where it is crossed by the supraorbital artery. The whole margin of the orbit is subcutaneous and can thus readily be palpated. The two nasal bones can be palpated centrally projecting forwards and continuing as a cartilage down to the centre of the nose. Below this can be palpated the upper part of the maxilla investing the upper teeth.

Lateral aspect [Fig. 4.2c and d]

The **temporal** [*tempus* (L) = time (pertaining to the passing of time and the greying of the temples)] **bone** forms the central area on the side of the skull. Posteriorly it articulates with the occipital bone, superiorly with the **parietal bone** and anteriorly, with the sphenoid [*sphen* (Gk) = a wedge] and zygomatic [*zygoma* (Gk) = a yoke or bar] bones.

The anterior section of the lateral aspect consists of the frontal bone and the maxilla, with the lateral part of the ethmoid [*ethmos* (Gk) = a sieve] just projecting between the sphenoid and frontal bones. Inferiorly the mandible [*mando* (L) = I chew] articulates by its **condyle** with the under surface of the temporal bone just anterior to the **external auditory meatus** [*meatus* (L) = a passage].

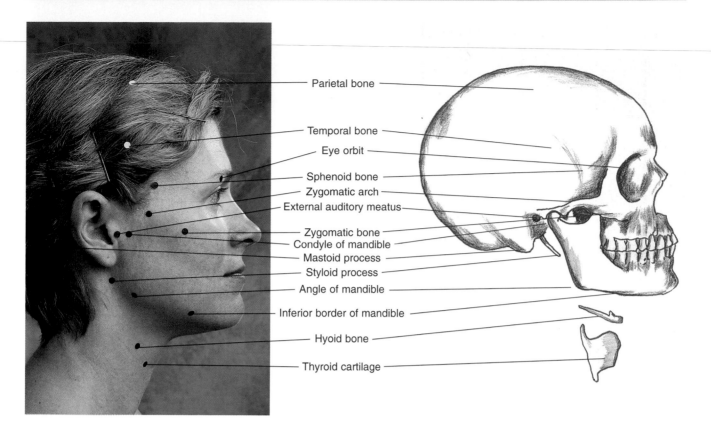

Fig. 4.2 (c), (d)   The skull (lateral aspect)

Palpation

The external auditory meatus is an obvious land-mark on the lateral side of the head. The little finger can be pressed deep into this opening to be sur-rounded by its bony walls. The pinna lies around three sides, while the tragus is the pointed area of soft tissue overlapping the meatus from the front. Running horizontally forwards just anterior to the tragus [*tragos* (Gk) and *tregus* (L) = a goat (possibly pertaining to the shape of a goat's beard)], a bony bridge can be palpated (the zygomatic arch). This forms the point of the cheek at the front where it joins the zygomatic bone (Fig. 4.2c, d). The arch is formed partly from the temporal and partly from the zygomatic bones.

Below the posterior part of the zygomatic arch anterior to the tragus a small tubercle can be pal-pated. This is the most lateral part of the condyle of the mandible. If the subject opens the mouth, this bony prominence can be felt, first rotating then moving forwards and downwards over the articular eminence of the temporal bone.

Some 7 cm directly below the condyle of the mandible, the angle of the mandible can be identi-fied, being more prominent in men than in women as it is slightly everted. The inferior border of the mandible can be traced forward to a raised vertical line centrally at the front, where it joins the bone of the opposite side. A small tubercle (the mental tubercle) can be palpated on the inferior border either side of this line.

The anterior and lateral surfaces of the mandible are subcutaneous and can be traced posteriorly as far as the angle where it is hidden by the powerful muscles of mastication. The lower border is thick-ened all round, giving a concave appearance to the anterior surface. Below the zygomatic bone the maxilla can be palpated, with the teeth and gums easily identifiable through the flesh of the cheek and the upper lip.

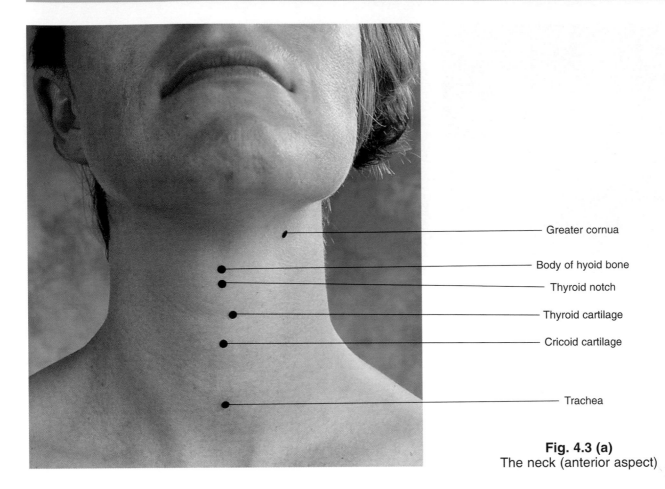

Greater cornua

Body of hyoid bone

Thyroid notch

Thyroid cartilage

Cricoid cartilage

Trachea

Fig. 4.3 (a)
The neck (anterior aspect)

The neck

Anterior aspect [Fig. 4.3a and b]

A series of midline structures run down the anterior aspect of the neck, being part of the respiratory tract. Just below the mandible is the small horseshoe-shaped hyoid bone [*hyoeides* (Gk) = U-shaped, i.e. shaped like the Greek letter upsilon]. Below, the thyroid [*thyreos* (Gk) = a shield] cartilage, formed from two cartilaginous plates fused at their anterior, but notched centrally above (the thyroid notch), projects slightly forward, particularly in the adult male, to form the 'Adam's apple'.

Behind the sternal notch lie the upper rings of the trachea [*trachys* (Gk) = uneven]. Interestingly, Aristotle mistakenly thought that this structure was an uneven surfaced artery. Between the upper ring and the thyroid cartilage lies the thicker and stronger signet-shaped ring of the cricoid cartilage [*krikos* (Gk) = a ring].

The larynx, formed mainly from the thyroid and cricoid cartilages, lies centrally at a level with the third to the sixth vertebral bodies and between the two sternomastoid muscles which are converging from above downwards.

The mandible, hyoid bone, thyroid and cricoid cartilages, and the upper part of the trachea, are all linked by muscle and ligaments and provide the tube for air to enter the lungs – 'the wind pipe'.

Palpation

It is quite unpleasant, and often frightening, to have these structures palpated by another person. It is therefore advisable to perform the palpation on yourself.

Place the fingers and thumb of one hand on either side of the mandible halfway along its inferior border (see page 153), and then slide your fingers and thumb down on to the sides of the throat. Some 3–5 cm below the mandible, the hyoid bone can be felt lying almost horizontal. It will appear as a horseshoe-shaped structure, rounded and thicker

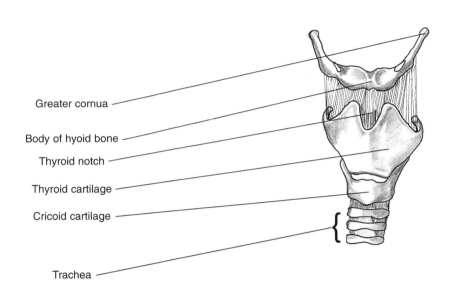

Greater cornua

Body of hyoid bone

Thyroid notch

Thyroid cartilage

Cricoid cartilage

Trachea

Fig. 4.3 (b)
Bones of the neck (anterior aspect)

anteriorly and becoming pointed on either side posteriorly as it curves upwards slightly. This is the greater wing (*cornua*). Gentle pressure applied to either side will confirm its bony consistency.

Continue down the sides of the neck from the hyoid. After crossing a small space (felt as a depression), the broad flat lamina of the thyroid cartilage on either side is encountered. Each lamina is angled medially so that they meet in the midline anteriorly. A marked projection (the laryngeal prominence), more pronounced in men, will be found superiorly in the midline. This projection is commonly referred to as the 'Adam's apple'. If your finger is now placed on the anterosuperior aspect of this prominence a small space can be palpated, concave upwards; this is the thyroid notch.

Trace down the sides of the thyroid cartilage for about 4 cm to a line just above the level of the medial ends of the clavicles. Here, after crossing another small space, a further ring-shaped structure will be

palpated. This is the cricoid cartilage and it presents with a small tubercle at its centre.

Below the cricoid cartilage and deep in the suprasternal (jugular) notch, the cartilaginous rings of the upper part of the trachea can be palpated.

Each of the structures identified above can be taken between the finger and thumb of the same hand and carefully moved from side to side for a distance of about 1 cm. However, too much side movement can lead to tenderness in this part of the neck. During swallowing, each of the structures rises and then falls approximately 1 cm.

On either side of these central structures the sternocleidomastoid (sternomastoid) can be palpated, particularly if the supine subject tries to raise the head off a pillow. These muscles are widely spaced at the level of the hyoid bone but become much closer together as they approach the level of the clavicles.

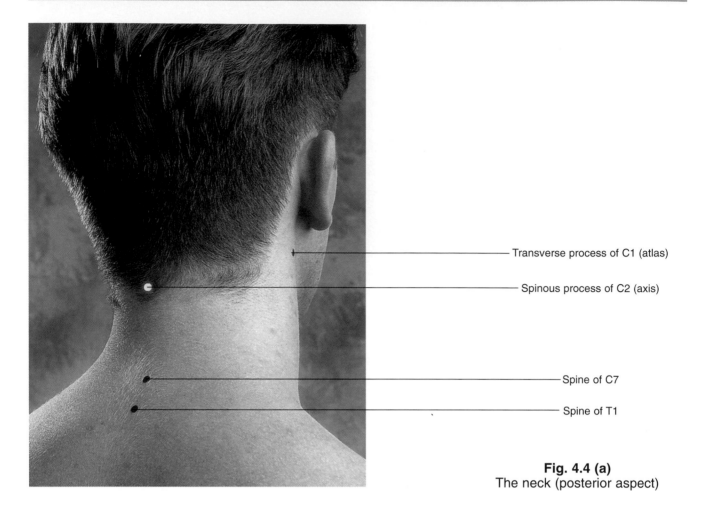

Transverse process of C1 (atlas)

Spinous process of C2 (axis)

Spine of C7

Spine of T1

Fig. 4.4 (a)
The neck (posterior aspect)

Posterior aspect [Fig. 4.4]

There are seven cervical vertebrae. Except for C1 (the atlas [derived from *atlao* (Gk) = I sustain]), C2 (the axis [*axis* (L) = a pivot or axle]) and C7, they all exhibit similar characteristics: small oval bodies, large vertebral canal, long laminae, a bifid spine and a broad transverse process with a foramen transversarium.

C1 does not possess a body, but has two lateral masses to support the weight of the head transferred via the occipital condyles. It has a posterior tubercle instead of a spine, and its transverse processes are wide and relatively pointed.

C2 has a tooth-like process projecting superiorly from its body, the dens or odontoid [*ódous* (Gk) = tooth) peg, a large prominent spine and small transverse processes. The seventh cervical vertebra is noted for its long non-bifid spine (vertebra prominens).

Palpation

Palpation of the neck is generally best carried out with the subject in the prone or supine position, achieving optimum relaxation. The natural curvature of the cervical spine is with the concavity backwards, thus adding to the difficulty of palpation.

With the subject lying prone, the forehead resting on the backs of the hands, the chin tucked in slightly and the neck straight, begin the palpation by finding the external occipital protuberance (see page 151), with the raised crescentic superior nuchal lines curving laterally. Running inferiorly and under the back of the skull from the protuberance, the external occipital crest can be palpated, ending at a deep hollow, which is level with the tubercle of the atlas (not palpable). The hollow is bounded below by the large prominence of the spine of the axis; this is approximately 3 cm below the external occipital protuberance. The spine is easy to find and can be

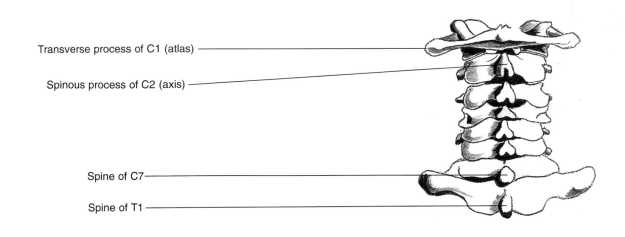

Transverse process of C1 (atlas) ————————

Spinous process of C2 (axis) ————————

Spine of C7————————

Spine of T1 ————————

Fig. 4.4 (b)
Bones of the neck (posterior aspect)

used for identification and location of other bony features.

Below, the spines of C3, 4 and 5 are closely packed together due to the curvature of the spine at this point. The spine of C3 lies close under the spine of C2 and is therefore difficult to palpate, the spine of C4 often being mistaken for that of C3.

Progress now to the lower part of the cervical spine, where two spinous processes can be felt projecting clearly. They are close together and rigid to the touch. The lower of the two is the spine of T1, that just above the spine of C7. The spine of C6 stands out clearly above that of C7 and can at times be mistaken for it. Differentiation between the spines of C6 and C7 can be carried out by asking the subject to extend the head and neck while keeping your finger on the spine of C6. It tends to move forward, causing it to disappear from beneath the palpating finger, while the spine of C7 remains stationary. Just above the spine of C6, that of C5 is identifiable, being very close to that of C4. It would be expected that flexion of the neck would improve identification. Unfortunately, except for the spines of C7 and T1, this is not the case as the tightening ligamentum nuchae hides the spines. The spines of C3, 4, 5 and 6, although difficult to identify separately, appear broad due to their bifid nature (Fig. 4.4).

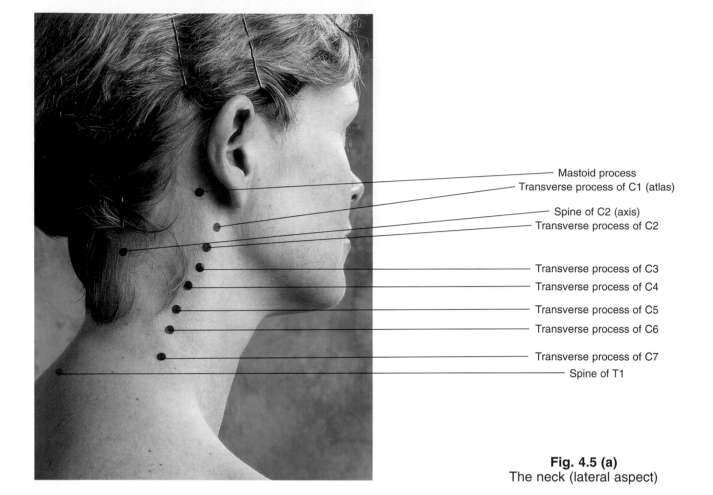

- Mastoid process
- Transverse process of C1 (atlas)

- Spine of C2 (axis)
- Transverse process of C2

- Transverse process of C3
- Transverse process of C4

- Transverse process of C5
- Transverse process of C6

- Transverse process of C7
- Spine of T1

Fig. 4.5 (a)
The neck (lateral aspect)

Lateral aspect [Fig. 4.5]

Although the transverse processes of the cervical vertebrae appear to project well out to the side, they are in fact quite difficult to palpate and identify. It is possible to palpate the tip of the transverse process of C1 between the angle of the mandible and the tip of the mastoid process. In some subjects the transverse process of C1 is not only palpable, but visible, as a small prominence. In others, it is difficult to identify even on deep palpation. This region can be quite tender if too much pressure is applied, and care must be taken to avoid the long and narrow styloid process just deep and anterior to the mastoid process.

The other transverse processes, with the exception of C2, present a double point laterally, the anterior and posterior tubercles, but owing to muscle attachments and fascial coverings they are not easy to distinguish. With the subject in prone lying, the line of the transverse processes can be identified from the back by easing the fingers into the side of the neck some 2 cm anterior to the tips of the spines. With care, the lower articular pillar of the vertebra above can be palpated immediately medial to each posterior tubercle. This is at the inferior limit of the facet (zygapophyseal) joint. Pressure on this tubercle will produce compression of the facet joint, whereas pressure just below the tubercle will produce an anterior movement of the lower articular pillar and slight gapping of the joint surfaces.

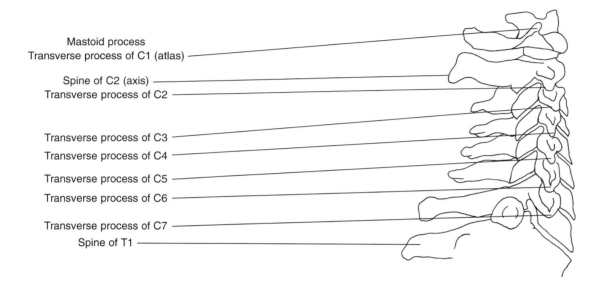

Mastoid process
Transverse process of C1 (atlas)
Spine of C2 (axis)
Transverse process of C2
Transverse process of C3
Transverse process of C4
Transverse process of C5
Transverse process of C6
Transverse process of C7
Spine of T1

Fig. 4.5 (b)
Bones of the neck (lateral aspect)

Normally the thick muscles covering the transverse processes need to be moved aside to facilitate palpation. More 'feel' of the transverse processes is available if the subject adopts a supine position with the occiput cradled in the hands of the examiner who stands at the head of the plinth facing the subject's feet. With the fingers of either hand resting on the posterolateral part of the neck, the head is moved from side to side, the axis of movement being an anteroposterior axis through the lower skull. Apply gentle pressure to the transverse process with your fingers on the opposite side to that being examined. This opens up the side of interest with the space between the transverse processes increasing, facilitating their identification. The facet joints of this side are also being gapped, causing a greater convexity to the side being examined. It will be noticed that slight rotation to the opposite side will occur during this movement (see Fig. 4.7a, b). This technique can be used from C1 down to T1. In the lower section of the neck these transverse processes can be palpated from the front, although it is slightly uncomfortable. Occasionally, the costal element (the anterior segment of the transverse process) of C7 projects more anterolaterally than usual and can be palpated 2 cm above and 2 cm lateral to the medial end of the clavicle. This is often referred to as a 'cervical rib'.

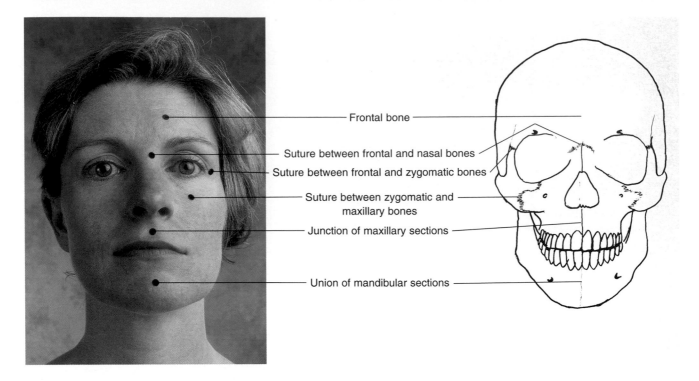

Fig. 4.6 (a), (b)
The joints of the head (anterior aspect)

The labels in the figure read:
- Frontal bone
- Suture between frontal and nasal bones
- Suture between frontal and zygomatic bones
- Suture between zygomatic and maxillary bones
- Junction of maxillary sections
- Union of mandibular sections

JOINTS

The skull [Fig. 4.6]

Most of the plates of bone which contribute to the vault of the skull are united by fibrous joints in the form of sutures. These are often visible on the surface and were described and palpated in the section on bones (see pages 150, 151). Other suture lines which can be palpated are those between the parietal and temporal bones, between the temporal and zygomatic bones and between the two halves of the mandibles.

The first suture lies at the upper edge of the squamous portion of the temporal bone. It arches convexly upwards from the depression just lateral to the eye orbit to just anterior to the upper part of the pinna of the ear. If the subject clenches the teeth the temporalis muscle can be palpated contracting above the zygomatic arch (see page 153). At the curved upper part of this muscle, the line of the suture can be identified.

The second suture can be palpated approximately halfway along the zygomatic arch. If the finger is run anteroposteriorly, the suture can be felt as a raised ridge crossing the arch vertically. The third can be palpated between the two halves of the mandible, running vertically downwards from the centre of the lower lip to the inferior border between the two mental tubercles. It is often marked by a sharp ridge.

Accessory movements of the joints of the skull

In the unborn child and infant these plates of bone can allow considerable movement and, on occasions, even override each other. There is slight movement throughout childhood and early adult life, but from the twenties through to middle age there is gradual fusion of the various sutures, beginning with the sagittal suture (Palastanga *et al.*, 1998). Some authorities believe that the movement of one plate of bone on another influences the structures below and can be used as a therapeutic technique.

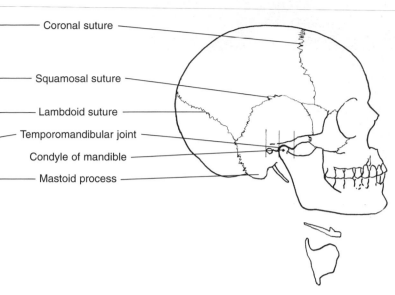

Coronal suture

Squamosal suture

Lambdoid suture

Temporomandibular joint

Condyle of mandible

Mastoid process

Fig. 4.6 (c), (d)
The joints of the head (lateral aspect)

The *temporomandibular joint* [*Fig. 4.6c and d*]

This is a bicondylar articulation taking place between the mandibular fossae of the temporal bone and the condylar processes of the mandible, the two joints being linked by the mandible.

Palpation

From the tragus of the ear, trace forwards under the posterior section of the zygomatic arch for 2 cm, where a small tubercle on the condyle of the mandible can be palpated. The line of the joint lies just above this tubercle, running forwards for approximately 2 cm concave downwards posteriorly and convex downwards anteriorly. If the subject opens the mouth, the line of the joint becomes clearer as the condyle first rotates and then moves forward on the under surface of the temporal bone.

Accessory movements

This joint is capable of many physiological movements, mainly involved in mastication. Its only true accessory movement, however, is distraction. This can be produced by placing the thumbs in the mouth on the lower molar teeth on both sides, with the fingers of each hand supporting the underside of the mandible from outside. Downward pressure is then applied to the teeth via the thumbs, using the fingers to hold the anterior part of the mandible stationary. This creates the necessary leverage to pull the condyles away from the temporal bone. Complete relaxation of the muscles of mastication is essential for any gapping to occur.

Fig. 4.7 (a)
Right lateral movement of the
cervical spine

Fig. 4.7 (b)
Left lateral movement of the
cervical spine

The cervical spine [Figs 4.7 and 4.8]

With the exception of the joints between the occiput
and C1, and C1 and C2, the cervical vertebrae articulate by a series of fibrous discs centrally, synovial
zygapophyseal joints between the articular processes laterally, and synovial uncovertebral joints
between the lateral margins of adjacent vertebral
bodies.

The occipital condyles either side of the foramen
magnum articulate with the facets on the superior
surface of the atlas (C1) as a bicondylar joint. The
atlas articulates with the axis (C2) via plane joints
either side of the dens and a single central pivot joint
between the dens and the anterior arch of the atlas,
in front, and with the transverse ligament, behind.
All of these are synovial joints.

Palpation

It is difficult to palpate any joints in the cervical
region owing to their depth and location. Movements of many can be achieved by pressure on the
bones that take part, but actual joint lines are normally impossible to determine and feel.

Find the articular pillars of C2–C7 lying 2 cm
lateral to the spines (see pages 158–159). With deep
but sensitive palpation, the lines of the lower zygapophyseal joints can be detected level with the tip of
the spinous process of the same vertebra.

Fig. 4.7 (c)
Anterior movement of the cervical spine

Fig. 4.7 (d)
Posterior movement of the cervical spine

Accessory movements

Traction on the cervical spine (C2–C7), either mechanically or manually, is a true accessory movement, as it is a movement that the subject cannot perform alone. It can be carried out in extension, flexion, rotation or any combination of these, depending on the results required. It produces parting of the surfaces of the zygapophyseal and central joints with a stretching of the disc, the surrounding ligaments and muscles. There will be a decrease in the pressure within the disc, and an increase in the size, particularly in flexion, of the intervertebral foramen, through which the cervical nerves emerge.

Traction on the joints between the occiput, C1 and C2 is best obtained when the neck is slightly extended. Its use, however, is normally restricted as it can produce undesirable and dangerous effects, due to the complex nature of these joints, particularly concerning the ligaments around the dens. The ligaments remain taut in all movements, thereby maintaining the relationship of the dens with the atlas and occiput. Accessory movement, necessary for gliding to occur, is only possible because of the precise curvatures of the articular surfaces.

With the subject lying supine, a sideways movement of the whole neck can be achieved by holding the head between the two hands and moving it from side to side while maintaining its longitudinal position (Fig. 4.7a, b).

A similar movement forwards and backwards can be achieved by placing one hand over the forehead and the other hand behind the occiput and moving the head forwards and backwards, again maintaining its longitudinal position (Fig. 4.7c, d).

Using a sagittal axis, passing through the nose, the side-to-side movement can be localized to the joints between the condyles of the occipital bone and the lateral masses of the atlas. Using a frontal axis through the centre of the skull, localized forward and backward gliding can also be achieved (Fig. 4.7c, d).

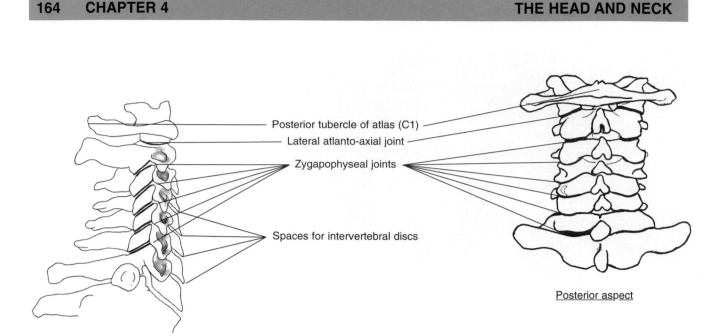

Posterior tubercle of atlas (C1)

Lateral atlanto-axial joint

Zygapophyseal joints

Spaces for intervertebral discs

Posterior aspect

Lateral aspect

Fig. 4.8 (a), (b)
Joints of the cervical spine

Other movements of the cervical vertebrae, often considered to be accessory movements, are very similar to normal physiological movements. Nevertheless, certain elements are exaggerated and therefore worthy of note.

With the subject lying prone, forward gliding of a whole vertebra on its neighbour can be achieved by pressure applied with the thumbs on the tip of the spinous process. Movement is greatest around C4 and least between C7 and T1. Pressure on the spine of C2 produces no movement between C1 and C2, as the dens is in contact with the anterior arch of C1; however, slight forward gliding will be achieved between the occiput and C1, due to the two bones moving together.

Pressure on the inferior articular pillar of C3–C7 produces a forward gliding of the inferior articular surface and a slight gapping of the superior zygapophyseal joint in a rotation-type movement. If a similar pressure is applied to the posterior aspect of the transverse process of C1, similar gliding of the lateral mass of that side against the occipital condyle and upper facet of C2 occurs.

With the subject lying supine, side-to-side movement of the vertebrae can be produced by cradling the head in the palms, as described on pages 162 and 163, with the fingers of one side applying pressure to the transverse process of the chosen vertebra. The fingers of the opposite side will then feel the transverse processes opening up, as an accompaniment to the gapping of the zygapophyseal joint.

Rotation of one vertebra on another can be taken to its limit by carefully fixing the lower vertebrae with the fingers and thumb and rotating

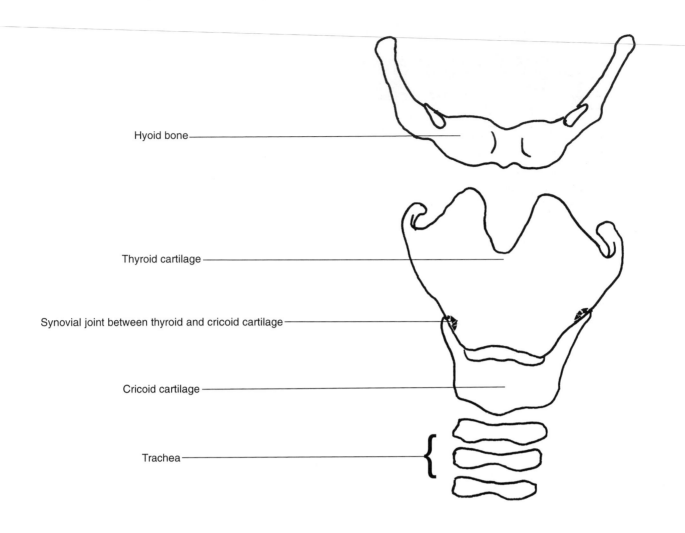

Hyoid bone

Thyroid cartilage

Synovial joint between thyroid and cricoid cartilage

Cricoid cartilage

Trachea

Fig. 4.8 (c)
Anterior structures of the neck

the head with the other hand. These movements can be produced between any two cervical vertebrae, and even to some extent between the occiput and C1, producing gapping of their surfaces.

Most accessory movements of the cervical spine are difficult to perform without a great deal of knowledge and practice. It can be highly dangerous for an unskilled therapist to employ these procedures in this area, and it is recommended that the student must be carefully monitored by an experienced practitioner, who should test for contra-indications prior to any movement being performed.

For further information, it is suggested that the reader consults the literature on manipulation and mobilization (Grieve, 1986; Maitland, 1991).

Anterior aspect of the neck

The hyoid bone and the thyroid and cricoid cartilages can all be moved from side to side approximately 1 cm using the finger and thumb alternately. They are linked by muscle and ligaments to the mandible and temporal bone above and the upper part of the trachea below.

Between the inferior cornua of the thyroid cartilage and the arch of the cricoid cartilage are small synovial joints which can be located just above the posterior projections of the cricoid cartilage. These possess a capsule and can, at times, give pain and distress when they become inflamed or degenerated.

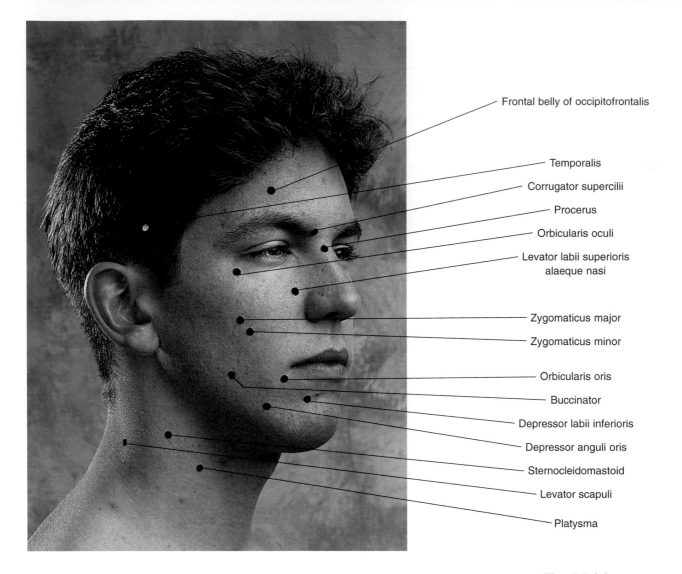

Frontal belly of occipitofrontalis

Temporalis

Corrugator supercilii

Procerus

Orbicularis oculi

Levator labii superioris
alaeque nasi

Zygomaticus major

Zygomaticus minor

Orbicularis oris

Buccinator

Depressor labii inferioris

Depressor anguli oris

Sternocleidomastoid

Levator scapuli

Platysma

Fig. 4.9 (a)
Muscles of the head and neck
(lateral aspect)

MUSCLES

Muscles of facial expression [Figs 4.9–4.11]

The muscles associated with the skull are mainly situated anteriorly, where they produce facial expressions, and laterally, where they produce the movements of mastication. The muscles are, however, very difficult to palpate unless they are contracting. Most muscles of the face arise from broad bony and fibrous attachments and pass to the fascia deep to the skin.

Their attachments at both ends are normally highly complex, sending fibres to blend with surrounding muscles, thus influencing the action which produces the many expressions possible in the human face. Because of this complexity only the basic attachments will be given in this text, but enough to demonstrate the action of the muscle.

Palpation

The muscle bellies of occipitofrontalis (Figs 4.9, 4.10a, b) attach superiorly via a fibrous aponeurotic sheet which passes over the scalp. Anteriorly the muscle attaches to the upper margin of the fascia over the eye orbit and posteriorly to the superior nuchal line. If the subject raises and lowers the eyebrow several times, the scalp can be felt moving forwards and backwards, with the posterior and anterior bellies contracting alternately.

Corrugator supercilii (Fig. 4.10c, d) can be palpated above the nose at the medial end of the eyebrow. If the subject frowns, short almost vertical ridges are produced as the muscle contracts.

Orbicularis oculi (Fig. 4.10e, f) closes the eye. The muscle can be palpated easily if the subject closes the eye and, with the examiner's fingers gently resting on the eyelids, the subject then squeezes the

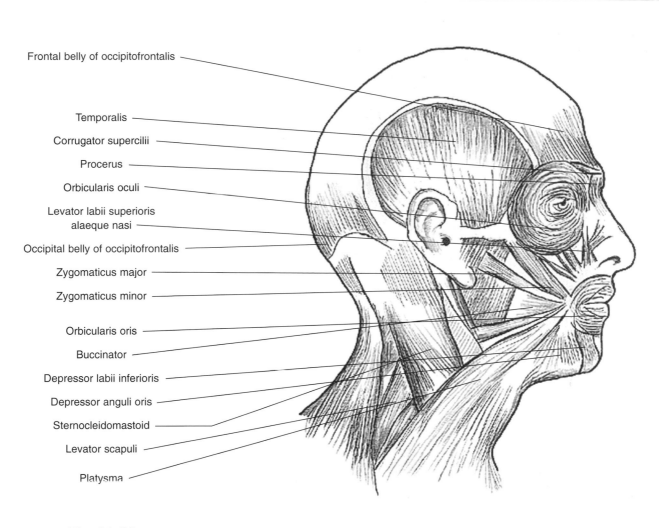

Frontal belly of occipitofrontalis

Temporalis

Corrugator supercilii

Procerus

Orbicularis oculi

Levator labii superioris
alaeque nasi

Occipital belly of occipitofrontalis

Zygomaticus major

Zygomaticus minor

Orbicularis oris

Buccinator

Depressor labii inferioris

Depressor anguli oris

Sternocleidomastoid

Levator scapuli

Platysma

Fig. 4.9 (b)
Muscles of the head and neck
(lateral aspect)

eyes shut tightly. A hard muscular covering can be felt.

If the fingers are placed over the corner of the nose and the upper lip when the subject sneers, the contraction of levator labii superioris alaeque nasi (Fig. 4.10g, h) can be felt. The alae of the nose will also be raised and move apart while the upper lip is raised at its centre.

When the subject smiles, the corners of the mouth are drawn upwards and laterally. This movement is produced by contraction of levator anguli oris and zygomaticus major and minor (Figs 4.9 and 4.11a, b) all of which are palpable between the angle of the mouth and the zygomatic bone (the point of the cheek).

Depressor anguli oris (Fig. 4.11c, d) can be palpated just below the angle of the mouth, particu-

larly when it is drawn downwards, as in the expression of sadness. Contraction of depressor labii inferioris (Fig. 4.11c, d) is palpable between the lower lip and the chin. It curls the whole lower lip downwards, thereby exposing the lower teeth.

If the lips are closed tightly, the hard ring of muscle surrounding the mouth, orbicularis oris (Fig. 4.11e, f) can be palpated and when the subject tries to blow through the closed mouth, contraction of buccinator (Fig. 4.11e, f) can be felt in the cheeks.

If the teeth are now clenched together, as in a 'snarling' expression, platysma (Fig. 4.11g, h) can be palpated anywhere between the mandible and the superior part of the chest. This muscle appears to expand the neck volume and is also brought into action when resistance is given to hands being tightened around the neck.

Occipitofrontalis

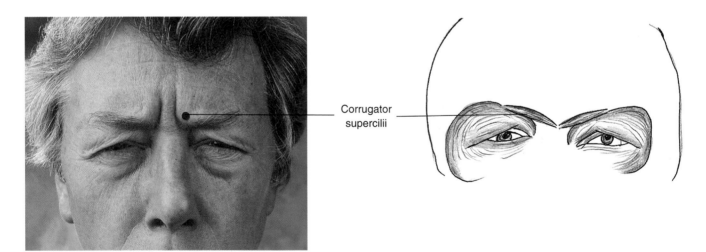

Fig. 4.10 (a), (b)
Muscles raising the eyebrows (surprise)

Frontal belly attaches to the fascia over the upper eye orbit. Posterior belly attaches to the lateral two-thirds of the superior nuchal line. Both bellies attach superiorly to the aponeurosis covering the scalp.

Corrugator supercilii

Fig. 4.10 (c), (d)
Muscles drawing the eyebrows together (frowning)

Medially attaches to bone at the medial end of the superciliary arch. Laterally attaches to the skin over mid point of the eye orbit.

Orbicularis oculi

Fig. 4.10 (e), (f)
Muscles closing the eyes

Elliptical muscle attaching to the bone surrounding the eye orbit.

Levator labii superioris alaeque nasi and levator labii superioris

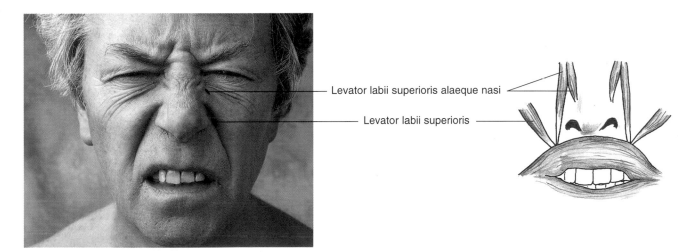

Fig. 4.10 (g), (h)
Muscles raising the upper lip and opening the nasal cavity (sneering)

Levator labii superioris alaeque nasi attaches above to the maxillary bone and below to the greater alar cartilage and skin covering it.

Levator labii superioris attaches above to the maxilla and zygomatic bone and below to the upper lip halfway between the angle of the mouth and the mid point.

Levator anguli oris

Levator labii superioris
Levator anguli oris

Fig. 4.11 (a), (b)
Muscles raising the corners of the mouth (smiling)

The levator anguli oris attaches above to canine fossa just below the infraorbital foramen of maxilla and attaches below to the corner of the mouth.

Depressor anguli oris and depressor labii inferioris

Depressor anguli oris
Depressor labii inferioris

Fig. 4.11 (c), (d)
Muscles pulling the corners of the mouth and lower lip downwards (indicating sadness)

Depressor anguli oris attaches to the mental tubercle of the mandible below and to the angle of the mouth above.

Depressor labii inferioris attaches below to the oblique line close to the mental foramen and above to the centre of the lower lip.

Orbicularis oris and buccinator

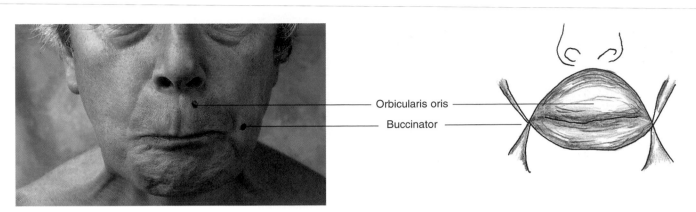

Fig. 4.11 (e), (f)
Muscles closing or pursing the lips

Orbicularis oris is a highly complex raphe of fibres surrounding the mouth composed of eight blending sections and functionally acting in four quadrants. In addition it receives fibres from all the surrounding muscles.

Buccinator basically attaches to the molar area of the maxilla and mandible. Its fibres pass forwards blending with the orbicularis oris, its upper fibres into the upper lip, its lower fibres into the lower lip, but its middle fibres crossing at the corners of the mouth.

Platysma

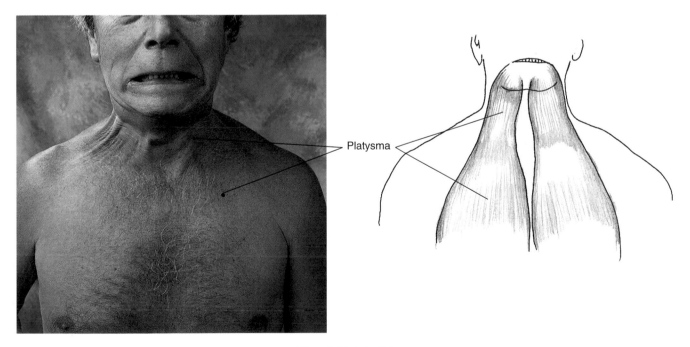

Fig. 4.11 (g), (h)
Muscles drawing fascia around the mouth downwards (protecting the structures in the neck and producing a snarling expression).

Attaches below to the fascia covering the upper part of pectoralis major and deltoid. Above it attaches to the inferior border of the mandible with some of its lateral fibres passing over to the lower lip and its medial fibres crossing over to the opposite side.

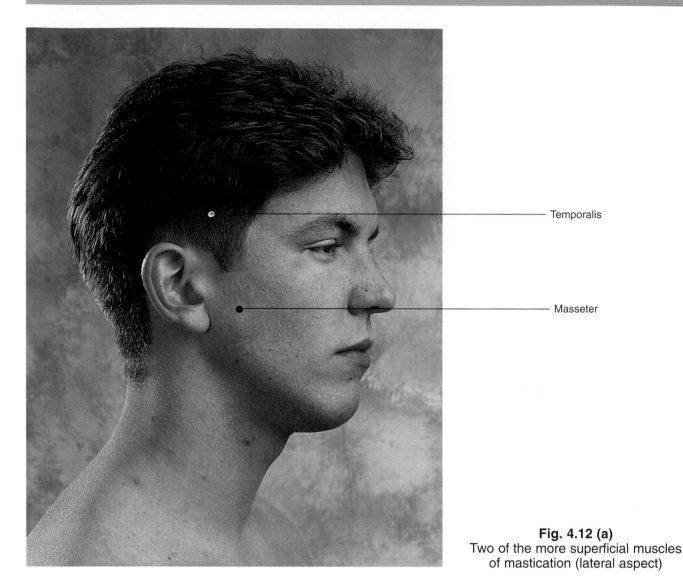

Temporalis

Masseter

Fig. 4.12 (a)
Two of the more superficial muscles
of mastication (lateral aspect)

Muscles of mastication [Fig. 4.12]

These are powerful muscles situated more deeply on the lateral side of the face. Temporalis is a fan-shaped muscle attaching above to the lateral side of the temporal bone, reaching as high as the suture between it and the parietal bone. The muscle passes down under the zygomatic arch to the coronoid process of the mandible. Masseter attaches above to the zygomatic arch, its fibres passing downwards and backwards to attach to the lateral surface of the mandible close to its angle.

The medial and lateral pterygoid lie deep to the upper part of the ramus and coronoid of the mandible. The medial pterygoid attaches above to the medial side of the lateral pterygoid plate and palatine bone to pass downwards and backwards to the medial side of the ramus and angle of the mandible. The lateral pterygoid attaches above to the lateral side of the lateral pterygoid plate and the temporal bone and passes backwards to attach to the neck of the mandible and the capsule and disc of the temporomandibular joint.

Palpation

With the fingers placed just above the zygomatic arch, alternately clench and relax the teeth. Although hidden to a certain extent by the thick fascia which covers it, the contraction of the fan-shaped belly of temporalis can be palpated. Passing almost vertically deep to the zygomatic arch to the mandible, its fibres become too deep to palpate.

The same action with the fingers over the side of the mandible just above and in front of the angle enables the powerful masseter muscle to be felt contracting and relaxing. A series of ridges can be palpated, indicating the direction and power of its fibres. In some subjects, particularly lean males, the coarse muscle fibres can be seen crossing the side of the jaw obliquely. The lower fibres can be traced as far as the lower border of the mandible, inferiorly, and the anterior end of the zygomatic arch superiorly.

Parietal bone

Temporalis

Zygomatic arch

Masseter

Angle of the mandible

Fig. 4.12 (b)
Two of the more superficial muscles
of mastication (lateral aspect)

Palpation of the medial and lateral pterygoid muscles is impossible, as they are too deeply situated.

It will be noted that the temporalis and the masseter muscles are concerned with closing the mouth and with powerful biting. Although the mandible acts as a third-order lever in the initial bite, as the food moves backwards between the molars it changes so that the food is first in line with the muscle pull and then nearer to the temporo-mandibular joint than the muscles. The mandible then becomes a second-order lever, with its decrease in range but increase in power. It is at this point that the act of chewing takes place.

Give the subject a piece of steak to eat, for example, and while he or she is doing so place your fingers over the posterior part of the cheeks. As the steak makes its way backwards, the muscles contract harder and the jaw moves from side to side in a grinding action utilizing the pterygoid muscles. If the steak is tough, these muscles will ache.

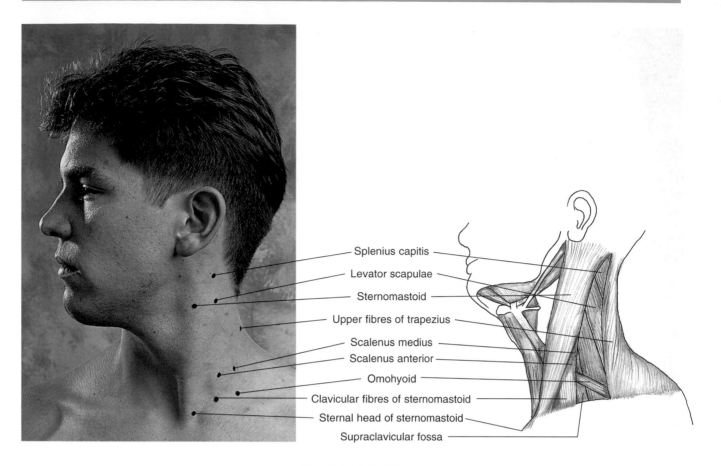

Splenius capitis
Levator scapulae
Sternomastoid
Upper fibres of trapezius
Scalenus medius
Scalenus anterior
Omohyoid
Clavicular fibres of sternomastoid
Sternal head of sternomastoid
Supraclavicular fossa

Fig. 4.13 (a), (b)
Muscles of the neck (lateral aspect, posterior group)

Muscles of the neck [Fig. 4.13]

The neck is surrounded by layers of muscle. These vary in their function which may include moving the neck itself, moving the head, mastication, swallowing and moving the shoulder girdle. Some are involved in a combination of several of these functions.

The more superficial muscles tend to be the more powerful and are therefore easier to find and palpate. However, because of their size they do tend to cover the smaller, deeper muscles.

Some of the muscles are only attached to different parts of the vertebral column, some attach the column to the head and thoracic cage. Others, usually the longer, attach to the head and the thoracic cage. All the attachments are complex, but have a direct bearing on the resultant movement and function. All attachments are essential knowledge in anatomy, and further study must be made beyond this palpation and surface marking text (see *Anatomy and Human Movement*, Palastanga et al.,1998; *Gray's Anatomy*, Williams et al., 1995).

Palpation

With the subject sitting, place your hands over the posterosuperior area of the neck, halfway between the occiput and the acromion process. When the subject raises the pectoral girdle, as in a shrugging movement, the powerful upper fibres of trapezius (Fig. 4.13a, b) can be felt contracting. The muscle can be traced superiorly to its aponeurotic attachment to the medial third of the superior nuchal line, external occipital protuberance and the sides of the ligamentum nuchae. Inferiorly it can be traced to its attachments to the posterior border of the lateral third clavicle, medial border of the acromion and lateral part upper lip of the spine of the scapula. The central muscular fibres sometimes appear to be stringy and are often quite tender, particularly after a period of sustained activity.

Sternomastoid (sternocleidomastoid) (Fig. 4.13a, b) attaches to the mastoid process above, and the upper surface of the medial end of the clavicle and upper border of the sternum below. To palpate the muscles, place your fingers over the lower attachment. When the subject turns the head to the

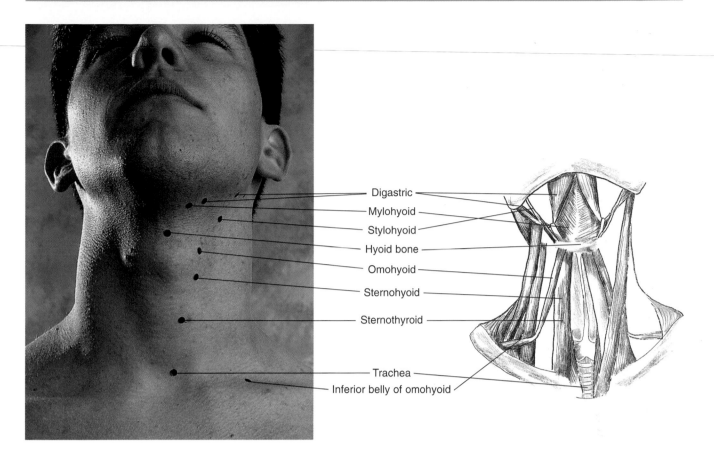

Digastric
Mylohyoid
Stylohyoid
Hyoid bone
Omohyoid
Sternohyoid
Sternothyroid

Trachea
Inferior belly of omohyoid

Fig. 4.13 (c), (d)
Muscles of the neck (anterior aspect, anterior group)

opposite side, two distinct attachments can be felt, one more cord-like from the sternum and the other more aponeurotic from the clavicle. These appear to twist on each other as they are traced upwards. The thick strap-like sternomastoid stands away from the neck when contracted. It becomes cord-like again as it approaches and attaches to the mastoid process, spreading as a sheet to the lateral part of the superior nuchal line. Both sternomastoid muscles contract strongly and are easily palpable if the subject raises the head when lying supine. (Contraction of both sternomastoid and trapezius can be produced by resisting movement of the head and neck to the same side – lateral flexion – or rotating the head to the opposite side.)

The scalene muscles (Fig. 4.13a, b) lie just behind and deep to sternomastoid, and with the subject seated can be palpated deep in the hollow between it and the upper fibres of trapezius in the posterior triangle of the neck. These cord-like muscles, running down to attach to the first and second ribs, appear to be continuously contracted while the head

is in the upright position. During coughing, it is often possible to palpate the inferior belly of the omohyoid muscle (Fig. 4.13a, b) as it crosses the lower anterior part of the posterior triangle of the neck. Posterosuperior to this is scalenus anterior, and a little higher, scalenus medius. On elevation of the pectoral girdle, the fibres of levator scapulae can be palpated nearer the top of the posterior triangle (Fig. 4.13a, b).

During swallowing, the muscles between the mandible, hyoid, thyroid cartilage and sternum contract and relax. Consequently, if the fingers are placed on either side of the throat between the mandible and the hyoid during swallowing, mylohyoid can be observed contracting and lifting the hyoid bone (Fig. 4.13c, d).

Sternohyoid is difficult to palpate during swallowing, but in yawning its fibres can be observed on either side of the thyroid cartilage passing downwards towards the sternum.

Fig. 4.14 (a), (b)
Cutaneous supply of the head and neck (lateral aspect)

NERVES [Fig. 4.14]

The cutaneous innervation of the face, including forehead, is by the cranial nerves, mainly by the ophthalmic, maxillary and mandibular branches of the trigeminal. The occipital, temporal and posterior part of the parietal regions are supplied by the greater auricular, and greater and lesser occipital, branches of the cervical plexus. The neck is supplied almost entirely through the anterior and posterior rami of the cervical nerve roots, via the transverse cutaneous and supraclavicular branches of cervical plexus (Fig. 4.14a, b). The muscles of facial expression are supplied by the facial nerve (cranial VII), the muscles of mastication via the mandibular branch of the trigeminal (cranial V). All the muscles of the neck are supplied by the cervical nerve roots via the cervical or brachial plexuses. Some of these roots receive communication from other cranial nerves, for example the glossopharyngeal (cranial IV), accessory (cranial XI) and hypoglossal (cranial XII).

Palpation

Very few nerves are palpable in the head and neck region. Usually only the terminal branches reach the surface and even these are difficult to find. Posteriorly it is possible to palpate the greater occipital nerve (root value C2) as it passes vertically to supply the skin over the back of the skull as far forwards as the vertex (Fig. 4.14a, b). This cord-like structure can be palpated over the lower part of the occipital bone approximately 3 cm from the midline. Pressure on the nerve either by the examiner's fingers or muscle tension due to poor posture, or long periods of continuous contraction, can lead to unpleasant sensations and headaches. Care should, therefore, be taken with this examination procedure. Massage to relieve the tension of the muscles surrounding the nerve can produce almost immediate relief from the resulting headache.

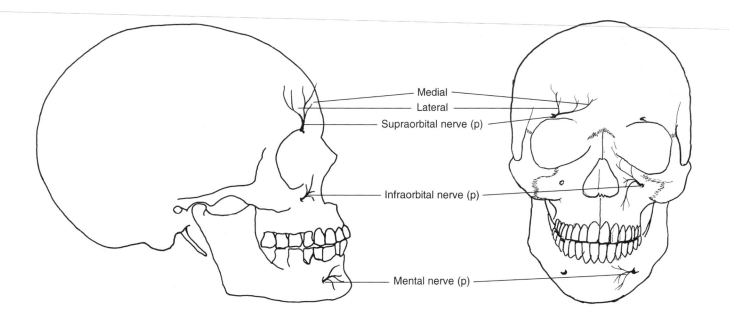

Fig. 4.14 (c), (d)
Cutaneous branches emerging onto the face (lateral and anterior aspect) (p, palpable)

Pressure on the **supraorbital nerve** as it crosses the superomedial rim of the orbit and on the **infra-orbital nerve** as it emerges from the maxilla just below the centre of the eye orbit (Fig. 4.14c, d) causes discomfort over these areas and the area supplied by the nerves. They are, however, quite difficult to palpate.

On the anterior surface of the mandible, approximately 1 cm lateral to the midline and approximately 1 cm above the inferior border, the **mental nerve**, a continuation of the inferior dental nerve, emerges on to the surface (Fig. 4.14c, d). The nerve is often palpable in this region, and if pressure is applied to the area an unpleasant feeling is experienced by the subject. It is worth noting that this is the area which appears to become numb first when the dentist gives an anaesthetic injection for drilling the bottom teeth. Just above the central part of the clavicle in the supraclavicular fossa, a series of 'cord-like' structures can be palpated running downwards and laterally. These are the trunks of the brachial plexus emerging from between scalenus anterior and scalenus medius before passing deep to the clavicle to enter the axilla. Pressure in this area will cause discomfort locally and possibly also result in a 'tingling', pain or numbness over the distri-bution of these nerves in the upper limb.

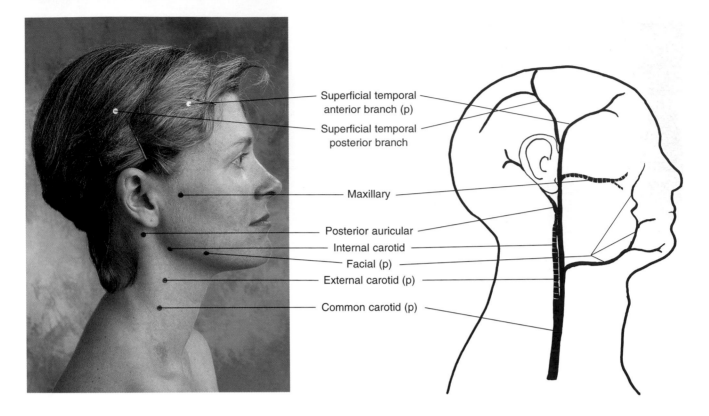

Fig. 4.15 (a), (b)
Main arteries of the head and neck, lateral aspect (p, palpable)

ARTERIES [Fig. 4.15]

The left common carotid artery arises from the arch of the aorta, while the right is a division of the brachiocephalic artery. They pass up on either side of the neck deep to sternomastoid to the level of the upper border of the thyroid cartilage, where each divides into the internal and external carotid arteries.

The former passes superiorly, anterior to the upper three transverse processes, to enter the skull through the carotid canal. Each supplies the cerebral hemisphere, orbit and nose of its own side.

The external carotid artery passes vertically from the upper border of the thyroid cartilage, deep to the parotid gland behind the ramus of the mandible, where it divides into the superficial temporal and maxillary arteries (Fig. 4.15a, b).

Palpation

The common carotid artery can be palpated on either side of the thyroid cartilage deep to sternomastoid. The muscle has to be moved laterally so that the fingers can be slipped from the anterior aspect into the cleft between the cartilage and the muscle. On the lateral side of the upper part of the thyroid cartilage, close to the greater cornua of the hyoid bone, the pulsations of the artery, as it divides, can easily be palpated. This point is important for checking the pulsations of the carotid arteries and is worth spending some time practising.

Between the tragus of the ear and the neck of the mandible the pulsations of the superficial temporal artery can be felt. If the fingers are placed above the upper limit of temporalis again the superficial temporal artery can be palpated. The maxillary artery, just below the zygomatic bone, is not quite so obvious as it is covered by muscle and fascia, although to the practised professional it is palpable running anteriorly.

The facial artery (Fig. 4.15a, b) can be palpated as it crosses the lower border of the body of the mandible, halfway between the angle of the mandible and the mental tubercle. With care, it can be traced upwards to the corner of the mouth and

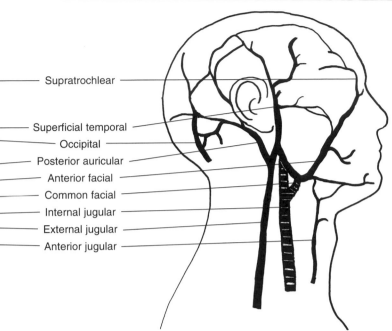

Fig. 4.16 (a), (b)
Veins of the nead and neck (lateral aspect)

cheek. Finally, above the eye the pulsations of the supraorbital artery can be palpated as it crosses the medial superior margin of the orbit. It is at this point that injuries, particularly in the sport of boxing, occur. The artery is often ruptured and large quantities of blood pulse out on to the eye and face. It is worth remembering that if pressure were applied to this point for just a few minutes, this loss of blood would cease and the area could be cleaned up, exposing the injury which is usually just a minor trauma.

VEINS [Fig. 4.16]

The veins of the head, neck, and face are divided into two main groups: (a) those that drain the exterior of the cranium and deep tissues of the face, and (b) those that drain the brain, the neck and the superficial areas of the face. The former mainly drain into the external jugular vein, while the latter mainly drain into the internal jugular.

Palpation

None of these veins is easy to palpate. The lower part of the external jugular contains two sets of valves 4 cm apart, the lower as it joins the subclavian vein. The valves do not prevent regurgitation of blood, and the area between the two sets often bulges and is termed 'the sinus'.

The surface marking of the external jugular is from the angle of the mandible to the middle of the clavicle.

The surface marking of the internal jugular vein can be marked by a broad line drawn from the lobe of the ear to the medial end of the clavicle. It also contains a valve at its junction with the subclavian vein and is often distended just above; however, this lies deep to sternocleidomastoid and cannot be palpated.

5

The thorax

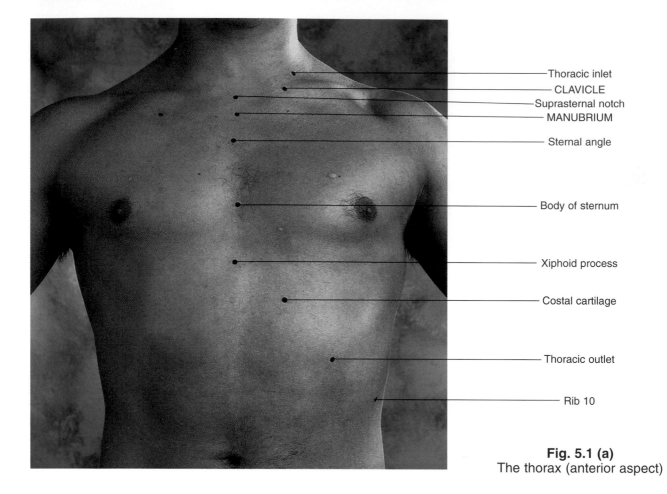

Thoracic inlet
CLAVICLE
Suprasternal notch
MANUBRIUM
Sternal angle
Body of sternum
Xiphoid process
Costal cartilage
Thoracic outlet
Rib 10

Fig. 5.1 (a)
The thorax (anterior aspect)

BONES

The thoracic cage

The bony structure of the thoracic cage consists of the sternum [*stereos* (Gk) = solid, hard], anteriorly, the twelve thoracic vertebrae [vertebra (L) = joint; from verto-I turn] posteriorly, the first being the smallest and the twelfth the largest (Figs 5.2–5.4), and the twelve ribs on either side linking the vertebrae with the sternum. The sternum is angled forward at the manubriosternal joint and angled backwards at the xiphisternal joint, forming a concavity backwards. The ribs are concave inwards and the vertebral column is concave forwards in this region. This forms a large cavity for the protection of vital organs such as the heart and lungs.

The rib spaces are filled with a musculofibrous sheet made up of the intercostal muscles and membrane forming a sealed unit in front, to the sides and behind. There are, however, openings at the top and bottom. The former is smaller and consists of the first thoracic vertebra posteriorly, the first rib on either side and the manubrium anteriorly. This is termed the 'thoracic inlet'. Below there is a much larger opening, termed the 'thoracic outlet', which consists of the twelfth thoracic vertebra posteriorly,

the xiphoid anteriorly and the costal cartilages of ribs 7, 8, 9 and 10, the tip of rib 11 and the full length of rib 12.

The sternum

The sternum lies centrally at the front of the chest and comprises three flat plates of bone, the manubrium [*manubrium* (L) = a handle; the sternum, as a whole, resembles a sword] superiorly, the body centrally and the pointed xiphoid [*xiphos* (Gk) = a sword] process inferiorly. The xiphoid usually remains cartilaginous until approximately the age of 40 years.

The clavicle and scapula

The clavicle lies almost horizontal, articulating with the superolateral part of the manubrium. Posterolaterally the scapula rests on the second to eighth ribs, with the acromion at the lateral end of the spine articulating with the lateral end of the clavicle at the acromioclavicular joint (Fig. 2.7).

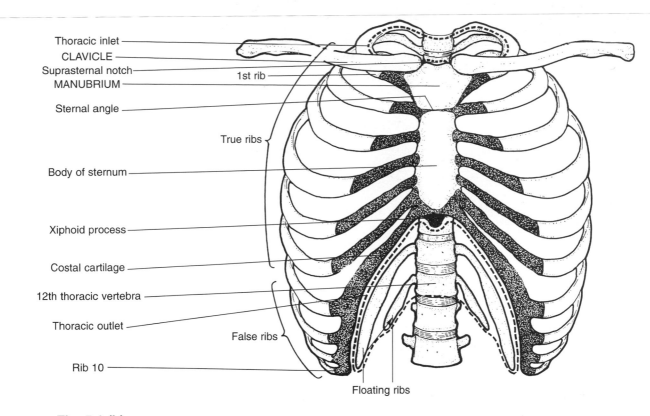

Thoracic inlet
CLAVICLE
Suprasternal notch
MANUBRIUM
1st rib
Sternal angle
True ribs
Body of sternum
Xiphoid process
Costal cartilage
12th thoracic vertebra
Thoracic outlet
False ribs
Rib 10
Floating ribs

Fig. 5.1 (b)
Bones of the thorax (anterior aspect)

Palpation

Find the suprasternal notch at the upper border of the manubrium (Fig. 5.1a, b). On either side, the medial ends of the clavicle project above the line of the manubrium. Just below the medial end of the clavicle, the manubrium appears to be enlarged laterally. This is actually the anterior end of the first rib and, with careful palpation, the joint between it and the manubrium can be located running vertically, concave laterally 1 cm below and 1 cm lateral to the medial end of the clavicle. Trace down the anterior surface of the manubrium until you find a raised horizontal line; this is where it joins the body of the sternum at the manubriosternal (sternal angle) joint (Fig. 5.1a, b). The reflex angle between the manubrium and body of the sternum is of the order of 200°, changing some 5–7° between full inspiration and full expiration. On either side of the manubriosternal junction the costal cartilages of the second

ribs can be palpated, with the lateral border of the manubrium just above.

Continue to trace down either side of the sternum and identify the third to sixth ribs and their costal cartilages, with the lateral border of the sternum lying between their medial ends. The sternum narrows inferiorly and usually dips inwards to join the cartilaginous xiphoid process. The costal cartilage of the seventh rib usually articulates with the sternum at the xiphisternal junction. The whole of the sternum is subcutaneous and is commonly used to take samples of bone marrow. The xiphoid process varies in its formation; it may appear to be pointed, double pointed or even rounded. Normally it projects forwards and therefore can easily be palpated. Occasionally it projects downwards and backwards and is then difficult to palpate.

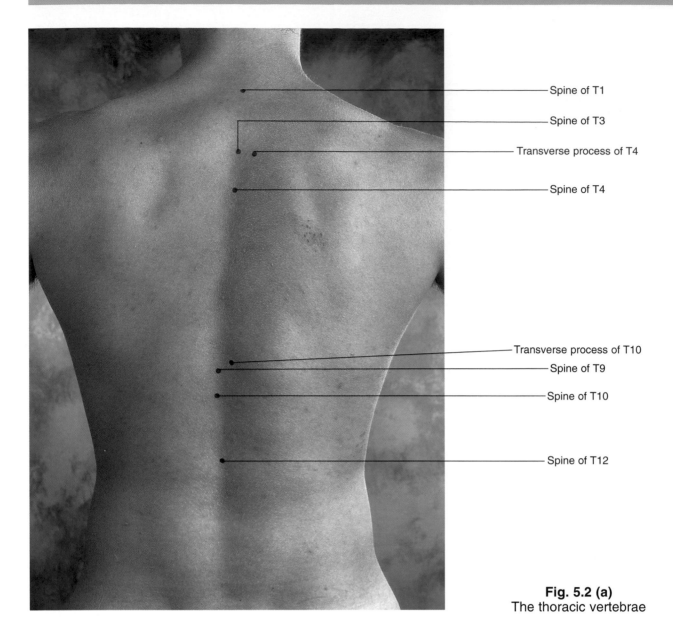

Fig. 5.2 (a)
The thoracic vertebrae

The vertebrae

The thoracic part of the vertebral column can only be palpated posteriorly, where it presents spines and transverse processes. However, these either overlap each other or are covered with strong, thick muscles and fascia, proving difficult even for the experienced palpator to identify with ease.

The spines form a line of tubercles down the midline of the thorax. They are not uniform in length, but pass downwards and backwards with a tendency to overlap the spine below. Those near the upper part of the thorax have their tips level with the upper surface of the vertebral body below, while the lower half have longer spines which reach to the lower border of the vertebra below. The tip of the spine of T3 is roughly level with the root of the spine of the scapula, and that of T7 level with the inferior angle of the scapula. The spine of T12 is not typical, as it is squared posteriorly and resembles that of a lumbar vertebra; it is level with the disc between T12 and L1. Accurate location of these spines must therefore be carried out by palpation, normally, counting down from an identifiable point above or below.

The transverse processes are much more difficult to palpate as they are covered by strong, thick muscles even in the thinner subject. The tips of the transverse processes are level with the upper border of their own vertebral body (Fig. 5.2).

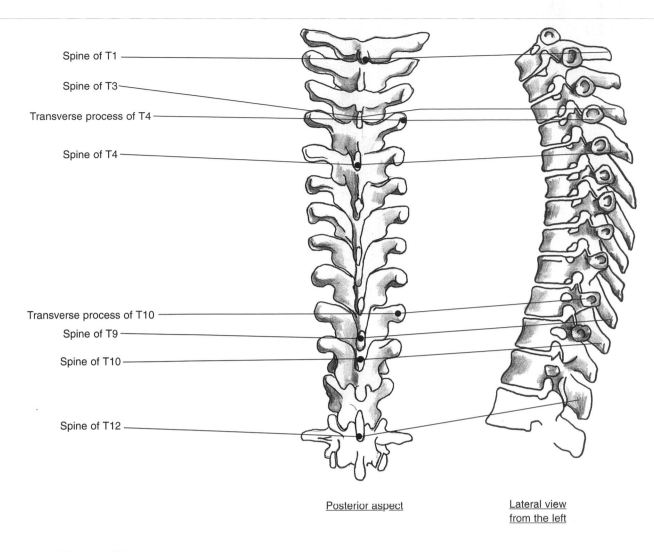

Spine of T1
Spine of T3
Transverse process of T4
Spine of T4
Transverse process of T10
Spine of T9
Spine of T10
Spine of T12

Posterior aspect

Lateral view
from the left

Fig. 5.2 (b)
The thoracic vertebrae

Palpation

With the subject in slump sitting, and rounding the back by placing the chin on the chest, the tips of the spines become more identifiable. Find the spines of C7 and T1, these being the two most prominent spines at the base of the neck.

With great care, count down the tips of the spines, being sure to mark the upper spine with the fingers of one hand while seeking the spine below with the other. Each spine will appear quite pointed until the level of T12, where a flattened appearance is noted, being similar to that of a lumbar spine. If palpation is difficult, use the technique suggested on page 5, where the fingertips are moved rapidly up and down the spine, in a scanning manner. This type of palpation is a useful method of locating and mapping structures which lie below the surface. It is rarely used, as it gives the impression of merely moving the skin on the underlying structures. It amounts to the building up of a total picture by adding together many disparate bits of information.

Use the pads of all fingers of one hand, the most sensitive if possible, to sweep across an area, allowing the fingers to move the skin and superficial fascia on the deeper structures. The palpator will be building up a picture in a similar manner to the scanning beam of a video camera. The other hand will be used to mark certain points and mark from where the previous information was obtained. Finer palpatory techniques can then be used on selected areas.

The lateral tips of the transverse processes lie 3 cm lateral and parallel to the spines. The tip of the spine, however, lies 1 cm below the level of the transverse process of the vertebra below. This measurement remains constant because the shorter spines in the upper thorax are compensated for by the transverse processes being slightly raised. Lateral to the tips of the transverse processes is a groove marking the line of the costotransverse joints.

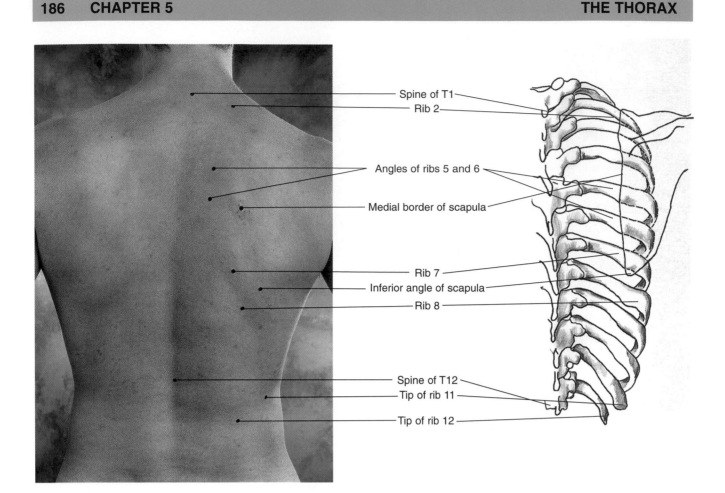

Fig. 5.3 (a), (b)
The ribs of the right side (posterior aspect)

The ribs

There are 12 ribs on either side, convex outwards, the eighth being the longest and the twelfth the shortest. The upper seven ribs articulate with the vertebral bodies and transverse processes posteriorly by the facets on their heads and tubercles. The first, tenth, **eleventh** and **twelfth** ribs have only one facet, the rest two. The eleventh and twelfth ribs have no tubercles. The ribs articulate with the sternum anteriorly via a varying length of costal cartilage. These are termed **'true' ribs**. The three ribs immediately below that are the eighth to tenth, which articulate anteriorly via their costal cartilage with the costal cartilage above, and are termed **'false' ribs**. The two lowest ribs do not articulate with their transverse process posteriorly and are free anteriorly and are therefore termed **'floating' ribs** (Fig. 5.1).

Palpation

To enable the back muscles to relax, the subject is best examined in a prone-lying position. Just lateral to the tip of each transverse process the posterior section of each rib can be palpated, being separated from the transverse process by a depression. With the subject's arm hanging over the side of the couch (i.e. the pectoral girdle in protraction), find and trace the first to tenth ribs laterally. The rib angle lies approximately 3–4 cm lateral to the tips of the transverse processes and can readily be palpated in the mid-thoracic region, becoming less clear above and below. The first rib does not possess an angle and those of the eleventh and twelfth ribs are slight if present.

Each rib, together with the intercostal spaces above and below, can be traced anteriorly to where it joins the sternum. The second to seventh or eighth

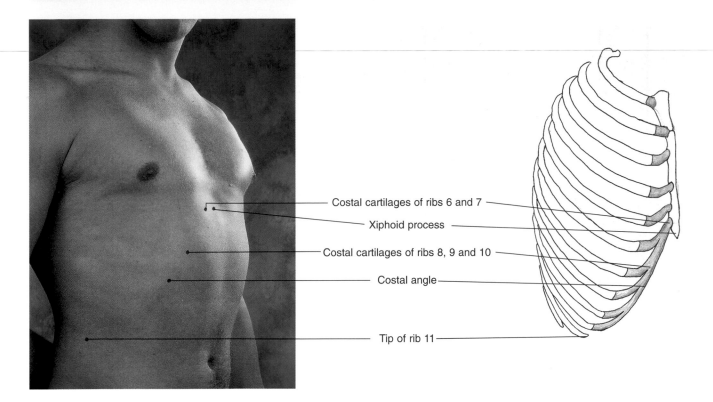

Costal cartilages of ribs 6 and 7

Xiphoid process

Costal cartilages of ribs 8, 9 and 10

Costal angle

Tip of rib 11

Fig. 5.3 (c), (d)
The ribs of the right side (lateral
aspect)

ribs are usually hidden posterolaterally by the scapula, while the eleventh and twelfth ribs only exist posterolaterally.

The first rib is the most difficult to palpate. It lies deep to the clavicle anteriorly, and deep to trapezius and levator scapulae posteriorly. If deep pressure is applied immediately below the clavicle, 1 cm lateral to its medial end, the junction of the rib with the manubrium can be palpated.

Above the middle of the clavicle in the supraclavicular fossa, it is possible, using deep pressure, to feel the lateral border of the first rib, but this area is particularly tender and may produce unpleasant reactions in the upper limb due to pressure on the trunks of the brachial plexus and subclavian artery.

Posteriorly, the neck and tubercle of the first rib can be palpated running downwards and laterally approximately 2 cm lateral to the tip of the spine of the seventh cervical vertebra. This, however, is dependent on the thickness of the upper fibres of trapezius.

The costal cartilages at the anterior end of the eighth to tenth ribs form the anterior part of the costal margin, running superomedially to join the xiphoid process. At the level of the ninth costal cartilage an angle and projection are formed, the 'costal angle'. This lies on a level with the trans-pyloric plane, in common with the spine of L1 and the tip of the twelfth rib. Just above the twelfth, the eleventh rib can easily be identified, ending in a point just anterior to the mid-axillary line.

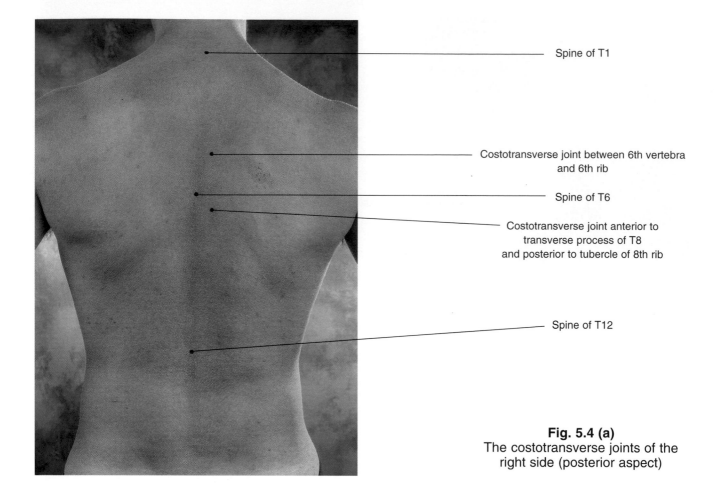

Spine of T1

Costotransverse joint between 6th vertebra and 6th rib

Spine of T6

Costotransverse joint anterior to transverse process of T8 and posterior to tubercle of 8th rib

Spine of T12

Fig. 5.4 (a)
The costotransverse joints of the right side (posterior aspect)

JOINTS

The thoracic vertebral column [Fig. 5.4]

The joints of the thoracic vertebral column are similar to those in the cervical region except that there are no uncovertebral joints and there are facets on the side of the bodies and tubercles (except eleven and twelve), for the articulation of the ribs. The vertebral bodies articulate centrally, by a series of intervertebral discs, which are complex cartilaginous symphyses made up of an outer ring of fibrous bands passing obliquely from one body to the other (the annulus fibrosus) and a central nucleus (the nucleus pulposus) composed of a soft highly hydrophilic substance. These discs are supported by many ligaments including the very strong anterior and posterior longitudinal ligaments.

On either side there are the **zygapophyseal joints** (Fig. 5.4d, e) between the articular facets, two above and two below. In addition there are the **costovertebral joints** (Fig. 5.4c), between the heads of the ribs and the side(s) of the body of the vertebrae and the **costotransverse joints**, between the tubercle of the rib and the transverse process (Fig. 5.4a–c). The zygapophyseal, costovertebral and costotransverse joints are all synovial, surrounded by a capsule which is lined with synovial membrane and supported by ligaments. (For detailed study refer to Palastanga et al., 1998.)

Palpation

All but the costotransverse and possibly the zygapophyseal joints are impossible to palpate. The costotransverse joints lie in the furrow between the transverse processes and the ribs and can be located either by following backwards along the line of a known rib to the point where it is obscured by the transverse process or by finding the tip of the spinous process of a known vertebra and tracing out laterally to the furrow mentioned above. Due to the length of the spines in the thoracic area the transverse process you can feel is that of the vertebra below.

The joints between the articular facets lie at the upper edge of the lamina as it meets the lamina above. The joint is virtually impossible to palpate, but the lamina can be traced a little laterally from the spines if the model is completely relaxed in prone lying and the fingers are slipped down the side of the spinous process. It must be remembered, however, that the lamina you feel is that of the vertebra below. The use of quick, gliding movements of the fingers (see page 5) and positioning the model with the spine in flexion will aid palpation.

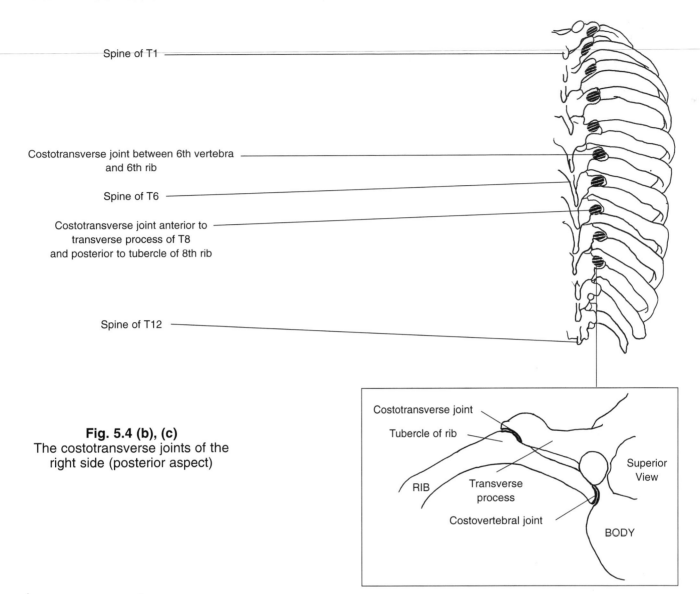

Fig. 5.4 (b), (c)
The costotransverse joints of the
right side (posterior aspect)

Accessory movements

As stated above, pressure on the lamina of one vertebra can part the zygapophyseal joint surfaces above and compress those below on the ipsilateral side (Fig. 5.4c).

Posterior-to-anterior pressure applied to the tip of the spine causes it to act as a lever, parting the upper zygapophyseal joint and compressing the lower (Fig. 5.4f, g). Pressure applied to the lateral side of the spinous process causes rotation of the body of the vertebra to the opposite side, resulting in gapping of the upper zygapophyseal joint on the side to which the spine is moved, but compressing the lower joint. It has the opposite effect on the joints of the ipsilateral side.

Traction on the thoracic intervertebral joints is difficult to produce, resulting in virtually no movement. However, movement certainly occurs, to a limited extent, during lumbar or cervical traction.

Laterally, the heads of the ribs articulate with the bodies of the vertebrae and the tubercles of the ribs articulate with the transverse processes of the vertebrae (Fig. 5.4).

With the subject lying prone, pressure on the angle of the rib will part the costotransverse joint. If the thumbs are moved a little medially to an area just lateral to the joint, the gapping is increased. However, if the pressure is applied even more medially, it will encroach upon the back of the transverse process, producing exactly the opposite effect and resulting in compression of the costotransverse joint (Fig. 5.4c).

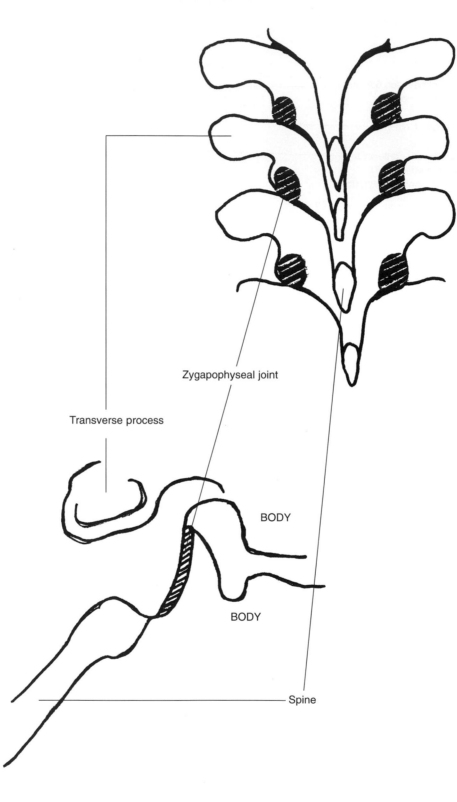

Posterior aspect

Shaded area shows joint surface deep to
inferior articular processes

Zygapophyseal joint

Transverse process

BODY

BODY

Spine

Lateral aspect

Fig. 5.4 (d), (e)
Zygapophyseal joints of thoracic spine. Shaded
areas show joint surface deep to inferior articular processes

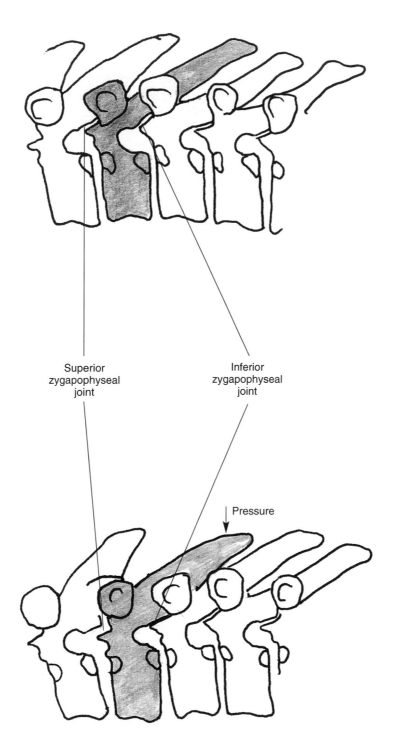

Superior
zygapophyseal
joint

Inferior
zygapophyseal
joint

Pressure

Fig. 5.4 (f), (g)
Vertebrae in horizontal position showing effect of
pressure on spine in direction of arrow

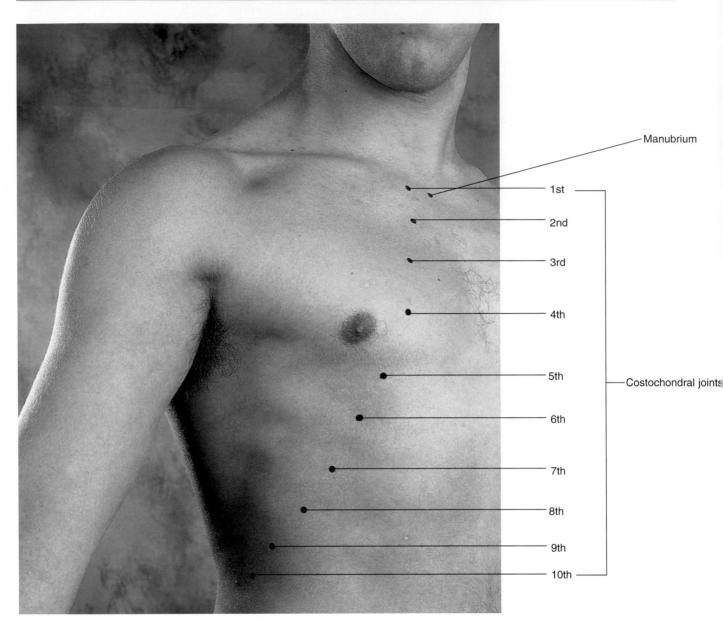

Fig. 5.5 (a)
Costochondral joints of the right side (anterior aspect)

The joints of the anterior end of the ribs

Anteriorly, the upper seven ribs articulate with the sternum via their costal cartilages. These are termed true ribs. The costal cartilages of ribs eight to ten articulate with the costal cartilage above, and are termed false ribs, and the two lower ribs are only capped with costal cartilage and do not link up with the sternum, and are termed floating ribs. There are three sets of joints in this area, namely, the costochondral, the interchondral and the sternocostal joints.

The costochondral joints

These joints are really the junction between the rib and its anterior end which has not yet ossified. The rounded end of the cartilage fits into the depressed roughened end of the rib. Its periosteum is continuous with its perichondrium.

Palpation

The costochondral joints (Fig. 5.5a, b) can be identified, in some subjects, lying approximately 3 cm lateral to the sternum at the second rib, progressing to some 12 cm from the xiphoid at the seventh rib and approximately 18 cm from the xiphoid process at the tenth rib. Pressure on the anterior surface of these joints can often be unpleasant and too much palpation may lead to a very tender area which may last for some time.

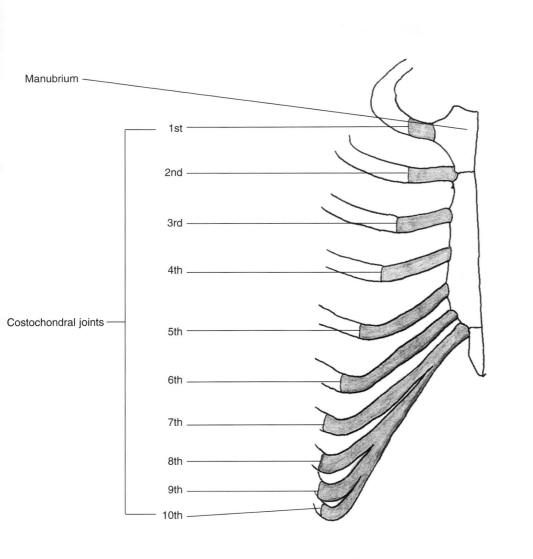

Manubrium

Costochondral joints

1st
2nd
3rd
4th
5th
6th
7th
8th
9th
10th

Fig. 5.5 (b)
Costochondral joints of the right side (anterior aspect)

Accessory movements

With the subject lying supine and applying pressure to the sternal area of the chest, quite marked compression can be achieved. This is due in part to the flexibility of the ribs and costal cartilage and in part to the slight gliding and bending movements occurring between the costochondral, interchondral, sternocostal and intersternal joints.

Movement of each individual joint can be achieved by applying pressure, normally with two thumbs, to the rib or to the costal cartilage close to either side of the joint. The movement is minimal in some joints, such as that of the first and second ribs with the sternum, but quite considerable lower down the thorax, particularly at the interchondral joints.

Some of these joints can be traumatized and become inflamed, usually following a blow on the chest or stress on the rib cage due to resting heavily against a beam or bar. This causes an acute pain over that area of the chest. If the pain is over the area of the heart, it may erroneously be associated with a heart attack.

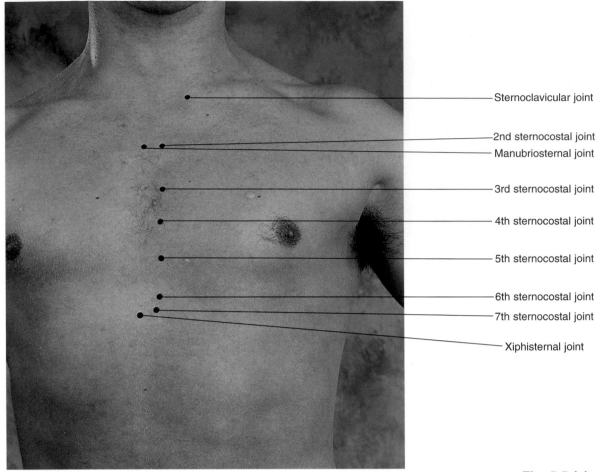

Sternoclavicular joint

2nd sternocostal joint

Manubriosternal joint

3rd sternocostal joint

4th sternocostal joint

5th sternocostal joint

6th sternocostal joint

7th sternocostal joint

Xiphisternal joint

Fig. 5.5 (c)
Joints of the sternum (anterior
aspect)

The sternocostal (chondrosternal) joints [Fig 5.5c and d]

These are the joints between the anterior rounded end of the costal cartilages of the upper seven ribs and the small hollow cavities on the side of the sternum.

The first articulates with the side of the manubrium just below the clavicular notch. It is a synarthrosis, having a similar structure to a symphysis and therefore forms a fairly rigid union. It is close to the midline of the body, a location where most symphyses are found.

The second to the seventh are all synovial joints, being surrounded by a capsule which is lined with synovial membrane and supported by ligaments that radiate from the front of the cartilage on to the anterior aspect of the sternum (the sternocostal radiate ligaments). The second costal cartilage joins the sternum at the side of the manubriosternal joint and has the extra support of an interosseous ligament which attaches to the disc of the manubriosternal joint. The seventh costal cartilage joins a small shallow facet formed by the lower part of the sternum and the xiphoid process. It is supported front and back by costoxiphoid ligaments. This synovial joint is often replaced by a symphysis.

Palpation

At the side of the manubriosternal joint, 4 cm below the sternal notch, the articulation of the second costal cartilage, the manubrium (Fig. 5.5b) and body, can be palpated as a small V- shaped notch, with the concavity facing laterally. Below this, on either side, the third to seventh ribs and their costal cartilages can be palpated as they articulate with the lateral border of the sternum at the costosternal or chondrosternal joints. The section of the sternum between each costal cartilage is concave laterally, being the anterior limit of the intercostal spaces. The joint between the first rib and the manubrium lies 1 cm below, and 1 cm lateral to, the medial end of the clavicle and is more difficult to identify; nevertheless, the anterior limit of the rib can be palpated.

The costal cartilage of the eighth to tenth ribs can be identified articulating medially, with the costal cartilage above, at the interchondral joints and forms the costal margin.

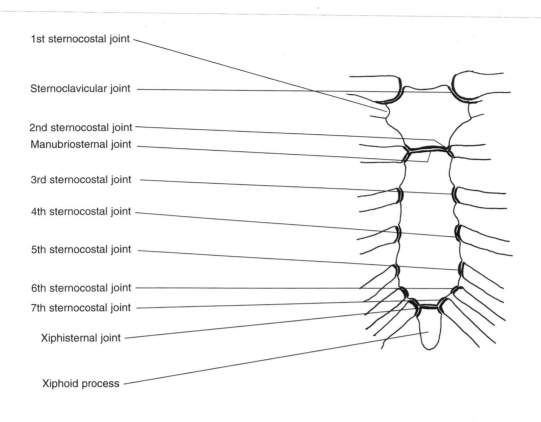

1st sternocostal joint

Sternoclavicular joint

2nd sternocostal joint
Manubriosternal joint

3rd sternocostal joint

4th sternocostal joint

5th sternocostal joint

6th sternocostal joint

7th sternocostal joint

Xiphisternal joint

Xiphoid process

Fig. 5.5 (d)
Joints of the sternum (anterior
aspect)

Joints of the sternum

The sternum is composed of three segments: the manubrium superiorly, the body centrally, and the small, pointed xiphoid process inferiorly. The joints between these sections are secondary cartilaginous symphyses.

Palpation

The manubriosternal joint is easy to identify (Fig. 5.5c, d) as it is some 7 cm below the upper border of the sternum at the sternal angle. It is level with the articulation of the second costal cartilage with the sternum.

The joint between the body and the xiphoid process (Fig. 5.5c, d) is more difficult to palpate, although the body and the xiphoid are both easily identifiable.

Accessory movements

There is very little accessory movement of the manubriosternal joint, although pressure on either the body or the manubrium, close to the joint, will produce slight angling of the two sections. At the xiphisternal joint, however, the xiphoid process can normally be moved backwards some considerable distance by pressure applied to its anterior surface. This produces an angling at the joint.

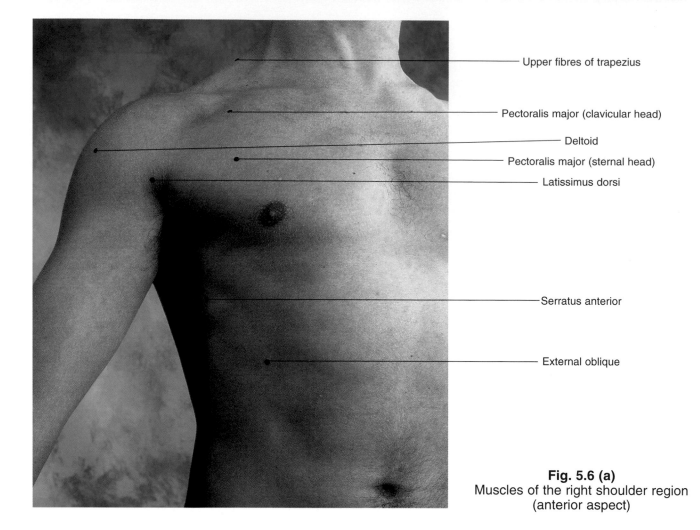

Upper fibres of trapezius

Pectoralis major (clavicular head)

Deltoid

Pectoralis major (sternal head)

Latissimus dorsi

Serratus anterior

External oblique

Fig. 5.6 (a)
Muscles of the right shoulder region
(anterior aspect)

MUSCLES

The anterior aspect of the chest

The muscle that dominates the upper part of the chest is pectoralis major. Lying deep to it are pectoralis minor and the upper intercostal muscles. In the lower part of the chest, rectus abdominis and the external oblique muscle of the abdomen have their upper attachment (see Fig. 6.5).

The pectoralis minor is a triangular muscle with its base attaching to the third, fourth and fifth ribs at approximately the mid-clavicular line and its apex attaching to the coracoid process of the scapula. It is very difficult to palpate. The intercostal muscles attach to the lower border of the rib above and to the upper border of the rib below. They are easier to palpate in the lower region of the chest (see page 199). The external oblique muscle attaches above to the external surface of the lower border of the lower eight ribs. You will be able to feel the contraction of the muscle if you place your fingers under the lower border of the rib cage, on the right, just lateral to the costal angle and ask the sitting model to turn to the left. The rectus abdominis attaches above to the fifth, sixth and seventh costal cartilages just lateral to the sternum. Place your fingers just below the rib cage just lateral to the xiphoid process and ask the sitting

model to lean backwards. Immediately the powerful contraction of the muscle will be palpated. (See also pages 228, 229.)

Pectoralis major

Pectoralis major (Figs 5.6 and 5.7) is a large, thick triangular muscle situated on the upper anterior area of the chest wall. It is composed of two main groups of fibres, clavicular and sternal. The clavicular fibres attach medially to the anterior surface of the medial half of the clavicle and its sternal fibres attach to its side of the sternum, the anterior surface of the upper seven costal cartilages and the upper part of the aponeurosis covering the abdominal muscles. Both sets of fibres pass laterally, leaving a small space between them, and join together laterally to form a bilaminar tendon which attaches to the lateral lip of the intertubercular groove. The lower sternal fibres tend to fold up behind the upper fibres to form the double bilaminated tendon. The muscle forms a pleasantly shaped lower border, which becomes the anterior border of the axilla laterally.

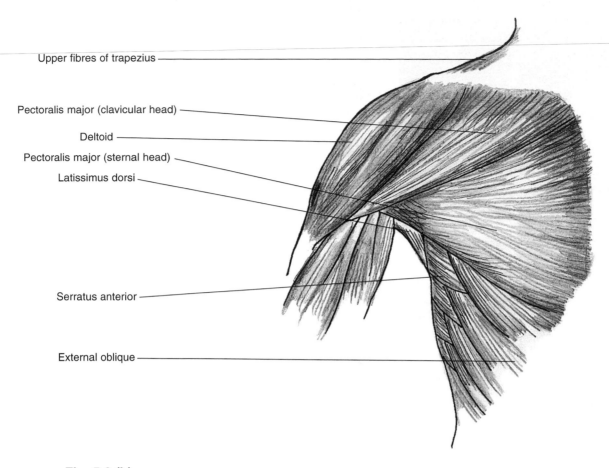

Upper fibres of trapezius

Pectoralis major (clavicular head)

Deltoid

Pectoralis major (sternal head)

Latissimus dorsi

Serratus anterior

External oblique

Fig. 5.6 (b)
Muscles of the right shoulder region
(anterior aspect)

Palpation

Pectoralis major is easily recognizable and palpable in even the less muscular subject. If the subject presses the hands against the iliac crest, the whole of the muscle contracts. The lower border of the anterior wall of the axilla is rounded, due to the lower sternal fibres of pectoralis major twisting upwards posterior to its upper fibres. The muscle can be traced medially and inferiorly on to the anterior aspect of the chest as far down as the costal cartilage of the seventh rib and xiphoid process.

The bulk of the muscle forms a rounded shape on the upper anterior chest wall and is the muscle that men try to develop to give a pleasant shape to the upper part of the chest. It is almost entirely covered by the breast in the female, particularly in its lower section. If the arms are flexed against resistance, the clavicular fibres can easily be identified, just below the medial half of the clavicle, as a column of muscle standing clear of the chest wall (Fig. 5.7a, b) passing downwards and laterally.

During extension against resistance from the flexed position, the lower sternal fibres become apparent as a thick triangular shape forming the lower boundary of the muscle (Fig. 5.7c, d). To observe the two sets of fibres clearly, the subject's arm should be held at about 45° of flexion and he or she should then be asked to first raise and then pull down the arm against resistance. The tendon can be traced laterally to its attachment to the humerus.

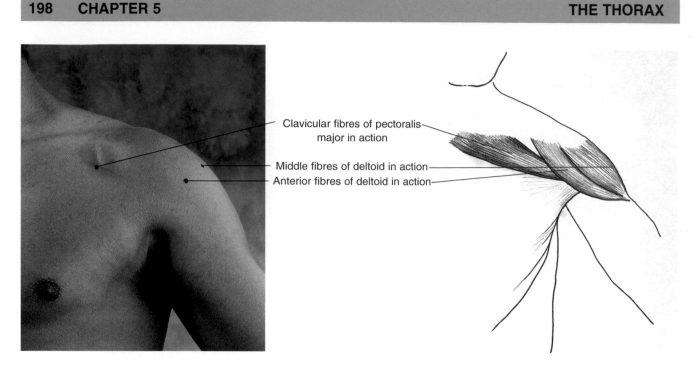

Clavicular fibres of pectoralis major in action

Middle fibres of deltoid in action

Anterior fibres of deltoid in action

Fig. 5.7 (a), (b)
Clavicular fibres of pectoralis major and deltoid of left shoulder (anterior aspect)

Functional anatomy

It is interesting to note that pectoralis major has two functionally distinct sets of fibres, a bilaminal tendon, and is supplied through two nerves (lateral and medial pectoral). In addition, it is involved in two actions which appear to oppose each other. The clavicular fibres will flex and the sternal fibres will extend the shoulder joint. In prone kneeling, both sets of fibres act to stabilize the upper trunk posture, preventing sway either forwards, backwards or from side to side; and in crawling, the limb is taken forwards by the clavicular fibres and backwards by the sternal fibres. This important muscle must have had a greater importance in our evolution, and recognition of its residual function may help in its re-education.

In patients suffering from respiratory embarrassment, pectoralis major may be used as an accessory muscle of inspiration. In this case the arms have to be fixed, as in gripping a post or beam, thus fixing the lateral attachment of the muscle to the humerus. The medial attachment of the muscle may then be used to expand the chest a little more.

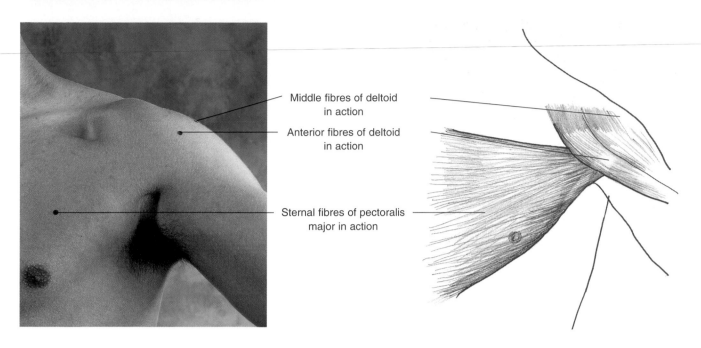

Fig. 5.7 (c), (d)
Sternal fibres of pectoralis major and deltoid of left shoulder (anterior aspect)

Comparative anatomy

The pectoralis muscle(s) also play an important role in the animal, bird, fish, reptile and insect worlds. In the quadruped it acts as a stabilizing muscle for the forelimb in the standing position, similar to that in the human prone kneeling position, and because of its shape takes part in both the propulsive and recovery phase of the forelimb in locomotion. It also acts as a sling for the thorax holding it up between the two limbs. In the bird and insect it creates the enormous thrust for take-off and flight, while at the same time controlling the intricate movements of the wings. In the fish it controls the fine movements of the pectoral fin in a comparatively simple up-and-down motion, but occasionally may have fibres which are extended into the neck region. The pectorals in the forelimb of a reptile normally have the adaptability of being functional in water and on the land.

Biceps brachii and coracobrachialis

Running vertically from the coracoid process (see pages 13, 17), the combined tendon of the biceps brachii and coracobrachialis can be palpated just below the coracoid process but is soon hidden by the broad tendon of the pectoralis major. It emerges below and can be identified passing down into the antero-medial aspect of the arm and splitting into its anterior (bicipital) and posterior (coracobrachialis) section.

The intercostals

If the fingers are placed between the ribs, a tight membranous sheet can be palpated. This consists of the external and internal intercostal muscles and their covering fascia. These are best palpated just below the pectoralis major and slightly lateral to the line of the nipple. On muscular subjects they are more hidden by larger, more superficial muscles.

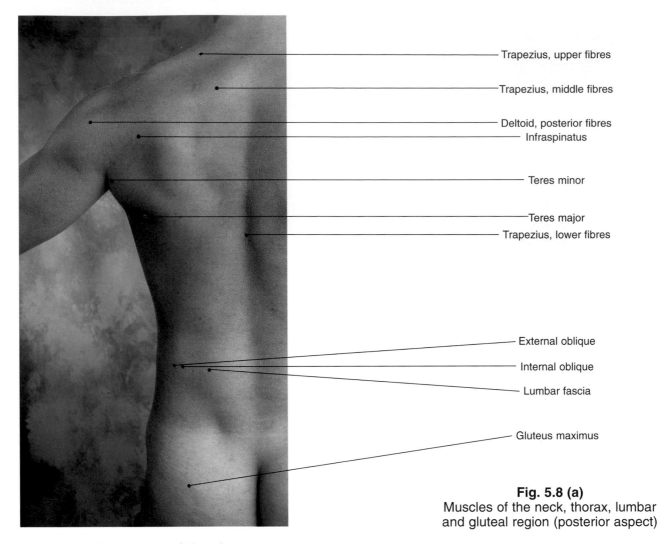

Trapezius, upper fibres

Trapezius, middle fibres

Deltoid, posterior fibres
Infraspinatus

Teres minor

Teres major
Trapezius, lower fibres

External oblique

Internal oblique

Lumbar fascia

Gluteus maximus

Fig. 5.8 (a)
Muscles of the neck, thorax, lumbar
and gluteal region (posterior aspect)

The posterior aspect of the chest

Trapezius [Fig. 5.8a and b]

The two trapezius muscles cover most of the posterior aspect of the neck and upper thorax connecting the skull, ligamentum nuchae, seventh cervical and all the thoracic spines to the lateral end of the clavicle, acromion and superior border of the spine of the scapula. Their upper fibres can be palpated halfway between the external occipital protuberance and the acromion process, forming the pleasant contour of the upper lateral aspect of the shoulder. Its middle fibres can be palpated between the upper border of the spine and the lower cervical and upper thoracic regions. The lower fibres are more difficult to identify as they pass from the lower thoracic spines to the medial end of the spine of the scapula. The upper fibres are easier to identify if the shoulder girdle is raised, the middle fibres if the shoulder girdle is retracted and the lower fibres if the shoulder girdle is depressed.

Levator scapulae and the rhomboids

These muscles lie deep to the trapezius. Levator scapulae attaches above to the transverse processes of the upper four cervical vertebrae and below to the upper part of the medial border of the scapula. The rhomboid muscles attach above to the lower part of the ligamentum nuchae, the spine of the seventh cervical vertebra and the spines of the upper five thoracic vertebrae. They pass downwards and laterally to attach to the lower two-thirds of the medial border of the scapula. These muscles add bulk to the area between the scapula and lower neck and can be palpated in this region when the shoulders are raised and braced back.

Supraspinatus and infraspinatus

Supraspinatus arises from the supraspinous fossa of the scapula, passing laterally to the top of the greater tuberosity of the humerus. Infraspinatus arises from the infraspinous fossa, passing laterally to the posterior aspect of the same tuberosity.

When the subject begins to raise the arm from the side, supraspinatus can be identified just above the spine of the scapula in the supraspinous fossa. Below the spine, infraspinatus can be felt contracting when the arm is laterally rotated.

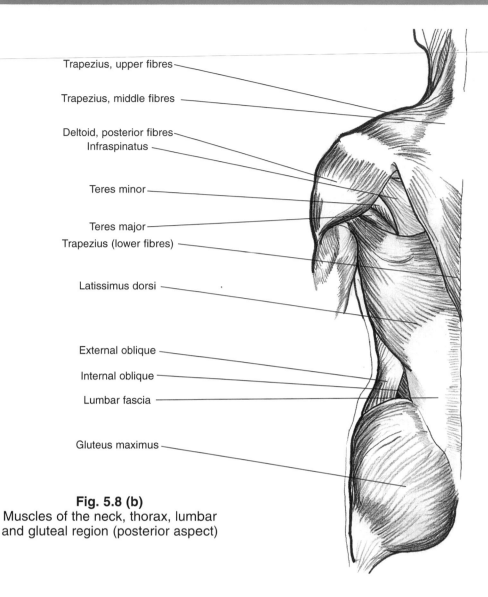

Trapezius, upper fibres

Trapezius, middle fibres

Deltoid, posterior fibres
Infraspinatus

Teres minor

Teres major
Trapezius (lower fibres)

Latissimus dorsi

External oblique

Internal oblique

Lumbar fascia

Gluteus maximus

Fig. 5.8 (b)
Muscles of the neck, thorax, lumbar
and gluteal region (posterior aspect)

Teres major and latissimus dorsi

These two muscles are triangular in shape and cover the lateral border of the scapula, **teres major** actually arising from the border. **Latissimus dorsi** comes from an extensive attachment to the spines of the lower six thoracic vertebrae, the thoracolumbar fascia and the posterior section of the iliac crest. It passes over the inferior angle of the scapula, taking a few fibres of origin, and then twists under the axilla, with teres major, to attach to the floor of the intertubercular groove with teres major attaching to its medial lip.

If the arm is extended against resistance from a flexed position, teres major and latissimus dorsi can be felt contracting. The triangular bulk of teres major lies over the lateral border of the scapula, while the tendon of latissimus dorsi can be traced, laterally and forwards, forming the posterior wall of the axilla. This tendon can be traced to its muscle fibres medially over the dorsum of the chest and lumbar area and can readily be identified if the subject coughs.

Serratus anterior [Fig. 5.6a and b]

Serratus anterior is a flat but powerful muscle attaching to the whole of the medial border of the scapula. Passing deep to the scapula, it attaches anteriorly to the lateral aspect of the first to eighth ribs at the mid-axillary line. Most of the muscle is concealed beneath the scapula, but palpation of its anterior attachment to the ribs is possible. If, during protraction, the fingers are placed behind the mid-axillary line but in front of the scapula, its anterior attachment to the ribs can be identified. Care must be taken to observe the contraction when the pectoral girdle is retracted and begins to move forwards. Once the lateral border of the scapula has passed beyond the mid-axillary line, the muscle is hidden.

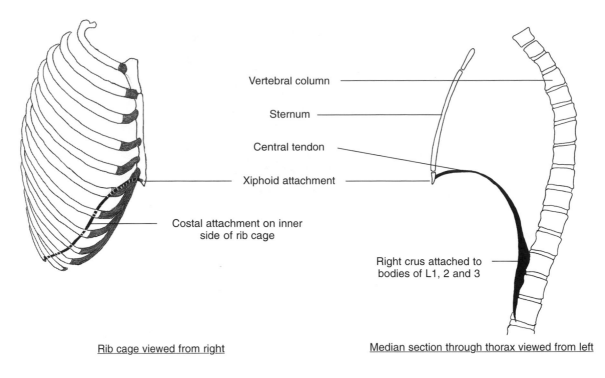

Vertebral column

Sternum

Central tendon

Xiphoid attachment

Costal attachment on inner
side of rib cage

Right crus attached to
bodies of L1, 2 and 3

Rib cage viewed from right

Median section through thorax viewed from left

Fig. 5.9 (a), (b)
Attachments of the diaphragm

The diaphragm [Figs 5.9 and 5.10]

The diaphragm is a musculotendinous sheet separating the thoracic and abdominal cavities. It forms
a double cupola within the thorax, with the heart
resting upon its central tendinous part. Anteriorly it
attaches to the xiphisternum, laterally to the inner
aspect of the lower six ribs on a line with the inner
surface of the costochondral joints, and posteriorly
to the vertebral column. It is the main muscle of
inspiration and moves according to the state
of respiration. It is therefore more useful to indicate
its surface markings after full expiration and then
after a deep inspiration. The attachments to the
xiphisternum, ribs and vertebral column remain
constant, but the two cupolae and central tendon
vary in height. It must also be remembered that the
position of the diaphragm is influenced by other factors: it lies at a higher level with respect to the rib
cage when lying supine than when standing; its
downward movement is restricted by food and gas
in the stomach, and by increased pressure in the
abdominal cavity, for example during pregnancy; in
side lying it is pushed up into the thoracic cavity on
the lower side by the contents of the abdomen; and
in prone lying the liver tends to restrict its downward movement on the right side.

On full expiration, the right cupola rises to the
level of the fourth rib, the left to the fourth intercostal space and the central tendon to the level of the

fifth costal cartilage. On full inspiration, which may
produce a 6 cm descent of the cupolae, the diaphragm may reach the level of the sixth or seventh
ribs. In quiet respiration, the diaphragm normally
only moves up and down 1–2 cm.

The attachment of the diaphragm to the inside of
the chest wall can be marked by an oblique line
drawn from the xiphoid process, anteriorly, downwards and laterally slightly concave downwards. It
follows the line of the sixth costal cartilage attaching
to the inner surface anterior end of the sixth to tenth
ribs (Fig. 5.9a). It then attaches to the inner surface of
the eleventh and twelfth ribs with its vertebral
attachment being marked by a line running down
the lateral side of the bodies of the first and second
lumbar vertebrae on the left and the first to third
lumbar vertebrae on the right (Fig. 5.10b). These can
be marked by two vertical lines, 2 cm lateral to the
first and second lumbar spines on the left and the
first to third lumbar spines on the right.

Palpation

It is impossible to palpate the diaphragm. On full
inspiration there is a bulging of the abdomen
between the two costal margins. Although this is
produced by the diaphragm, it is actually the upper
section of the abdominals

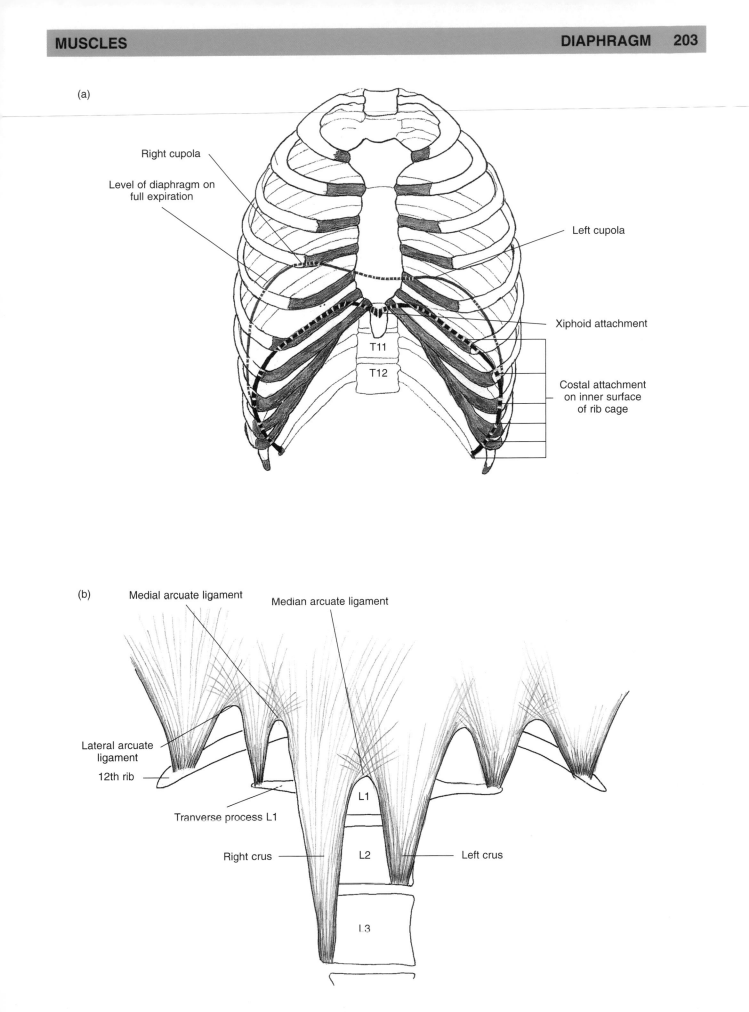

Fig. 5.10
The diaphragm. **(a)** The rib cage (anterior aspect). **(b)** Attachments of diaphragm to the vertebrae and 12th rib (anterior aspect viewed from inside rib cage)

Anterior aspect

Posterior aspect

Fig. 5.11 (a), (b)
Cutaneous nerve supply to the thorax

NERVES [Figs 5.11 and 5.12]

The only nerves that become superficial in the thoracic region are those that supply the skin covering the ribs and intercostal spaces. By the time they reach the surface they are fine filaments and impossible to palpate.

Each **intercostal nerve** passes around the inside of the rib cage deep to the **internal intercostal muscle**, normally giving off a **lateral branch** at approximately the mid-axillary line. The area of skin supplied by each nerve usually includes that covering the rib above and below, including the **external intercostal muscle** passing between. Therefore there is an area of overlap of the cutaneous nerves, so that the loss of sensation from one nerve only leaves an area of paraesthesia not anaesthesia.

Below the sixth rib the nerves continue obliquely around the abdominal wall in the same direction as the ribs between which they commenced.

In the condition herpes zoster (shingles), the sensory component of an individual thoracic nerve is often affected by the virus and this leads to small pustules appearing over the area supplied by this particular nerve. The patient presents with a strip around the chest or abdomen following the line of its distribution (Fig. 5.11). Although this condition commonly appears to affect a single thoracic nerve it may affect any nerve in the body.

Fig. 5.12 (a), (b)
The course and distribution of a typical intercostal nerve

Apex
Sternal angle
Anterior borders of lungs
Left lung
Transverse fissure
Cardiac notch
Left oblique fissure
Right oblique fissure
Pleural cavity
Attachment of pleura

Anterior aspect

Fig. 5.13 (a)
The lungs

STRUCTURES WITHIN THE THORACIC CAGE

Although the structures contained within the thoracic cage are almost totally hidden by the ribs, sternum and vertebral column, it is of some importance to be able to indicate the surface markings of the major organs and vessels. Owing to considerable movement during life, no surface marking can be constant; nevertheless, each organ stays within certain boundaries. These will be indicated by the markings given.

The lungs [Fig. 5.13]

The lungs almost totally fill the thorax either side of the heart. The apex of each lung can be palpated, on deep inspiration, as it rises behind the middle third of the clavicle. These are the only areas of the lungs which are palpable and may prove to be elusive in some individuals. Each lung takes on the shape of the deep surface of the rib cage and intercostal muscles, being convex laterally and concave medially and inferiorly. Each lung presents anterior, posterior and inferior borders medially. The borders

divide the lung into lateral, medial and inferior surfaces.

Surface markings

The surface markings of the anterior borders of the two lungs differ slightly. Both descend from the apex of the lung, behind the sternoclavicular joint of the appropriate side, to come together behind the sternal angle. They then pass downwards close to the midline until the level of the fourth costal cartilage, where the left anterior border passes laterally in a C- shaped curve concave medially (the cardiac notch) to reach the inferior border behind the sixth costal cartilage in the mid-clavicular line. The right medial border passes straight downwards, reaching the inferior border at the sixth chondrosternal joint (Fig. 5.13a).

The posterior borders of both lungs pass vertically downwards in front of the necks of the ribs, approximately 2 cm either side of the spines of

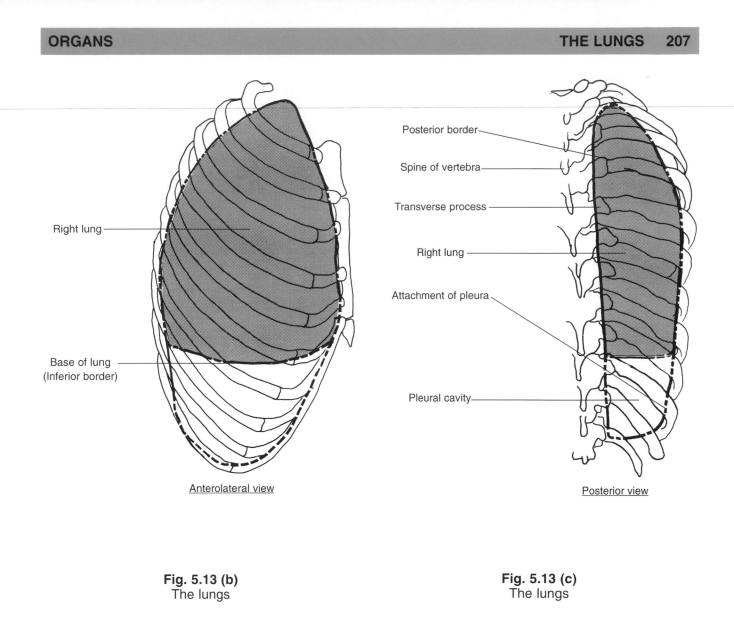

Fig. 5.13 (b)
The lungs

Fig. 5.13 (c)
The lungs

the vertebrae, from the apex of the lung to the level of the tenth rib (Fig. 5.13c).

The inferior border of each lung passes almost horizontally around the chest wall, being level with the sixth costal cartilage anteriorly, crossing the eighth rib in the mid-axillary line and the tenth rib posteriorly. The base of the right lung is usually slightly higher than the left owing to the presence of the liver below it (Fig. 5.13a–c).

Parietal pleura lines the thoracic cage of each side and covers each lung in parts. The lower part of this pleura, however, is prolonged downwards for some 5 cm below the lower border of the lung to the twelfth rib posteriorly, the tenth rib at the mid-axillary line and the sixth costal cartilage anteriorly. (Fig. 5.13a, c). This is termed the pleural cavity

The fissures of the lungs

Each lung is marked by an oblique fissure; the right lung, in addition, has a transverse fissure. These mark the junctions between the various lobes of each lung; the left therefore possesses two lobes, upper and lower, while the right possesses three, upper, middle and lower. Each oblique fissure can be marked on the chest wall by a line drawn obliquely downwards and forwards from a point 2 cm lateral to the spine of T3, crossing the mid-axillary line at the fifth rib, to reach the inferior border of the lung at the costal cartilage of the sixth rib, 7 cm from the midline (Fig. 5.13a). A good guide for the direction of this line is given by the medial border of the scapula when the arm is raised above the head.

Only the right lung has a transverse fissure, which marks the division of the upper and middle lobes. It is indicated by a line from the fifth rib in the mid-axillary line to the fourth costal cartilage 3 cm from the median plane, essentially running along the lower border of the fourth rib.

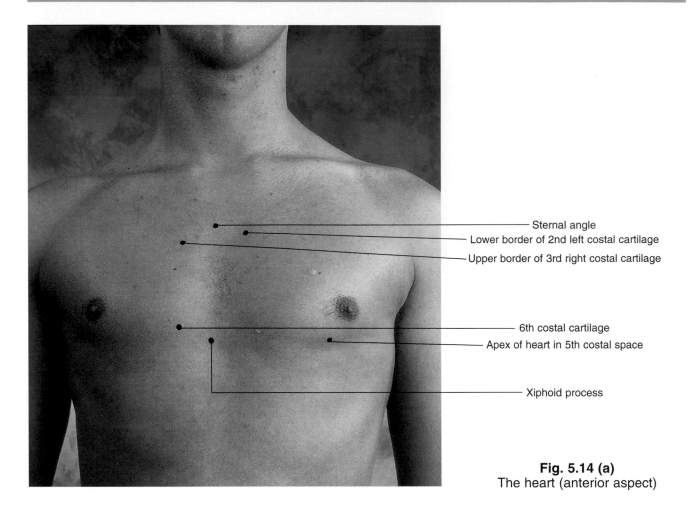

Sternal angle

Lower border of 2nd left costal cartilage

Upper border of 3rd right costal cartilage

6th costal cartilage

Apex of heart in 5th costal space

Xiphoid process

Fig. 5.14 (a)
The heart (anterior aspect)

The heart

The heart is a roughly cone-shaped double muscular pump situated behind the sternum with its apex downward and to the left and its base upward and to the right. It is composed of specialized contractile muscular tissue (myocardium) contained within a double layer of serous pericardium, which is joined around the area where the great vessels enter the heart. The outer layer of the pericardium is attached to the central part of the upper surface of the diaphragm and the inner layer is connected to the heart musculature. The two pumps, although pumping together, are completely separate and are often referred to as the 'left heart' and the 'right heart'. Each pump is composed of an upper receiving chamber called the atrium and a lower more powerful muscular chamber called the ventricle.

The heart is a rhythmically contractile tissue,

which is controlled by nerve impulses. The upper chambers or atria are completely separated from the lower ventricles by a fibrous non-conductive layer. The only communication between the two is by a bundle of specialized tissue.

Location

The position of the heart within the thorax is variable, to some extent, depending on the posture adopted, so that its surface markings are slightly higher when lying compared with standing and sitting.

The projection of the heart on to the anterior surface of the chest is as follows (Figs 5.14 and 5.15). The apex of the heart points downwards and to the left and can be palpated 9 cm from the midline in the fifth left intercostal space. The pulsations are

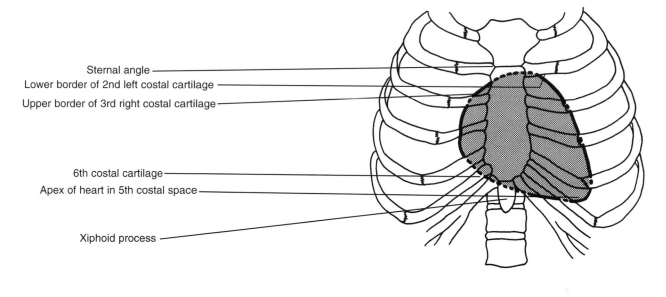

Sternal angle

Lower border of 2nd left costal cartilage

Upper border of 3rd right costal cartilage

6th costal cartilage

Apex of heart in 5th costal space

Xiphoid process

Fig. 5.14 (b)
The heart (anterior aspect)

enhanced if the subject is sitting and leans slightly forward, as the apex of the heart is pressed against the chest wall. The upper limit of the heart is marked by two points, one at the **lower border of the second left costal cartilage** 3 cm to the left of the midline, and the other at the **upper border of the third right costal cartilage** 3 cm to the right of the midline. The lower right border of the heart can be indicated on the lower border of the **costal cartilage of the right sixth rib** 3 cm from the midline. The boundaries are curved, joining the above points and making an area approximately the size of the individual's clenched fist.

Function

The heart is responsible for pumping the blood around the body. The deoxygenated blood enters the right atrium from the systemic circulation through the large veins, e.g. the inferior and superior vena cava. It is then pumped down into the right ventricle through the right atrioventricular, tricuspid, valve which then contracts, sending the blood into the lungs, passing via the pulmonary valve.

Oxygenated blood is received into the left atrium from the lungs and is propelled down into the left ventricle through the left atrioventricular (mitral) valve. When full, the left ventricle contracts, pumping the blood through the aortic valve into the aorta and back into the systemic circulation.

Equal volumes of blood must be expelled from the two ventricles at each stroke, the right into the lungs and the left into the systemic circulation. This will maintain an equal rate of flow in both systems.

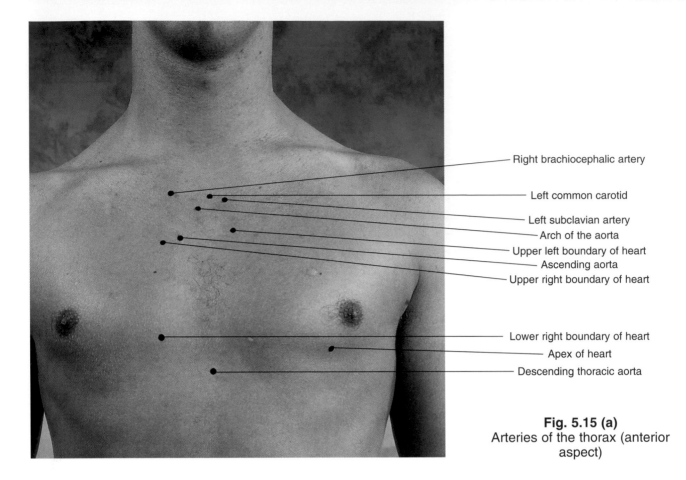

Right brachiocephalic artery

Left common carotid

Left subclavian artery

Arch of the aorta

Upper left boundary of heart

Ascending aorta

Upper right boundary of heart

Lower right boundary of heart

Apex of heart

Descending thoracic aorta

Fig. 5.15 (a)
Arteries of the thorax (anterior aspect)

Major arteries [Fig. 5.15]

The aorta

The aorta is the main artery carrying oxygenated blood to the body. It leaves the heart at the base of the left ventricle, immediately giving off the two coronary arteries which supply the heart itself with blood. It passes upwards, slightly forwards and to the right before arching backwards and to the left over the right pulmonary vessels. It then passes inferiorly through the thorax on the left side of the vertebral bodies, behind the heart. As it does so it gradually comes to lie more in the midline, finally leaving the thorax in front, but slightly to the left of the body of T12, passing between the two crura and behind the median arcuate ligament of the diaphragm.

Surface markings

The aortic valve lies deep to the sternum adjacent to the third intercostal space. From here the ascending aorta, a band 2.5 cm wide, passes upwards and to the right as far as the second right chondrosternal joint. The arch of the aorta then passes behind the sternal angle (and the lower part of the manubrium) over the heart, to end behind the second left costal cartilage. The descending aorta can be represented by a line extending from this point to its exit from the thorax just left of the mid-line and above the transpyloric plane, which is on a level with the tips of the ninth costal cartilages.

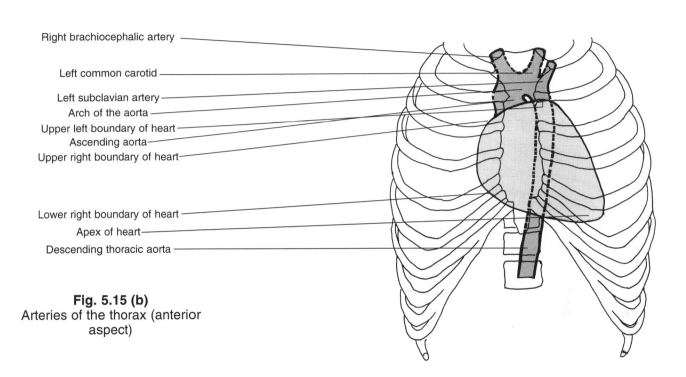

Right brachiocephalic artery

Left common carotid

Left subclavian artery
Arch of the aorta
Upper left boundary of heart
Ascending aorta
Upper right boundary of heart

Lower right boundary of heart
Apex of heart
Descending thoracic aorta

Fig. 5.15 (b)
Arteries of the thorax (anterior
aspect)

The brachiocephalic, left common carotid and left subclavian arteries

From the upper convexity of the arch of the aorta, three major vessels arise. The brachiocephalic (innominate) artery is anterior and to the right. Immediately behind and to the left is the left common carotid. Behind and to the left of the left common carotid is the left subclavian.

The brachiocephalic artery supplies oxygenated blood to the right side of the head and neck via the right common carotid artery through its internal and external branches. It also supplies blood to the right arm via the right subclavian artery. The left common carotid artery supplies blood to the left side of the head and neck via its internal and external branches. The left subclavian supplies blood to the left arm.

Surface markings

The brachiocephalic artery arises from the arch of the aorta behind the manubrium slightly right of centre and passes upwards, backwards and to the right for approximately 5 cm. It divides behind the right sternoclavicular joint into the right subclavian and right common carotid.

The left common carotid arises from the aorta just to the left of the mid point of the manubrium and passes upwards, backwards and to the left for approximately 4 cm to enter the neck behind the left sternoclavicular joint.

The left subclavian artery arises from the posterior part of the arch of the aorta behind the first intercostal space on the left, just lateral to the manubrium. It passes upwards and to the left for approximately 7 cm behind the first chondrosternal joint on the left to the inner borders of the left first rib. It passes over the rib *en route* to the left upper limb.

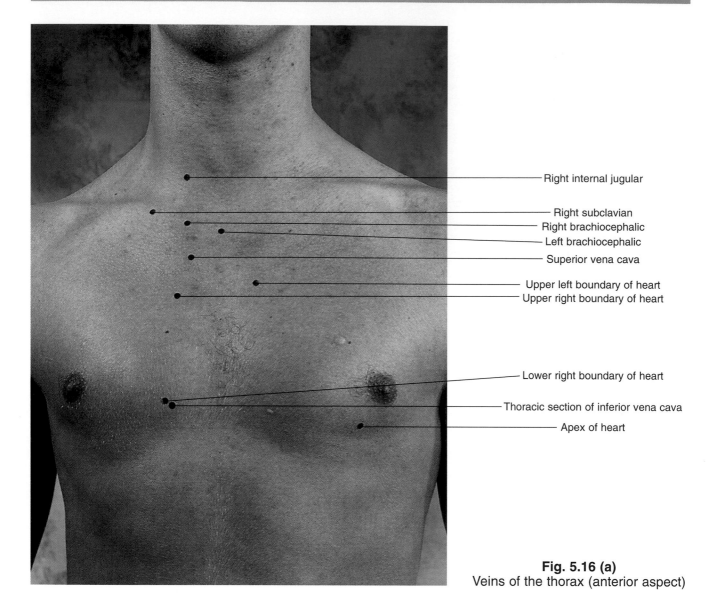

Right internal jugular

Right subclavian
Right brachiocephalic
Left brachiocephalic
Superior vena cava

Upper left boundary of heart
Upper right boundary of heart

Lower right boundary of heart

Thoracic section of inferior vena cava

Apex of heart

Fig. 5.16 (a)
Veins of the thorax (anterior aspect)

Veins [Fig. 5.16]

The large veins of the thorax are also situated deep within the thoracic cage and are impossible to palpate. Nevertheless, it is of some value to know where they lie in relation to palpable surface markings. It must, however, be remembered that the chest wall, the heart, diaphragm and lungs are all moveable structures and this will lead to small differences in their relationship to one another. Surface markings, therefore, will be as accurate as possible but a little leeway must be expected in this area.

Outline of network

Venous blood from the head, neck, both upper limbs and upper trunk enters the left and right brachiocephalic (innominate) veins. It then passes into the superior vena cava and thus into the upper part of the right atrium of the heart.

Venous blood from the two lower limbs and lower trunk passes, via the internal and external iliac veins, into the abdominal inferior vena cava, entering the thoracic cavity, for just a short distance forming its thoracic section. This empties into the lower part of the right atrium of the heart.

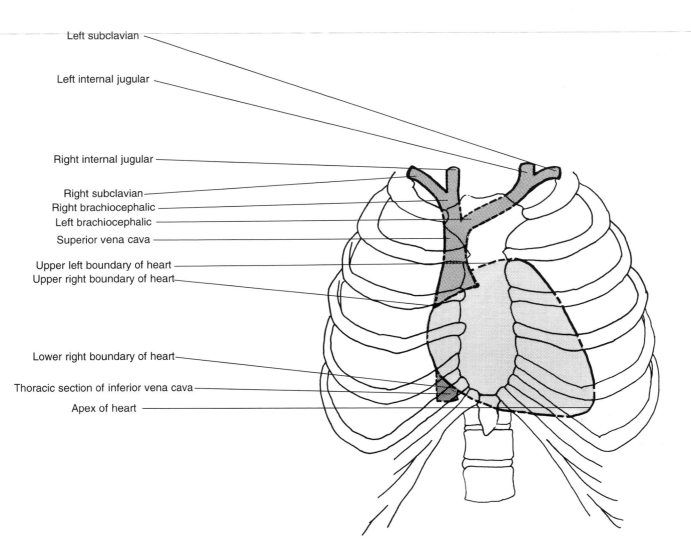

Left subclavian

Left internal jugular

Right internal jugular

Right subclavian
Right brachiocephalic
Left brachiocephalic
Superior vena cava
Upper left boundary of heart
Upper right boundary of heart

Lower right boundary of heart

Thoracic section of inferior vena cava

Apex of heart

Fig. 5.16 (b)
Veins of the thorax (anterior aspect)

Surface markings

In the upper thorax, the left and right brachio-cephalic (innominate) veins are formed by the internal jugular and the subclavian veins of their respective sides, just lateral to each sternoclavicular joint.

The left brachiocephalic vein passes downwards and to the right for approximately 6 cm to join the right brachiocephalic behind the sternal end of the first, right costal cartilage. At this point they form the superior vena cava.

The superior vena cava passes vertically downwards for approximately 7 cm from behind the costal cartilage of the first rib on the right to enter the right atrium behind the sternal end of the third costal cartilage.

In the lower thorax, the inferior vena cava enters the thoracic cavity through the upper fibrous part of the diaphragm, entering the lower part of the right atrium of the heart almost immediately, lying behind the sternal end of the sixth right costal cartilage.

6

The abdomen

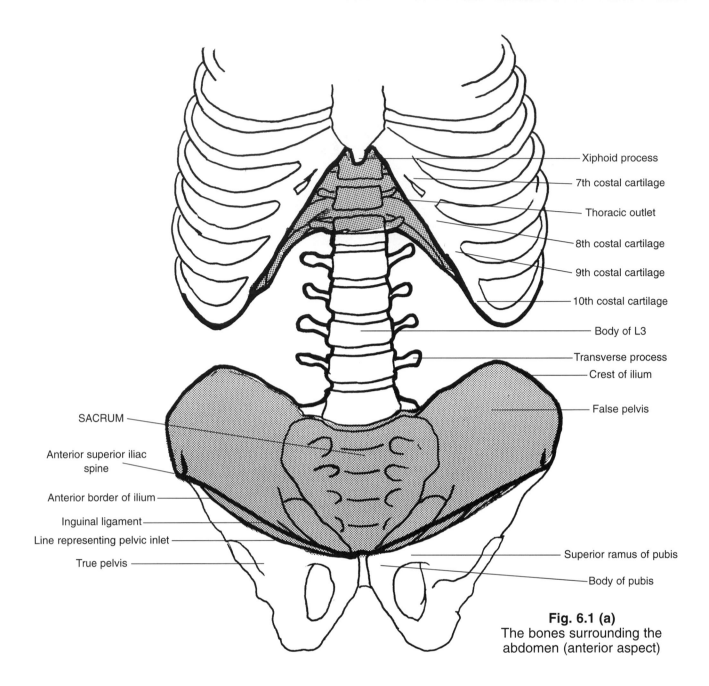

Fig. 6.1 (a)
The bones surrounding the
abdomen (anterior aspect)

BONES

The abdomen consists mainly of soft tissue contained within predominantly muscular walls. Its only bony features are the boundaries of the **thoracic outlet** above consisting of the **xiphoid process** at its centre in the front, the lower border of the **seventh, eighth, ninth** and **tenth costal cartilages**, the tip of the eleventh rib and the inferior border of the twelfth rib. Posteriorly, the body of the twelfth thoracic vertebra completes the ring. Below, the pelvic inlet comprises the pubis anteriorly, its **superior rami** on either side, the **anterior border** and the **crest** of the **ilium** and posteriorly the **base of the sacrum** The vertebral column forms its posterior boundary. It is, however, important to mark out these boundaries, as they provide useful landmarks for some of the organs it contains.

The thoracic outlet [Fig. 6.1a]

Palpation

Find the xiphoid process, which is the most inferior portion of the sternum. Trace along the costal margin beyond the costal angle (the ninth costal cartilage) to its lowest extremity, which is normally the **tenth rib**. Continuing posteriorly, the eleventh rib becomes evident, with its tip just anterior to the mid-axillary line, with the tip of the twelfth rib slightly lower and just posterior. The tip of the twelfth rib normally lies on the same level as the spine of the first lumbar vertebra.

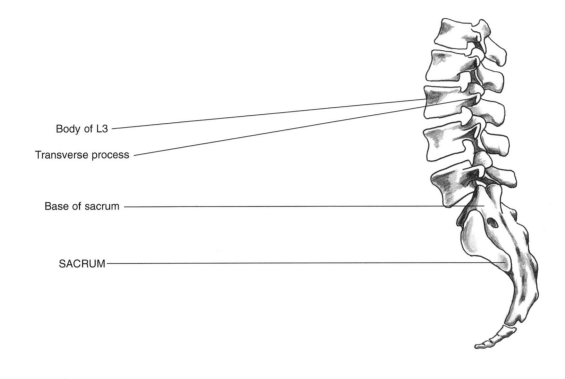

Body of L3

Transverse process

Base of sacrum

SACRUM

Fig. 6.1 (b)
The bones surrounding the
abdomen (lateral aspect, viewed
from left)

The pelvic girdle

Palpation

Identify the **anterior superior iliac spine** at the anterior extremity of the iliac crest. Trace the lateral lip of the iliac crest posteriorly, beyond the iliac tubercle to the posterior superior iliac spine and sacrum. Now, run the pads of your fingers down the central part of the abdominal wall to about 5 cm above the genitalia. The pubic tubercles become evident on either side, with each pubic crest running medially to a central space which marks the pubic symphysis. The bony ring is completed by the superior ramus of the pubis, which is difficult to palpate, and anterior border of the ilium, easily identifiable in its upper section. The **inguinal ligament** stretches above this region from the pubic tubercle to the anterior superior iliac spine.

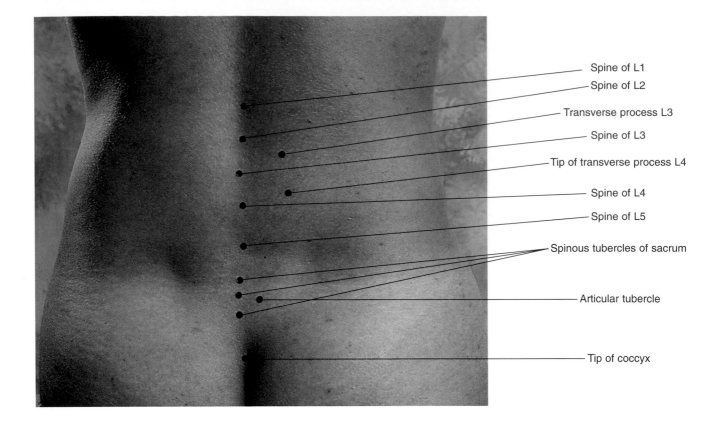

Fig. 6.1 (c)
Lumbar vertebrae and sacrum (posterior aspect)

The lumbar vertebrae

There are five lumbar vertebrae, with L1 being the smallest and L5 the largest. As in all other vertebrae, their bodies are anterior and their spines are posterior. Laterally, they present transverse processes, the fifth being much larger than the rest. Their upper articular processes face inwards and their lower facets face outwards, those of the fifth facing more anteriorly. There is a large neural canal in the lumbar region which is more triangular in shape.

Palpation

Lumbar vertebrae. Posteriorly the spines of the lumbar vertebrae project backwards and are individually identifiable. With the subject lying prone, place a firm pillow under the abdomen which flattens the lumbar lordosis. This makes the spines of the lumbar vertebrae become more pronounced, appearing as a line of flattened edges forming a crest down the centre of the lumbar region (Fig. 6.1c, d). The spines are continuous with those of the sacrum below and the thoracic vertebrae above.

Immediately above the central part of the sacrum is a hollow, due to the spine of the fifth vertebra being shorter and the body being situated slightly more anterior than the rest. The small gaps between the spines tend to disappear when the vertebral column is flexed, owing to the tension of the supraspinous ligament.

If deep pressure is applied approximately 5 cm lateral to the vertebral spines, beyond the bulk of the erector spinae muscles, the tips of the transverse processes, particularly of the first lumbar vertebra, can be palpated. These are quite thin compared with those of the thorax and may be tender to palpate.

The sacrum

The sacrum is composed of five fused vertebrae, with S1 being the largest and S5 being the smallest. The sacrum is triangular in shape, with its base uppermost. Evidence of the separate vertebral bodies is still clear on the anterior surface. A line of spinous tubercles can be seen running vertically down the centre of its posterior surface and it is marked on either side by articular tubercles. Laterally the sacrum presents large lateral masses beyond its neural foramina. The sacrum is tilted forwards above, with its lower section projecting backwards.

Spine of L1
Spine of L2
Transverse process L3
Spine of L3
Tip of transverse process L4
Spine of L4
Spine of L5
Spinous tubercles of sacrum
Articular tubercle
Sacral cornua
Sacral hiatus
Tip of coccyx

Fig. 6.1 (d)
Lumbar vertebrae and sacrum (posterior aspect)

Palpation

The sacrum. The posterior surface of the sacrum can be identified between the posterior borders of the two ilia. Its lower section projects backwards and is easy to palpate, while its upper section (the base) lies more anterior and is more difficult to examine. It has a central, vertical series of spinous tubercles, in line with the lumbar spines and the coccyx, accompanied on either side by a row of articular tubercles which are all palpable (Fig. 6.1c, d).

The coccyx

The coccyx comprises three or four rudimentary vertebrae normally fused into one bone, with the upper being the largest and the lowest being a very small tubercle of bone. Normally it is tilted, with its inferior tip pointing downwards and forwards.

Palpation

The coccyx. As this bone varies considerably in size and shape it may prove a little difficult to palpate. Several alternative methods can be employed:
1. Trace the spinous processes which run down the centre of the posterior surface of the sacrum

to approximately 2.5 cm below the level of the posterior inferior iliac spines (see pages 82 and 83). Here, the pointed lower end of the coccyx can be palpated.
2. Gently run your fingers up the cleft between the two gluteus maximus muscles until the hard bony tip of the coccyx is found.
3. Draw an equilateral triangle with its base on the two posterior inferior iliac spines of the ilium with its apex downwards. This point should be on the tip of the coccyx.

In many subjects the coccyx is angled forwards and the finger must be pressed deep into the cleft to identify the shape. Care must be taken as pressure on the bone can cause pain, particularly if the joints between it and the sacrum have been damaged at any time.

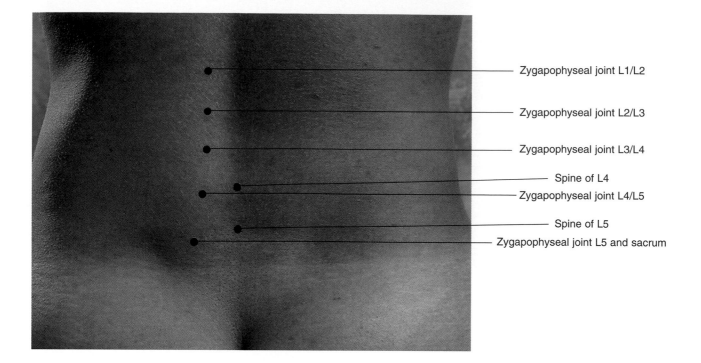

Fig. 6.2 (a)
Zygapophyseal joints of lumbar spine (posterior view)

JOINTS

The lumbar spine [Fig. 6.2]

The zygapophyseal joints are the most superficial in the lumbar region. They are nevertheless covered by thick, strong muscle, making the task of palpation extremely difficult. With the fingers pressed between the sides of the vertebral spines and the parallel-running column of muscle (sacrospinalis), the sides of the spines and in some subjects the laminae of each vertebra may be palpated. Each is a little higher than its corresponding spine, being almost totally hidden by the thick muscle layer.

Deep pressure through the muscle, using the tips of the thumbs, applies pressure to the posterior aspect of the zygapophyseal joints, which lie 1 cm lateral and slightly lower than the vertebral spine.

With great care and precision this pressure can be targeted on to the upper articular pillar of the vertebra below by moving lateral to the joint, or on to the lower articular pillar of the vertebra above by moving just medial to the joint. The lower facets of the vertebrae are convex anteriorly and fit snugly into the concave anterior edge of the upper facets of the vertebra below. Thus, anterior pressure on the lower vertebra causes its articular facet to glide forwards, slightly parting its anterior segments, whereas pressure on the upper vertebra pushes the lower facet into the socket, preventing any further movement (Fig. 6.2d, e).

Fig. 6.2 (b)
Zygapophyseal joints of lumbar spine (posterior view)

Accessory movements

Distraction (traction) of the joints of the lumbar spine is the only true accessory movement possible. All other movements of gliding, gapping and compression of the zygapophyseal joints, together with twisting and compression of the intervertebral discs, occur in the area during normal lumbar activities.

Traction can be applied to this area in many ways, either manually or mechanically. The lumbar column, however, can be placed in many different positions to achieve the therapeutic result required.

Extension of the lumbar spine tends to create a 'close-packed' position for the individual joints, as the articular surfaces come into full contact and ligaments become taut. This, therefore, is not a desirable position in which to achieve traction. All other positions towards flexion allow space for the joint surfaces to part or glide; however, in full flexion the ligaments again become taut, preventing the required movements. Traction in full flexion is almost impossible to apply. The optimum position in which to apply traction is midway between extension and flexion.

Simple traction can be applied to the lumbar spine by applying a distraction force to either the pelvis or the lower limbs, with the subject lying either supine or prone. It is preferable to place a pillow under the abdomen in the latter position to prevent extension. Manual traction can also be applied with the subject sitting or standing, by raising the upper trunk and allowing the pelvis and lower limbs to act as the traction force.

Mechanical traction can be applied in many positions of the lumbar spine, avoiding full extension and full flexion for the same reasons as outlined above. It may be applied continuously or intermittently over a set period of time. These therapeutic traction techniques are complex and need skill and knowledge of techniques and precautions. For further study, reference should be made to literature dedicated to this subject.

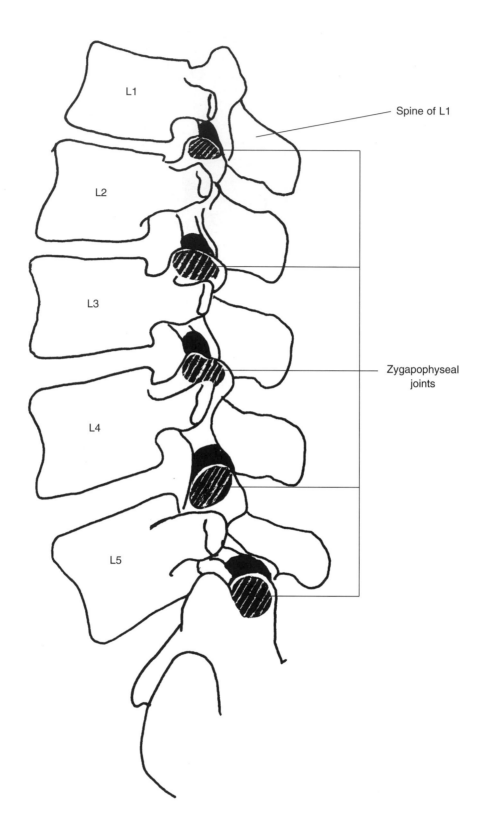

Fig. 6.2 (c)
Zygapophyseal joints of the lumbar spine (lateral aspect from left)

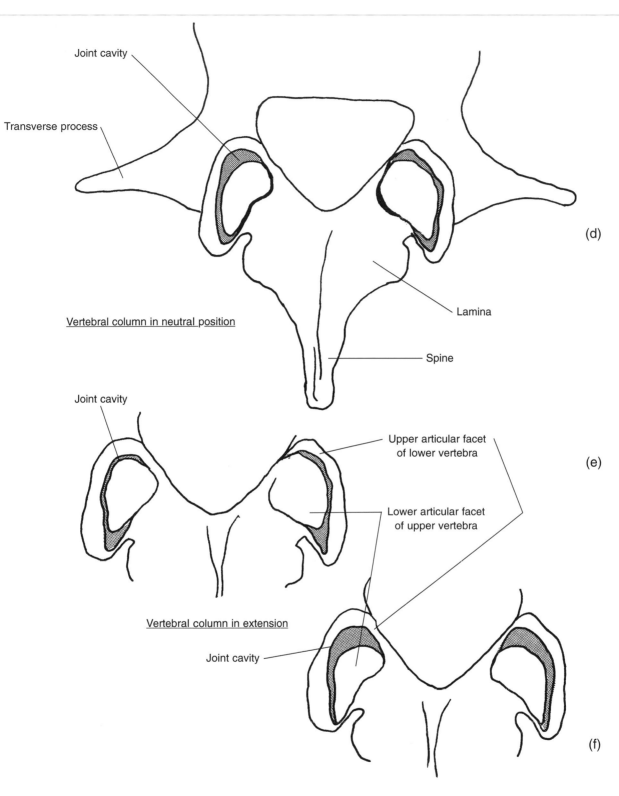

Fig. 6.2 (d)–(f)
Zygapophyseal joints of lumbar section of vertebral column (viewed from above)

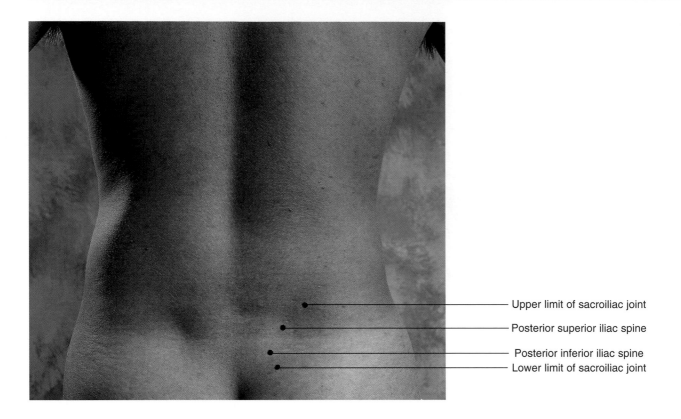

Upper limit of sacroiliac joint

Posterior superior iliac spine

Posterior inferior iliac spine
Lower limit of sacroiliac joint

Fig. 6.3 (a)
Sacroiliac joint (posterior aspect)

The pelvis [Figs 6.3 and 6.4]

Posteriorly, the sacrum articulates on either side with the ilium (innominate) bone at the sacroiliac joints (also discussed in Chapter 3). Anteriorly, the two pubic bodies articulate with each other at the pubic symphysis. The former is a very stable plane synovial joint supported by powerful interosseous and accessory ligaments. The latter is also stable, but is a secondary cartilaginous joint containing a modified disc of fibrocartilage. The sacroiliac joints allow a small degree of rotation of the sacrum, with respect to the innominate bones, about an axis through its interosseous ligament. Movement is more noticeable in young females, particularly during pregnancy and childbirth, reducing considerably after the third decade. In males, movement is negligible and virtually nil after the second decade.

The pubic symphysis allows a slight rocking and twisting to occur, which accompanies any movements which may occur at the sacroiliac joints.

The sacroiliac joint

Palpation

With the subject lying prone and the abdomen resting on a pillow, identify the posterior superior iliac spine. The sacroiliac joint lies 1 cm lateral and 1 cm anterior to this spine, on an oblique line extending above and below a further 2 cm. The line of the joint can also be marked by an oblique line passing downwards and medially, at an angle of approximately 25°, from a point 5 cm lateral to the spine of the fifth lumbar vertebra to a point just lateral to the posterior inferior iliac spine (Fig. 6.3b). It is impossible to palpate this joint.

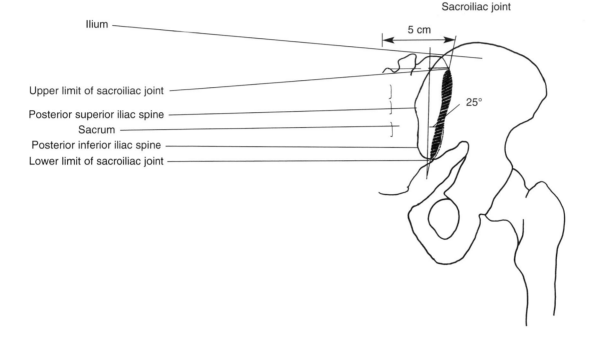

Fig. 6.3 (b)
Sacroiliac joint (posterior aspect)

Accessory movements

Little movement occurs at the sacroiliac joint, there being more in the young female and less in the middle-aged and elderly male (see above).

Rocking the sacrum around a frontal axis can be achieved in the prone subject by placing the heel of one hand over the apex and the heel of the other over the base of the sacrum. Alternate pressure applied to the apex and base produces a slight rocking movement of the sacrum between the two innominate bones. This movement can be increased locally on one side if one hand is placed on the apex of the sacrum and the other on the posterior aspect of the crest of the ilium. The opposite movement can be produced by placing one hand on the base of the sacrum and the other on the ischial tuberosity. The pressure applied to these two areas must be downwards and towards each other, in the same direction as the movement of each component. It is a difficult movement to obtain, and some skill and practice is necessary before it can be achieved.

The posterior aspect of the joint can normally be gapped or at least stressed by using the leverage of the femur. With the subject supine, flex the opposite knee and hip and roll the limb and pelvis towards you. When the pelvis is rotated approximately 45°, a downward and medial pressure toward the opposite hip joint can be applied to the femoral condyles. This technique is used in the examination and treatment of sacroiliac problems and is covered in greater detail in the manipulation literature.

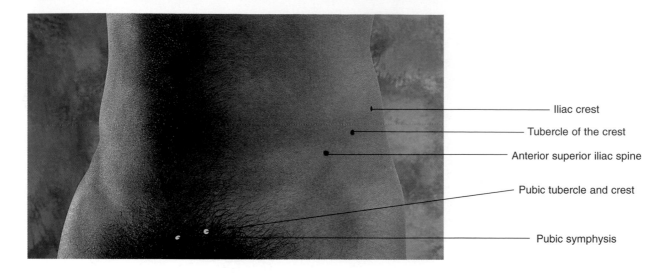

Fig. 6.4 (a)
The pelvis (anterior view)

The pubic symphysis

This joint is situated centrally at the lower aspect of the abdomen between the two **pubic bones** and just above the external genitalia. Locate the **pubic tubercles** on the upper border of the body of the pubis, either side of the midline. Between the two is a depressed line which can be traced downwards for about 2.5 cm. This indicates the anterior marking of the **pubic symphysis**, being the medial surfaces of the pubic bones separated only by the intervening interarticular disc.

Accessory movements

The slight twisting and gapping that occurs at this joint is due to stresses on the pelvis and sacrum which occur during movements at the sacroiliac and hip joint. With the subject lying supine, a slight gliding movement can be produced between the two bones by applying pressure to the anterior surface of the pubic body on one side only.

With the subject lying on the side, a downward compression force applied to the upper part of the ilium increases compression at the pubic symphysis, while also stressing the posterior sacroiliac ligament. With the subject supine, the two ilia can be stressed laterally by a downward and lateral pressure being applied to the two **iliac crests**. This produces a distraction force to the pubic symphysis and, in addition, an anterior gapping and stress on the anterior ligament of the **sacroiliac joint**

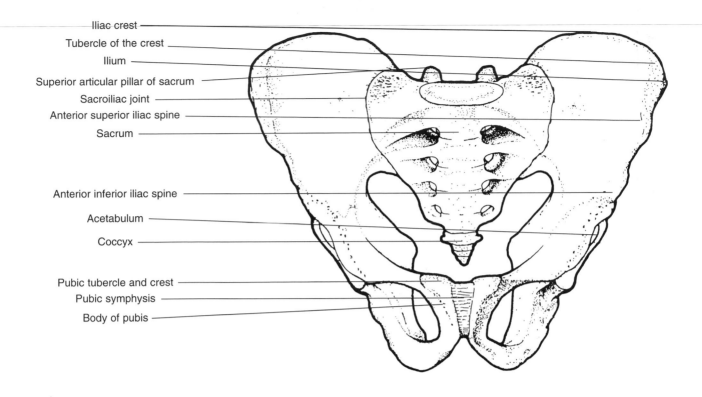

Iliac crest
Tubercle of the crest
Ilium
Superior articular pillar of sacrum
Sacroiliac joint
Anterior superior iliac spine
Sacrum
Anterior inferior iliac spine
Acetabulum
Coccyx
Pubic tubercle and crest
Pubic symphysis
Body of pubis

Fig. 6.4 (b)
The pelvis (anterior view)

Pubic symphysis
Pubic bones

Fig. 6.4 (c)
The pelvis (anterior view)

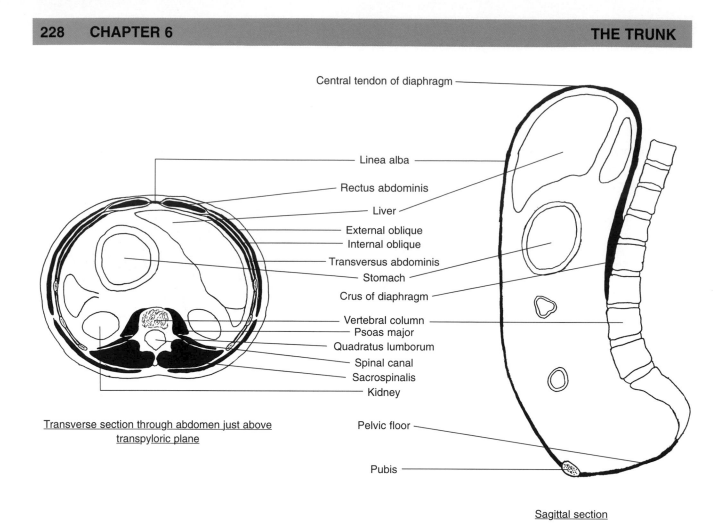

Transverse section through abdomen just above transpyloric plane

Sagittal section

Fig. 6.5 (a), (b)
The abdomen

MUSCLES

The abdominal muscles form a continuous wall around the abdominal viscera. The cavity so formed is enclosed by the **diaphragm** above; the **vertebral column** and **psoas major** posteroinferiorly; **quadratus lumborum** posterolaterally; the **internal** and **external oblique** abdominal muscles anterolaterally, supported on their deep surface by **transversus abdominis**; **rectus abdominis** anteriorly; and inferiorly by the muscles which form the **pelvic floor**, i.e. levator ani and coccygeus. Some of these muscles may be palpable when they are contracting, although they may not always appear distinct (Fig. 6.5).

Palpation

Identification of structures and muscles in this area is dependent, to a certain extent, on the physique of the subject. Subcutaneous fat in the superficial fascia covering the abdomen can hinder accurate identification.

With the subject lying supine, place both hands on the central area of the abdomen, one above and one below the **umbilicus**. If the subject now raises the head, a column of muscle can be palpated running down either side of the central depressed line (the **linea alba**) (Fig. 6.5a–d). Each muscle is narrow inferiorly and can be traced from the **pubic tubercle** and **crest** below to its broader superior attachment to the **fifth**, sixth and seventh **ribs**. The upper attachment is V-shaped, as the attachment to the fifth rib laterally is higher than that to the seventh costal centrally. The lateral border of each muscle is convex. The muscle is interrupted by three transverse depressed **fibrous intersections**, which are at

Anterior aspect

Anterolateral aspect

Fig. 6.5 (c), (d)
Muscles of the abdomen

the level of the xiphoid, the umbilicus and midway between the two. These appear as transverse grooves across the muscles.

Both the external and internal oblique muscles contract during flexion of the trunk, but each can be identified more easily if its action is resisted. To facilitate palpation of the right external oblique, resistance must be applied to oppose upper trunk rotation to the left. This can be achieved with the subject supine, by standing to the left side and applying resistance to the right shoulder, preventing the head and shoulder being lifted and turned to the left. Contraction of the muscle tightens the aponeurosis just above its attachment to the right iliac crest.

The internal oblique lies deep to the external oblique so that, during the same actions as outlined above (rotation to the left), the left internal oblique also contracts, palpable between the left iliac crest and the umbilicus.

Quadratus lumborum can be palpated either side of the vertebral column, between the twelfth rib above and the posterior part of the iliac crest below. It mostly lies deep to latissimus dorsi, but its anterior border can be palpated just posterior to the mid-axillary line. If the subject is lying prone and raises the head and shoulders, the muscle becomes easier to palpate.

In this region sacrospinalis (erector spinae) lies close to the spinous processes of the lumbar vertebrae, forming two firm columns of muscle passing from the posterior part of the iliac crest and sacrum below, to the angle of the ribs and transverse processes of the thoracic vertebrae. They become visible and palpable lateral to the lumbar spines when the subject raises the head and shoulders in a prone position.

Anterior view

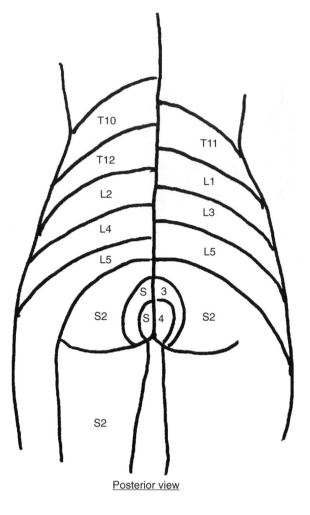

Posterior view

Fig. 6.6 (a), (b)
The cutaneous nerve supply

NERVES [Fig. 6.6a,b]

The nerve supply to the abdomen and lower limbs is derived from the thoracic 8–12, all five lumbar, all five sacral and the coccygeal nerve roots. The arrangement of these nerves is extremely complex (see *Anatomy and Human Movement*, Palastanga et al., 1998) and is dealt with here in outline only.

The thoracic nerves

Nerve roots T8–11 behave in a similar manner to intercostal nerves, supplying muscles in intercostal spaces and anteriorly contributing to the supply to the abdominal muscles. Their cutaneous branches follow the same general direction, supplying a band of skin running downwards and forwards.

The lumbar plexus

This is formed by part of T12 and L1–4. It supplies muscles of the lower abdomen, pelvis and front and inner side of the thigh. Its cutaneous supply is to the lower back and running downwards and forwards to the lower abdomen and the front and inner side of thigh and the inner side of the leg and foot.

The sacral plexus

Deriving its fibres from the ventral rami of L4, 5 and S1, 2, 3, 4, it supplies the muscles of the gluteal region, hamstrings, leg and foot. Its cutaneous supply is the gluteal region, back of the thigh, anterior, lateral and posterior aspects of the leg and plantar and dorsal aspects of the foot.

The coccygeal plexus supplies an area of skin around the anus
. The larger nerves of this region are situated deeply within the abdomen. Those of the lumbar plexus are formed within psoas major, while those of the sacral plexus mainly lie in front of the sacrum. All nerves that reach the surface of the abdominal and lumbar areas are too small to palpate. Nevertheless, these cutaneous nerves often influence their areas of distribution, with palpable signs such as changes in temperature and sweating. It is therefore important to study the plan of cutaneous distribution over the abdomen and lumbar area. There is, similar to the costal area, an overlap of root supply, each nerve covering an area of skin above and below.

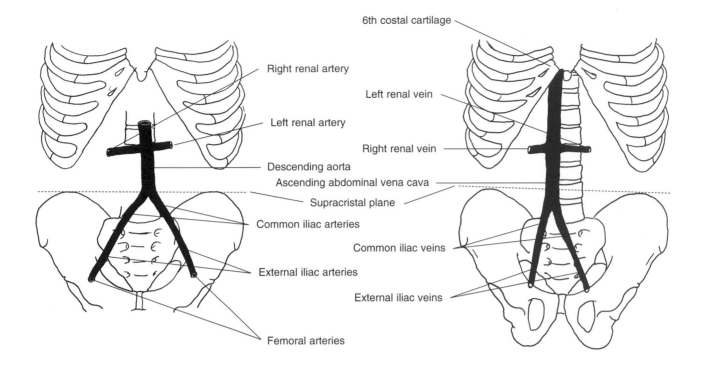

Fig. 6.6 (c)
Abdominal aorta and common iliac arteries

Fig. 6.6 (d)
Ascending abdominal vena cava and common iliac veins

ARTERIES [Fig. 6.6c]

All the larger arteries of the abdomen are also situated deeply within the abdominal cavity and are difficult or impossible to find. The pulsations of the abdominal aorta can be palpated in the supine subject if the fingers are pressed deeply to the left of the umbilicus, thereby compressing the abdominal aorta against the lumbar vertebral bodies. This technique is unpleasant for the subject, but can be improved by encouraging relaxation of the abdominal muscles. The abdominal aorta can be marked by a line drawn vertically from a point on the midline 2.5 cm above the transpyloric plane (see Fig. 6.7b) to a point just to the left of the midline 2.5 cm below the supracristal plane (Fig. 6.6c). Here it divides into the common iliac arteries which diverge from each other at an angle of approximately 37° to bifurcate again one vertebra below (lower border of the fifth lumbar vertebra) into the internal and external iliac arteries. The external iliac artery can be marked as it passes to the mid point of the inguinal ligament to be continued below the ligament as the femoral artery

VEINS [Fig. 6.6d]

Again, all the large veins of the abdomen are deep within the cavity and impossible to palpate. It is, however, quite important to know where the abdominal portion of the inferior vena cava commences and leaves the abdominal cavity. It commences at the junction of the two common iliac veins at the level of the fourth lumbar vertebra and progresses upwards and slightly to the right, first accompanied on its left by the abdominal aorta. It leaves the abdominal cavity by passing behind the liver and through the diaphragm at the level of T8 (Fig. 6.6d).

The vena cava can be marked by a line 2.5 cm broad, commencing at a point just to the right of the midline 2.5 cm below the supracristal plane (lower body of the fourth lumbar vertebra), to a point just above the sixth costal cartilage on the right, where it passes through the vena caval opening in the tendinous portion of the diaphragm (Fig. 6.6d).

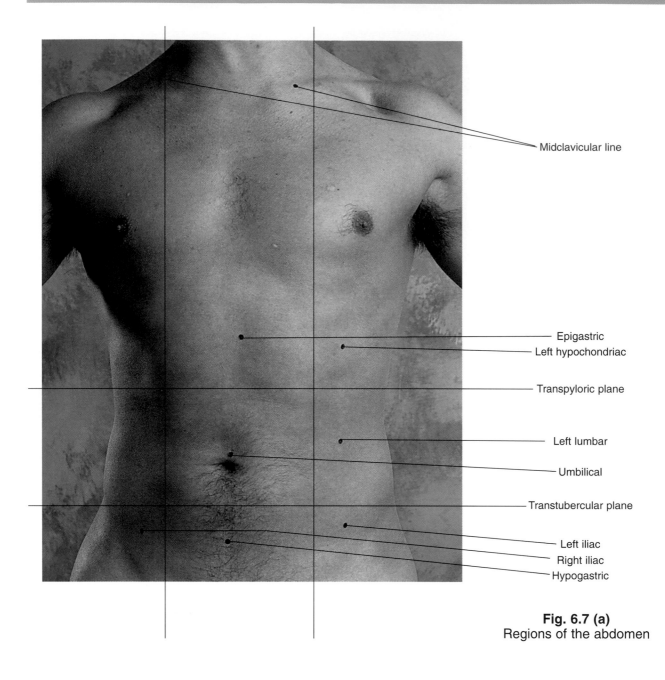

Fig. 6.7 (a)
Regions of the abdomen

Labels on figure: Midclavicular line, Epigastric, Left hypochondriac, Transpyloric plane, Left lumbar, Umbilical, Transtubercular plane, Left iliac, Right iliac, Hypogastric

STRUCTURES WITHIN THE ABDOMINAL CAVITY

For convenient location of viscera, the abdomen may be divided into nine regions by two vertical and two horizontal lines (Fig. 6.7a, b). Other methods of dividing the abdomen into regions also exist but will not be covered here (Keogh and Ebbs, 1984). The two vertical lines pass superiorly from the mid-inguinal point, which is halfway between the anterior superior iliac spine and the pubic tubercle, to the mid point of the clavicle. They are usually referred to as the midclavicular lines. The upper horizontal line is drawn level with the tip of the ninth costal cartilage: it crosses the tip of the twelfth rib and the spine of the first lumbar vertebra. This is known as the transpyloric plane, as it also passes through the pylorus of the stomach. The lower horizontal line is drawn across the abdomen between the tubercle of the crest of each ilium and is

known as the transtubercular plane (Fig. 6.7a,b). It crosses the vertebral column level with the upper portion of the body of L5, and may serve as a useful landmark when identification of lumbar vertebrae is necessary.

The three regions above the transpyloric plane are the right and left hypochondriac, with the epigastric centrally. The three regions between the transpyloric and transtubercular planes are the right and left lumbar, with the umbilical centrally, while the three lower regions are the right and left iliac, with the hypogastric centrally.

Organs in the abdominal cavity are normally quite movable, with some changing their shape and size according to their contents. This makes surface marking difficult and often unreliable. It is, however, important to be able to mark the areas in which

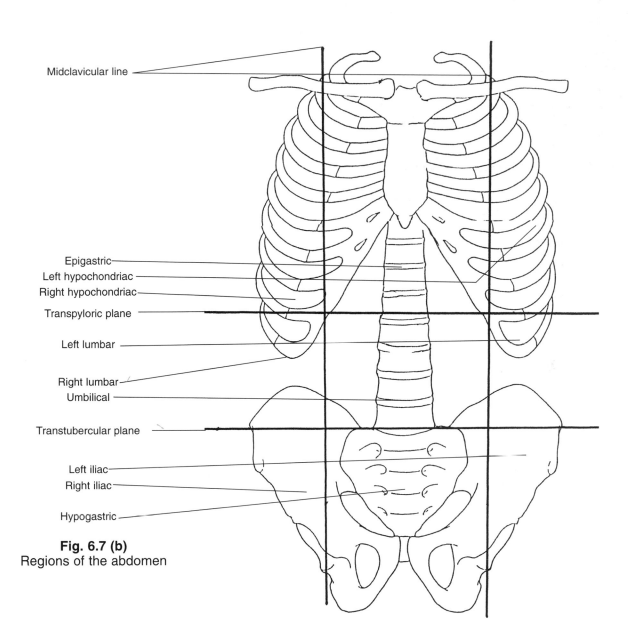

Midclavicular line

Epigastric
Left hypochondriac
Right hypochondriac
Transpyloric plane

Left lumbar

Right lumbar
Umbilical

Transtubercular plane

Left iliac
Right iliac

Hypogastric

Fig. 6.7 (b)
Regions of the abdomen

the particular organ lies and note any fixed sites where markings are constant.

General locations

The liver lies mainly in the right hypochondriac and epigastric areas.

The spleen is located mainly in the left hypochondriac and extends posteriorly into the epigastric area.

The pancreas lies on the transpyloric plane between the epigastric and umbilical areas. The gall bladder again lies on the transpyloric plane where it crosses the right midclavicular line.

The stomach varies considerably in size but is normally in the left hypochondriac and umbilical areas.

The duodenum is partly in the umbilical and partly in the epigastric areas, the transpyloric plane passing through its second part.

The small intestine lies mainly in the hypogastric area.

The caecum and appendix lie in the right iliac region.

The large intestine passes through the right iliac and lumbar, umbilical, left lumbar and iliac areas and passes down through the hypogastric area.

The kidneys lie partly in the epigastric and partly in the umbilical areas.

The bladder lies behind the two pubic bones and pubic symphysis.

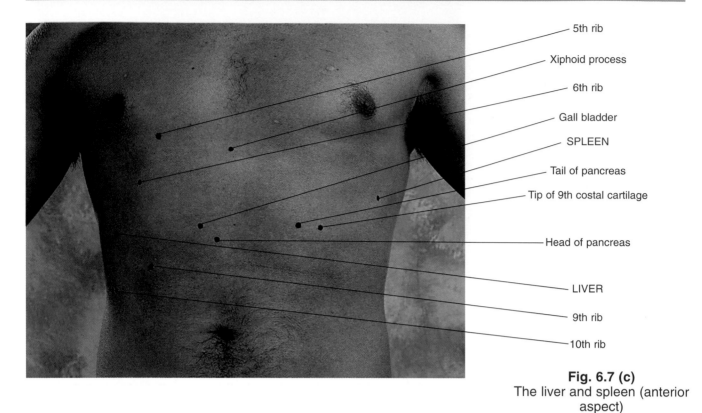

Fig. 6.7 (c)
The liver and spleen (anterior aspect)

The liver [Fig. 6.7c and d]

The liver is a large wedge-shaped organ situated mainly in the right hypochondriac and epigastric region of the abdomen just below the diaphragm. Its upper surface is moulded by the under surface of the diaphragm. The right side is thicker, narrowing as it passes towards the left. Posteriorly it is grooved by the inferior vena cava.

Surface markings

The position of the liver is fairly constant in healthy subjects. The upper boundary can be marked by a line drawn horizontally at the level of the xiphister-nal joint, extending some 7 cm to the left of the mid-line and all the way round the right side of the thoracic cage. Its lower border is an oblique line beginning 7 cm to the left of the midline, crossing the left costal margin at the eighth costal cartilage, reaching the right costal margin at the **ninth costal cartilage** and continuing around the costal margin.

The spleen [Fig. 6.7c and d]

The **spleen** [*splen* (L) = spleen] is a reservoir for blood. It is soft and highly vascular and is just deep to the lower left ribs below the diaphragm and behind the stomach. In addition to the storage of blood, it is part of the reticuloendothelial system. It contains phagocytes which engulf microorganisms, foreign particles and damaged cells. It is involved with the manufacture of white blood cells and in the infant it will also produce red blood cells.

The spleen lies under cover of the ribs, although it is an abdominal organ. This is due to the domes of the diaphragm rising into the thorax from its costal attachments.

The spleen lies posteriorly on the left side deep to the **ninth**, **tenth** and eleventh ribs, extending as far forwards as the mid-axillary line. It is approximately 10 cm long, 7 cm deep and 3–4 cm thick. Although it occasionally projects just below the costal margin, the spleen cannot usually be palpated unless it is enlarged to approximately three times its normal size. It is often ruptured in severe accidents where the chest is crushed and may well be overlooked. This will lead to large amounts of blood escaping into the abdominal cavity. The spleen can be removed without affecting the human body too seriously.

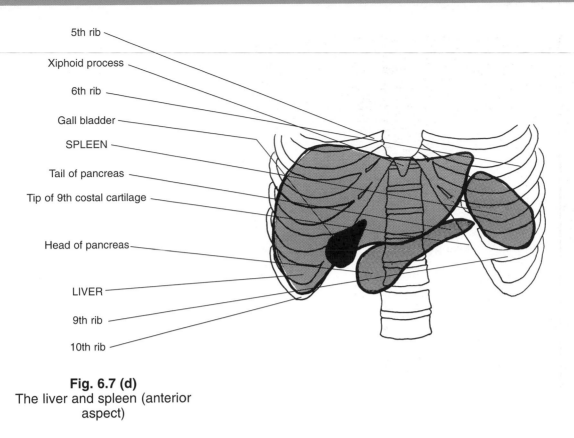

5th rib

Xiphoid process

6th rib

Gall bladder

SPLEEN

Tail of pancreas

Tip of 9th costal cartilage

Head of pancreas

LIVER

9th rib

10th rib

Fig. 6.7 (d)
The liver and spleen (anterior aspect)

The pancreas [Fig. 6.7c and d]

The pancreas [*pan* (Gk) = all, *keras* (Gk) = flesh] is a strangely shaped gland resembling a large tadpole, having a head to the right with a body and tail which narrows as it passes to the left. It is approximately 10 cm long and 4 cm broad at its head. It is situated anterior to the vertebral column, level with the body of the first lumbar vertebra. The head is surrounded by the four sections of the duodenum, the pylorus of the stomach lying anterior to the body. The pancreatic duct passes from the head to the right, emptying into the second part of the duodenum at a point on the transpyloric plane 2 cm to the right of the median line (Fig. 6.7c, d). Behind the body lie the superior mesenteric and splenic veins; just below, they form the portal vein. The head is related posteriorly with the inferior vena cava and the right crus of the diaphragm and the body lies just in front of the abdominal aorta. The tail is related to the spleen at its far left and with the stomach anteriorly. The pancreas is not palpable in the normal subject.

The gall bladder [Fig. 6.7c and d]

The gall bladder is a small reservoir, approximately 3 cm in diameter, with a short tail passing posteriorly. It is situated below the centre of the anterior border of the liver, projecting a little below the right costal margin deep to the costal angle level with the ninth costal cartilage (Fig. 6.7c, d). In the normal subject it is difficult to palpate. It discharges bile through the bile duct into the second part of the duodenum, which aids in the breakdown of fatty foods during digestion. Sometimes stones are formed in the gall bladder and are passed down the tortuous and sometimes narrowing tubes of the cystic and bile ducts. The blockage of these tubes causes acute pain and often irritates other structures in this area. If this is a recurring problem, the gall bladder can be removed (cholecystectomy)

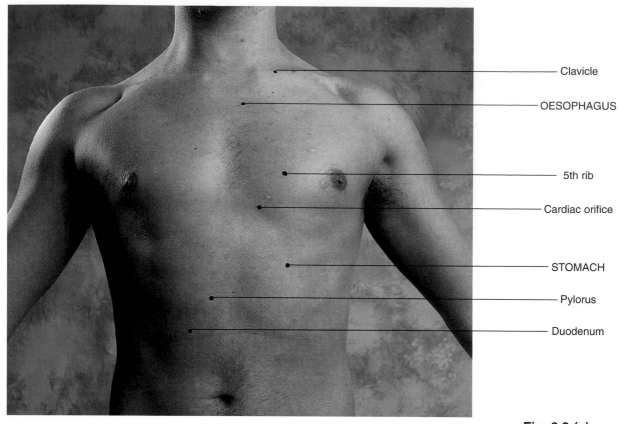

Fig. 6.8 (a)
The oesophagus, stomach and
duodenum

The stomach [Fig. 6.8]

The **stomach** [*stomachos* (Gk); the Greeks used this word for the gullet and the oesophagus, they later used '*gaster*' to denote the lower end] is a mobile, muscular, highly vascular container in the digestive system situated deep to the lower left rib cage, below the diaphragm, to the left of the liver and in front of the spleen. It receives food from the **oesophagus** [*oiso* (Gk) = I carry, *phagein* (Gk) = food] through its **cardiac orifice** into its upper part (the **fundus**) and after passing through the **body of the stomach** the partially digested food is passed on through the **pylorus** and **pyloric orifice** into the first part of the **duodenum**. It varies enormously in shape and size according to its contents. It is basically J-shaped, with its upper section being thicker and more expanded, while its lower end becomes narrower as it passes medially and slightly up-

wards, continuing as the first part of the duodenum.

A full stomach can be palpated as it extends below the rib cage on the left side and can be felt contracting and moving during the early part of digestion. An empty stomach is hidden beneath the rib cage.

Surface markings

Although the central section of the stomach varies in shape and size, its two openings – the cardiac and pyloric orifices – remain comparatively fixed. The former can be marked by a short oblique line, approximately 2 cm long, along the seventh costal cartilage 2.5 cm to the left of the midline, being level with the tip of the xiphoid process. The latter lies on the transpyloric plane 1.5 cm to the right of the

Clavicle

OESOPHAGUS

5th rib
Greater curvature
Cardiac orifice
The fundus
STOMACH
Lesser curvature
The body of the stomach
Pyloric orifice
Pylorus
Duodenum

T11

T12

L2

L3

L4

L5

Fig. 6.8 (b)
The oesophagus, stomach and
duodenum

midline. The fundus, or upper part of the stomach, may rise up as far as the fifth intercostal space 7 cm left of the midline or as far down as the tenth costal cartilage.

The **lesser curvature** of the stomach can be represented by a curved line, concave to the right, joining the cardiac and pyloric openings, while the **greater curvature** is represented by a line, convex to the left, joining the upper limit of the stomach at the fifth intercostal space to approximately the tenth costal cartilage (Fig. 6.8a, b).

The duodenum [Fig. 6.8]

The **duodenum** [*duoden arius* (L) = continuing twelve; Herophilus in 344 BC measured the duodenum as twelve finger breadths] is the contin-

uation of the digestive tract beyond the pylorus of the stomach. It is approximately 25 cm long, passing initially upwards, backwards and to the right for 5 cm as far as the costal margin (first part), and then downwards to the left for 7.5 cm, to reach the level of the tenth costal cartilage (second part), across the front of the body of L3, passing upwards and to the left for approximately 10 cm (third part), and finally ascending for 2.5 cm (fourth part) to become continuous with the jejunum at the duodenojejunal flexure at the level of L2, 2 cm left of the mid line. The common bile duct and pancreatic duct drain into the duodenum midway along its second part.

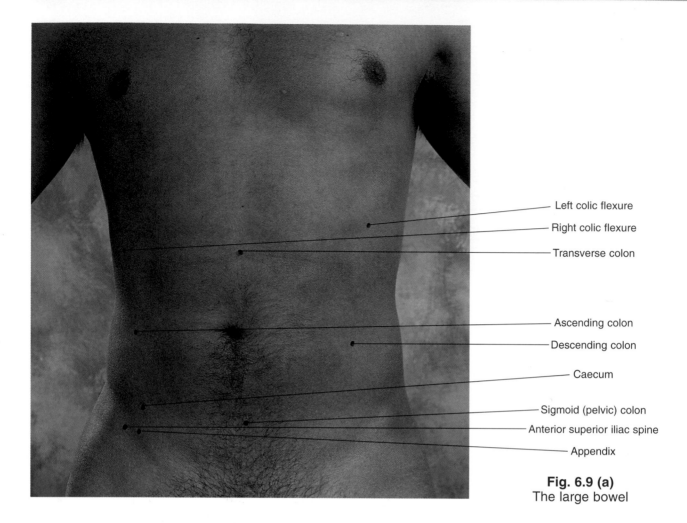

Left colic flexure
Right colic flexure
Transverse colon

Ascending colon
Descending colon

Caecum

Sigmoid (pelvic) colon
Anterior superior iliac spine
Appendix

Fig. 6.9 (a)
The large bowel

The small intestine

The small intestine is described in two parts, the first being termed the jejunum and the second, the ileum. The jejunum begins as a continuation of the duodenum (Fig. 6.8a, b) at the level of L2, 2 cm to the left of the midline and continues as the ileum which ends at its junction with the caecum (Fig. 6.9a, b) at the junction of the right mid-clavicular line with the transtubercular plane (drawn through the tubercles of the crest of the ilium). Each end is fixed in its position; the central portion, which may be up to 8 m long, is continually mobile. It is, however, contained within the confines of the large bowel.

The caecum [Fig. 6.9a and b]

The caecum [*caecus* (L) = blind; Galen confused the caecum with the appendix] is the first section of the large intestine and receives the contents of the small intestine. It fills the right iliac region of the abdomen, lying above the lateral half of the right inguinal ligament, with the appendix lying in the mid-clavicular line, 1.5 cm medial to the anterior superior iliac spine. The caecum and appendix are not palpable, but pressure applied to this region can be extremely painful, particularly if the appendix is inflamed.

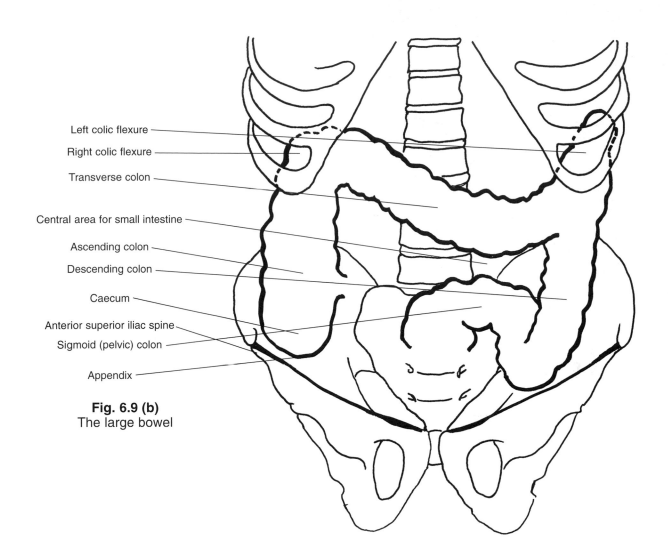

Left colic flexure

Right colic flexure

Transverse colon

Central area for small intestine

Ascending colon

Descending colon

Caecum

Anterior superior iliac spine

Sigmoid (pelvic) colon

Appendix

Fig. 6.9 (b)
The large bowel

The large intestine (large bowel)
[Fig. 6.9a and b]

For descriptive purposes, the large intestine is normally divided into four sections: ascending, transverse, descending and sigmoid (pelvic). It can be represented by a band, approximately 5 cm wide, but varies considerably according to its contents. The ascending colon commences in the right iliac region at the caecum and ascends through the right lumbar region, deep to the costal margin, to the level of the transpyloric plane, where it arches backwards and to the left, forming the right colic (hepatic) [*hepar* (Gk) = liver] flexure. The transverse colon passes from the colic flexure, across the umbilical region below the liver towards the spleen, where it turns downwards, forming the left colic (splenic) flexure just above the transpyloric plane. The descending colon passes through the left lumbar and iliac regions, turning backwards at the inguinal ligament to become the sigmoid [*sigma* (Gk) = letter C, *-oeides* (Gk) = shape, form] colon. This latter section passes backwards and downwards in an S-shaped curve to pass vertically downwards in front of the sacrum becoming the rectum. This is continuous with the anal canal and reaches the surface at the anus.

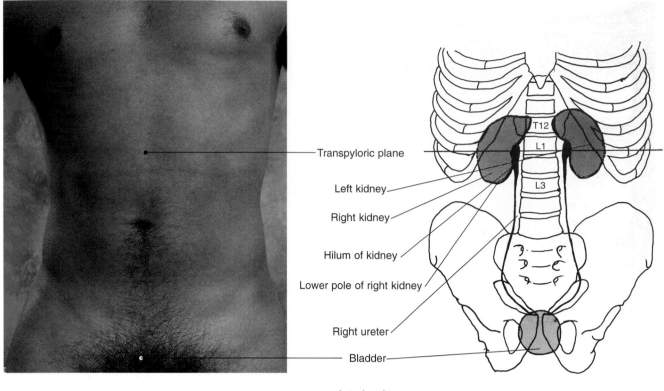

Fig. 6.10 (a), (b)
The kidneys, ureters and bladder

The kidneys [Fig. 6.10]

The kidneys are situated on the posterior abdominal wall anterior to quadratus lumborum behind the peritoneum. Each kidney lies obliquely with its anterior surface facing slightly laterally. The anterior relations of the right kidney are the right suprarenal gland and liver superiorly, the duodenum and right colic flexure inferomedially. The left kidney has the left suprarenal gland above, the tail of the pancreas and splenic vessels, the stomach and left colic flexure anteriorly, with the spleen postero-superiorly. Each kidney is related posteriorly to quadratus lumborum, the diaphragm, and the medial and lateral arcuate ligaments. The right kidney lies mainly in front of the twelfth rib, while the left lies anterior to the eleventh rib. Each kidney is approximately 11 cm in length, 6 cm broad and 3 cm thick. The hilum lies level with the spine of the first lumbar vertebra (the transpyloric plane), the right normally slightly lower than the left.

Surface markings

Each kidney can be located between two horizontal and two vertical lines, forming a rectangle either side of the vertebral column. The upper and lower limits of both kidneys lie between horizontal lines through the upper margin of T12 above and the L3 vertebra below. It may be easier to locate these lines if the following procedure is adopted: draw a horizontal line through the lower edge of the spine of L1; draw a second line 5.5 cm above this (i.e. level with the upper border of T12) and a third line 5.5 cm below (i.e. level with L3).

Because the two kidneys lie obliquely, the two vertical lines enclosing them are closer together than the width of the organ. Draw two vertical lines, one 3 cm and one 6.5 cm, lateral to the lumbar spines; these represent the medial and lateral margins of the kidneys.

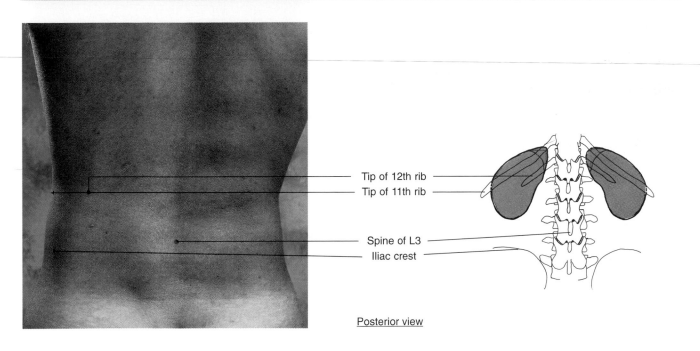

Posterior view

Fig. 6.10 (c), (d)
The kidneys

Palpation

The kidneys are well protected, lying anterior to the lower ribs and strong back muscles, below the diaphragm. The vertebral column, with the attachments of the crura of the diaphragm, lies between the two kidneys and the psoas major and minor lie behind them. The kidneys are protected in front by the large and small bowel and the powerful abdominal muscles. They are thus virtually impossible to palpate. However, the lower pole of the right kidney can be palpated with difficulty using deep pressure through a relaxed abdominal wall at a point just lateral to the vertical mid-clavicular line and just below the level of the tenth rib.

The bladder [Fig. 6.10a and b]

The bladder is a thin-walled muscular reservoir which varies in size according to the volume of fluid it contains. It is estimated that it is able to hold about 250 ml of urine before having to be emptied, but this estimate appears to be a little on the low side practically. Its volume obviously grows according to the frequency it is filled with large quantities of fluid.

The bladder is situated directly behind the two pubic bones and pubic symphysis, with its upper border reaching to the crest on either side. When full, however, it rises above the pubic rami by up to 5 cm.

The empty bladder is not palpable in the normal subject, but when full it can be felt as a soft swelling just above the pubic symphysis.

7

Conclusion

Conclusion

Although the major part of this book is devoted to the acquisition of anatomical knowledge through surface markings of underlying tissues, the main aim of the exercise was to promote the use of the hands to discover more information. If you have read the book and carried out the manoeuvres suggested, not only will you have acquired a thorough knowledge of the surface markings, but you will have developed your sense of touch and palpation. The knowledge you have gained, either directly or indirectly through the application of your palpation, can be stored for future use.

The ability you have acquired to palpate can be developed further by use. The more exploration you perform, the more skilled as a palpator you become. Its use can be extended beyond its application to anatomy. If you observe the care and handling that a carpenter engages before or while working on a piece of wood, the loving care that a dressmaker expresses when selecting material, the caressing that a potter exerts on a piece of clay or the delicate, careful touch a gardener employs in pricking out seedlings, you will realize that those engaged in this care are totally aware of the feel of their materials. One cannot say, however, that the materials have any feeling for the contact of the handler. This is, therefore, a one-way passage of information.

If you now consider the care with which a hairdresser handles the hair of a client, the careful smoothing and moulding that a tailor carries out when fitting a suit or the care and sensitivity that a physiotherapist employs when handling a painful limb, it is easy to see that the recipient has also acquired something more from the physical contact. Most of these recipients will express the feelings of some pleasure at this contact and would probably feel that there was some therapeutic or psychological influence.

The gripping of a hand, an arm around the shoulder or a touch on the elbow can all be comforting to a person under some stress and the meaning is often interpreted in the type of touch used. Feelings of assurance and sympathy can easily be passed on with no visual or auditory communication needed. Many times physical contact is the only communication when sight and sound are obliterated due to an overflow of emotion.

As stated in Chapter 1, these abilities to pass on information through physical contact can be a source of communication of many feelings such as love, hate, care, understanding, etc. Those who have the privilege of contact with others in a professional capacity use those skills in their therapeutic handling of patients already, some with the knowledge of their influence, some with limited knowledge and some with none.

This book is aimed at the greater use of palpation in assessment, care and therapy. There seems to be an area in which those skills are under-used and it is my opinon that this source of communication holds secrets of mind and body which are undervalued.

Develop your palpation to the full. Observe carefully the results of each contact and do not be surprised at the power that lies in this enormously potential communication skill.

References and further reading

Field, E.J. and Harrison, R.J. (1947) *Anatomical Terms: Their Origin and Derivation*, W. Heffer and Sons Ltd, Cambridge.

Grieve, G. (ed.) (1986) *Modern Manual Therapy of the Vertebral Column*, Churchill Livingstone, Edinburgh

Guyton, A.C. (1991) *Medical Physiology*, 6th edn, W.B. Saunders, Philadelphia, pp. 605–606

Keogh, B. and Ebbs, S. (1984) *Normal Surface Anatomy*, William Heinemann Medical Books Ltd, London.

Maitland, A.D. (1991) *Peripheral Manipulation*, 3rd edn, Butterworth-Heinemann, Oxford

Montague, A. (1978) *Touching: The Human Significance of the Skin*, 2nd edn, Harper and Row, New York

Palastanga, N., Field, D. and Soames, R. (1998) *Anatomy and Human Movement*, 3rd edn, Butterworth-Heinemann, Oxford

Sunderland, S. (1978) *Nerves and Nerve Injuries*, 2nd edn, Churchill Livingstone, Edinburgh, p. 355

Williams, P.L. *et al.* (eds) (1995) *Gray's Anatomy*, 38th edn, Churchill Livingstone, Edinburgh

Index